Psychological Stress

Psychological

Stress

psychoanalytic and behavioral studies of surgical patients

IRVING L. JANIS

Department of Psychology

Yale University

Reprinted by

ACADEMIC PRESS New York San Francisco London

A Subsidiary of Harcourt Brace Jovanovich, Publishers

ACADEMIC PRESS, INC.
111 Fifth Avenue, New York, New York 10003

United Kingdom Edition published by
ACADEMIC PRESS, INC. (LONDON) LTD.
24/28 Oval Road, London NW1

LIBRARY OF CONGRESS CATALOG CARD NUMBER: 74-10292

ISBN 0–12–380750–6

First Reprinting, 1974

PRINTED IN THE UNITED STATES OF AMERICA

To the memory

of

Dr. Alfred Gross

Preface

A philosopher once said that every man suffers throughout his entire life from a fatal disease—mortality. No cure for this disease is ever likely to be discovered, but hundreds of prescriptions have been offered, which hold forth the promise of easing people of the accompanying psychological pains. The writing of such prescriptions, together with speculations about the emotional consequences of man's physical vulnerability, has long been a preoccupation of religious leaders, moral philosophers, dramatists, and novelists. Only within the past twenty years or so have research workers in the human sciences begun to make systematic observations for the purpose of finding out how people feel, think, and behave at times when they are facing the threat of pain, serious injury, or death.

It is hardly surprising, therefore, to discover that various attempts to produce a "propositional inventory" of warranted scientific generalizations about stress behavior yield only a very meager list. About ten years ago, when I first began surveying the literature in this field, I became acutely aware of the lack of cogent, dependable evidence. There were, of course, many controlled laboratory experiments purporting to deal with stress behavior, but almost all of them dealt with extremely brief exposures to threat stimuli or measured only peripheral aspects of emotional excitement. The main source of difficulty, in my opinion, was that these carefully executed experiments had been carried out prematurely, before the significant variables in human stress behavior were adequately identified. Such experiments provide behavorial data which are generally quite reliable but of dubious value for extrapolating to the conditions of actual life stress.

In contrast to the tangential laboratory investigations were a large number of field studies of major disasters, focusing on the effects of prolonged exposure to powerful stress stimuli. But most of these studies proved to be extremely weak in precisely those respects where the laboratory studies were strong: They consisted mainly of impressionistic accounts interpreted by observers who had failed to make use of any systematic procedures for minimizing the biasing influence of their own *a priori* expectations, attitudes, or emotional blindspots.

The two types of shortcomings, posing the danger of being left with inconsequential or undependable findings, were very salient at the time when I decided to study surgical patients. The surgical ward of a large general hospital was selected as a good site for investigating stress behavior, partly because I surmised that both types of shortcomings could be averted. Since major surgery involves a profound threat to body integrity as well as a variety of severe deprivations, it seemed likely that a great deal could be learned about the processes of normal adjustment to life stresses. From the standpoint of collecting dependable evidence, a major consideration was that, during the period when surgical patients are confined to a hospital ward, it is feasible to conduct systematic interviews and to secure behavioral records made by a number of independent observers. Once I began the actual research, however, it soon became apparent that there are many methodological difficulties in working with surgical patients which prevent the evidence from being as unambiguous as I had originally hoped. From the findings presented in this book, the reader will be able to judge for himself the values and limitations of carrying out research with surgical patients.

With the cooperation of the surgery staff in a general hospital, I was able to obtain pertinent data for a series of intensive case studies. In this initial study, which included 30 surgical cases, several regularities were noted concerning the sequence of stress responses, the most important of which involved a striking relationship between the degree of fear manifested *before* the operation and the degree of stress tolerance manifested *after* the operation. In order to test the apparent relationship and to obtain further correlational data bearing on the influence of preoperative information about the impending stressful events, a second study was conducted with a much larger group of subjects. In the follow-up study, questionnaire survey data were obtained from several hundred young men who had undergone fairly recent surgical procedures. Finally, after the series of case studies and the questionnaire survey study had been carried out, another source of intensive case study data unexpectedly became available. After having completed the formal course of training as a postdoctoral research student in the New York Psychoanalytic Institute, I participated in a psychoanalytic research project at Yale University, under which auspices I conducted the psychoanalytic treatment of a psychoneurotic woman. Shortly after her second year of the treatment, the patient developed an organic disorder in her leg, which, on advice of several physicians, required surgery. Detailed observational records were kept concerning this patient's emotional reactions, fantasies, and free associations during all psychoanalytic sessions. The records from the sessions immediately preceding and following the surgical operation proved to be an extraordinarily rich source of clues concerning unconscious psychological processes that may underlie some of the widely observed phenomena in stress behavior. The depth-interview material was particularly helpful in suggesting explanatory concepts to account for a number of puzzling findings from the series of case studies and from the questionnaire survey.

In this book, all three sources of evidence are used to present as complete a picture as possible of the psychological aspects of surgery. The primary purpose is to highlight the *theoretical implications* by conveying what has been learned concerning the dynamics of human adjustment to stressful life events. Secondarily, an attempt has also been made to draw attention to some of the main practical implications with respect to three important types of problems:

(a) The formulation of policies of medical management which take account of the psychological needs of sick people;

(b) the improvement of diagnostic procedures relevant for predicting high or low stress tolerance; and

(c) the development of effective methods of psychological preparation which could be widely applied as part of a mental health program designed to reduce the disruptive emotional impact of many different types of potential disasters.

The writing of this book was facilitated by a Grant-in-Aid for Research in the Behavioral Sciences awarded by the Ford Foundation.

I wish to express my appreciation to Dr. Mark May who, as director of the Institute of Human Relations at Yale University, encouraged me to begin the study of surgical patients and provided research funds to facilitate the early phases of the research. It was through the helpful cooperation of Dr. Gustaf E. Lindskog, Professor of Surgery in the Yale Medical School, that it became possible for me to conduct interviews in the surgical wards of the Grace–New Haven Hospital and to have access to the behavioral records made by the hospital staff.

For invaluable help in connection with the psychoanalytic case research reported in the first part of this book, I am particularly indebted to the late Dr. Alfred Gross of the Yale Department of Psychiatry, who, as supervisory analyst, continually gave me the benefit of his insight and criticism over a period of four years. My participation in the psychoanalytic research project at Yale University was greatly facilitated by the excellent administrative arrangements worked out by Professor Fredrick C. Redlich, Chairman of the Yale Department of Psychiatry. I am also grateful to my former instructors at the New York Psychoanalytic Institute, and especially to Drs. Edith Jacobson, Rudolph Loewenstein, and the late Ernst Kris, with whom I have had the opportunity to discuss informally some of the main methodological problems that beset any research worker who attempts to make use of psychoanalytic interview data.

I have profited greatly from numerous discussions with Drs. William Kessen, Margaret Sommers, and the late Katherine Wolf, each of whom read the first draft of the entire book and gave extremely valuable criticisms which were extensively used in redrafting. Constructive criticisms concerning one or more chapters were also gratefully received from Drs. John Benjamin, Lawrence Z. Freedman, Ralph Greenson, Robert N. Hamburger, and Martha Wolfenstein.

I am grateful to Daniel Bell for his helpful advice on many problems concerning the presentation of the case material. Special thanks are due to Marjorie G. Janis for her valuable aid in editing the manuscript. I also wish to thank John Enright for assistance in compiling the bibliography and Cathy Janis for checking the bibliographic references in the galley proofs.

Chapter 2 of this book draws heavily upon a lecture on "The Psychoanalytic Interview as an Observational Method," presented at Syracuse University in April 1957 and shortly to be published by Rinehart and Company as a chapter in a book on *Assessment of Human Motives,* edited by Gardner Lindzey. I wish to thank Professor

Lindzey and the publisher for permission to use portions of the material in the present book. I also wish to acknowledge my thanks to the publishers of the following books for permission to use quotations:

Basowitz, H., H. Persky, S. Korchin, and R. Grinker, 1955. *Anxiety and Stress.* N. Y.: McGraw-Hill.

Deutsch, M., 1954, Field theory in social psychology. *Handbook of Social Psychology*, G. Lindzey (Ed.). Cambridge: Addison-Wesley.

Grinker, R. and J. Spiegel, 1945. *Men Under Stress.* Philadelphia: Blakeston.

Janis, I., 1951. *Air War and Emotional Stress.* N. Y.: McGraw-Hill.

Kardiner, A. and H. Spiegel, 1947, *War Stress and Neurotic Illness.* N. Y.: P. B. Hoeber.

Permission to use quotations has also been gratefully received from the publishers of the following journal articles:

Bernstein, S. and S. Small, 1951, Psychodynamic factors in surgery. *J. Mt. Sinai Hospital*, **17,** 938–958.

Ferraro, A., 1948. Somato-psychic factors in anxiety neurosis. *J.nerv. ment. Dis*, **107,** 228–242.

Kubie, L., 1947. Problems in clinical research (Round Table 1946). *Amer. J. Orthopsychiat.*, **17,** 196–203.

IRVING L. JANIS

July, 1958

Contents

Part One Psychoanalytic Observations and Theory

Part Two Behavioral Research

Part one

Psychoanalytic Observations and Theory

1.

Introduction

How do people react upon discovering that they will soon be exposed to serious dangers? What factors determine whether or not a person will act effectively when a crisis or catastrophe actually materializes? Why do some persons become panic-stricken, demoralized, or irrationally enraged during an episode of extreme environmental stress, whereas others, exposed to essentially the same disruptive stimuli, are able to control their emotional impulses? After a harrowing crisis is over, what factors determine whether the surviving victims will regain their normal level of emotional equilibrium rapidly or slowly, completely or incompletely? Systematic studies in the human sciences have not yet arrived at sufficient evidence to give anything more than rather sketchy, incomplete answers to these questions; nor is there any established body of theory that can be relied upon for dependable predictions as to how people will react under specified conditions of environmental stress.

Most behavioral scientists acknowledge that this constitutes a very serious lack in our present psychological knowledge, one which is being increasingly felt because of a growing practical need for dependable methods of building up stress tolerance. Government planners, civil defense authorities, and local community leaders want to know how to prevent maladaptive behavior in present day peacetime disasters and in any future wartime catastrophes resulting from nuclear weapons. Psychiatrists, social workers, and other social welfare personnel are seeking for information about ways and means of promoting mental health among people who are undergoing personal adversity. One psychoanalyst recently estimated that the average physician's ability to take account of his patient's psychological reactions to illness and surgery ". . . may be a greater factor in mental hygiene than the efforts of all analysts together, because the physicians meet a much broader sector of human beings and have thereby a much greater opportunity." (Braatoy, 1954.)

In addition to these urgent practical needs, there is a growing theoretical interest in the behavioral sciences oriented toward understanding how people react to unfavorable environmental situations. Here the main need is for facts and explanatory hypotheses that will help to elucidate the basic mechanisms of adjustment to stress, the determinants of disorganized emotional behavior, and the changes in affects, cognitions, and attitudes resulting from extreme changes in environmental conditions.

The Problem of "Objective" Anxiety

Theoretical problems concerning the causes and consequences of psychological stress have been formulated in somewhat different ways by scientists in three allied fields of research—psychoanalysis, psychosomatic medicine, and experimental social psychology. Freud, after having made most of his major psychoanalytic contributions, pointed out that, for psychoanalysts interested in understanding normal personality functioning, ". . . the investigation of the mental reaction to external danger is precisely a subject which may produce new material and raise fresh questions." (S. Freud, 1920, p. 8.) In his theoretical writings on personality development, Freud frequently referred to children's reactions to frightening surgical operations and medical examinations, calling attention to the way in which they "work through" unpleasant experiences in their repetitive activities, which involves transforming the passivity of the distressing experience into the activity of an aggressive game. Freud also took account of the repetitive nightmares of adults following traumatic danger experiences; he concluded that these observations made it necessary to add a new category of dreams motivated by a "belated attempt at mastery," thus modifying his original theory which held that all adult dreams can be explained as symbolic fulfillments of forbidden infantile wishes. (S. Freud, 1920, pp. 35–45 and 1923, p. 146.) However, it has been pointed out by Szekely (1954) and others that, although Freud's writings on the problem of anxiety supply some valuable hints about the dynamics of "objective anxiety" or "fear," his own empirical and theoretical investigations as well as those of almost all of his followers have been centered largely upon "neurotic" anxiety stemming from unconscious inner dangers. Most psychoanalysts continue to restrict their attention to only a very limited class of objective danger situations, notably those childhood events which involve threats of castration or object loss and which are regarded as generating neurotic anxiety in adult life.

Freud once said that objective anxiety ". . . seems to us an intelligible reaction to danger—that is, to anticipated injury from without," whereas neurotic anxiety is "altogether puzzling and, as it were, purposeless" (S. Freud, 1933, p. 114). But investigators who have observed the reactions of normal adults in circumstances of external danger often encounter phenomena that are by no means readily intelligible, some of which seem to be even more puzzling than the most extreme forms of chronic anxiety symptoms. In fact, the latter symptoms are now reasonably well understood, precisely because of the intensive concentration of psychoanalytic and psychiatric research on the problems of neurosis. It is quite amazing to notice how often the scientific writers who discuss human behavior in extreme situations attempt to explain the "normal" emotional impact of frightening external dangers solely on the basis of more or less dubious extrapolations from what is apparently well known about how neurotic personalities cope with the inner dangers that generate neurotic anxiety. Thus, at the present time, the problem of objective anxiety seems to be much more of a puzzle than the problem of neurotic anxiety.

Consider, for example, the emotional reactions of cancer patients who have found out about their condition and have been informed that they must undergo surgery in order to prolong their lives. Many of these people turn out to be more concerned about surgical injuries and about the disruption of their daily patterns of living than about dying from cancer, even though they know about their poor prognosis (Sutherland and Orbach, 1953). Similar paradoxical phenomena have been noted among noncancer patients. For instance, patients awaiting perilous abdominal operations sometimes show a disproportionately small degree of conscious fear, whereas those facing a relatively safe form of minor surgery display much more apprehensiveness (H. Deutsch, 1942). In many such instances the disproportion between the magnitude of the danger and the intensity of the emotional reaction does not appear to be a symptom of a psychoneurotic disorder but, rather, seems to be a nonpathological defense that characterizes the adjustive tendencies of clinically normal personalities under fear-provoking circumstances.

Related phenomena, including a variety of displaced fears, are encountered in many cases of so-called psychosomatic disorders. As some specialists in psychosomatic research have pointed out, the causal sequence may sometimes be the reverse of that commonly assumed by those physicians who have been trained to look into personality disturbances as possible causes, but not as possible consequences, of somatic illness.

> With all the recent advances of psychosomatic medicine one cannot fail, however, to recognize its unilaterality, i.e., the emphasis on the value of psychogenic mechanisms in the determination of somatic pathology, with neglect somehow, of the reverse process, i.e., the process of soma influencing the psyche, the process of somatic stimuli determining psychologic reactions. . . . efforts must be made to investigate with the same eagerness every mechanism of a somatic origin which may result directly or indirectly in bringing into action psychologic reactions, thus giving origin to clinical pictures in which the somatic dysfunction is the primary causative factor, followed by a complicating secondary, psychologic dysfunction. (Ferraro, 1948, p. 228.)

Finally, it should be noted that some recent experimental studies in social psychology have highlighted the need for more refined theoretical constructs to account for attitude change and social conformity under conditions of exposure to fear-arousing stimuli. For instance, there is now some evidence that leads us to reject the common assumption of a one-to-one correspondence between level of fear and acceptance of authoritative antidanger recommendations (Hovland, Janis, and Kelley, 1954). Although the arousal of a low level of fear may produce a marked increase in conformity, the arousal of a high level of fear may have a disruptive effect and give rise to a decrease in conformity. The emotional learning processes underlying the complex relationships between fear stimulation and attitude change remain to be explored in relation to the theory of fear as a learnable drive (Dollard and Miller, 1950) and in relation to various alternative theories, especially those which emphasize cognitive aspects of personality functioning (Bruner, 1951; Bruner and Postman, 1949; Scheerer, 1954).

Scope of the Inquiry

The present volume is devoted to psychological studies which were intended to fill in some of the main gaps in our current knowledge about psychological stress. It deals with one major class of stressful events—episodes of severe physical danger which are capable of arousing emotional tension in every normal human being to an extraordinarily high degree, disrupting habitual patterns of daily behavior, drastically impairing mental efficiency, and producing distressing subjective states of painfully unpleasant affect. The category "physical danger" is a very broad one, which includes all occurrences of psychological stress attributable to those external events or signs that produce anticipations of pain, body injury, or death.* In most such instances, portending signs are unambiguously perceptible long before the actual impact occurs. Everyone receives continual training from parents, educators, community leaders, peers, and the society at large which helps him to identify and appraise signs of physical danger and to act in such a way as to minimize the potential loss of life, limb, and physical functions. Thus, much of the present investigation is focused on anticipatory reactions occurring before the onset of a crisis. We shall see that such reactions often play a major role in determining how a person subsequently is able to cope with conditions of actual danger.

The set of scientific problems toward which the present inquiry is directed encompasses all three major phases of psychological stress that typically occur when a person is exposed to a situation of objective danger (Janis, 1954):

1. The *threat* phase, during which the person perceives signs of oncoming danger and/or receives communications of warning which are likely to arouse anticipatory fear.
2. The *danger impact* phase, during which a person perceives that physical danger is actually at hand and realizes that his chances of escaping intact depend partly upon the protective actions executed by himself or by other people who are in a position to help him.

* Note 1 at the end of this chapter contains additional discussion of the term "psychological stress" as it is used in the present volume. At various points throughout the book it is necessary to discuss technical questions or to elaborate on theoretical issues. These supplementary discussions are presented in the notes at the end of each chapter to avoid interrupting the main presentation. The notes are numbered consecutively and designated by the superscripts which appear in the text.

3. The *postimpact victimization* phase, during which the person perceives the losses he has sustained and, at the same time, undergoes some severe deprivations which continue for a varying length of time after the acute danger has subsided.

To obtain observational data pertinent for understanding the factors influencing behavior during each of the three successive phases, the author has conducted systematic studies of hospitalized patients who were required to have surgical operations. These studies constitute the empirical core for two main types of propositions which will be presented in this book: (*a*) descriptive generalizations concerning the observable determinants of various emotional reactions and patterns of overt stress behavior which occur when people are exposed to external dangers; and (*b*) theoretical formulations specifying psychodynamic processes which help to explain the descriptive generalizations.

A major goal of the research was to arrive at propositions that are likely to be broadly applicable to most people in contemporary society and that will pertain to behavior in a wide variety of danger situations. Accordingly, the main variables investigated in the surgery studies were selected on the basis of *uniformities* noted in the extensive observational reports currently available on how people in many different national and cultural subgroups tend to react to severe physical dangers—tornadoes, floods, industrial accidents, air raids, criminal assaults, concentration camp tortures, epidemics, acute illness, etc. Having selected the variables with an eye to generalizability, the author sought to discover why certain regularities occur in the reactions of people exposed to physical dangers. The general hypotheses formulated on the basis of the surgery studies are those which, in the judgment of the author, seem to have a reasonably good chance of proving to be valid; they specify how normal people in our society will react before, during, and after exposure to any crisis involving the actual or potential danger of body damage, whether it be a wartime bombing attack, a peacetime disaster, an incapaciting illness, or a catastrophic accident.

In searching for general laws of stress behavior, we obviously should not overlook the fact that there are wide individual differences in reactions to the same external danger stimuli and that we may find some significant differences in the emotional reactions displayed by different types of personalities. For example, Fenichel (1945, pp. 454–456) asserts that compulsive personalities frequently develop acute anxiety symptoms when they encounter severe environmental hardships, whereas persons burdened by chronically latent guilt may react to "real misery" by becoming less worried than usual.

One might also expect to find some consistent variations according to nationality, ethnic origin, socio-economic status, religious affiliations, and other characteristics associated with differences in cultural background. In recent years, a number of social scientists have called attention to some of the ways that various ethnic groups within the United States (e.g., Italian, Irish, Jewish, and "old" American) might differ in their reactions to stressful events (Wolfenstein, 1957; Zborowski, 1952). A person's social background presumably influences the way in which a painful experience is perceived and assimilated; it determines to some extent whether or not the person will admit his potential losses, whether he will have high or low confidence in the protective capabilities of the authorities, and whether he will freely express his emotional agitation or try to keep it hidden from others.

It seems likely, however, that despite whatever social and individual variations may exist, there are a large number of cause-and-effect relationships which will prove to be applicable to the stress behavior of all sectors of contemporary modern society and which might even prove to be valid cross-culturally. The attempt to arrive at such propositions constitutes the ultimate purpose of the author's research on psychological stress. Thus, the empirical observations from the studies of surgical patients are used primarily to discover and to assess (at least in a preliminary way) a set of hypotheses about major factors which determine how the average person in our culture will react to any situation of physical danger.

In analyzing the major empirical findings from the surgery studies, an effort was made to take account of the possibility that differences in stress reactions may sometimes reflect the influence of different social norms which prescribe "appropriate" behavior according to the person's age, social position, sex, and marital status. Whenever comparisons are made between a group of people behaving one way and others behaving in a different way, the two groups are equated on relevant social characteristics.

Thus, the questions which the present studies of surgery seek to answer pertain to psychological factors that may hold true irrespective of a person's social class or subcultural background. Under what circumstances is a hospitalized patient most likely to feel relatively secure about the outcome of his surgical experience and under what circumstances will the same patient tend to develop exaggerated fears of being mutilated or killed? What types of communications from the surgeon or from other medical authorities will enable the average surgical patient to cope most adequately with the psychological stresses of the postoperative period? What are the typical attitudes and expectations that develop during the preoperative period and how do they affect the likelihood that the patient will subsequently feel elated or depressed during the postoperative period? What aspects of the hospital environment influence the average surgical patient's capacity to control his aggressive reactions when he experiences the pains, discomforts, loss of motility, and numerous other deprivations that characterize the period of convalescence?

By studying the major *situational* factors affecting reactions to danger, one can hope to discover some of the typical response tendencies evoked by any form of external danger. Such research may furnish some outstanding landmarks which will make it somewhat easier for supplementary studies to map out the differences in stress behavior attributable to differences in: (*a*) personality predispositions; (*b*) social background; and (*c*) the source, magnitude, and quality of the danger.

Surgery as a Danger Situation

From a psychological standpoint, a major surgical operation constitutes a stress situation which resembles many other types of catastrophes and disasters in that the "victim" faces a combination of three major forms of imminent danger—the possibility of suffering acute pain, of undergoing serious body damage, and of dying. The following is one of the main working assumptions used in interpreting the evidence from the psychological studies of surgery: Any valid generalization about the effects of one type of severe physical danger is likely to be applicable to any other crisis or disaster if it entails the same basic threats of pain, injury, and annihilation.

Perhaps some of the factors which influence the way people react to physical dangers also influence their reactions to a variety of other fear-evoking occurrences, including separation from loved ones, career failures, unemployment, loss of status, and other such purely "social" crises. One might expect some marked parallels in the emotional responses evoked by social and physical dangers. In the present volume, however, no specific assumptions will be made as to the psychological similarities and differences between the two types of dangers.

Organization of This Book

The studies reported in this book approach the problems of psychological stress from three different observational levels. In Part I, a detailed account will be given of the emotional and cognitive processes revealed by a psychoanalytic case study of one surgical patient. The values and limitations of this "microscopic" approach and the procedures used for selecting variables that are likely to be prototypic for other persons will be discusssed in the next two chapters. Chapters 4 through 16 will describe the psychoanalytic findings and will present theoretical inferences drawn from the data in the light of available empirical evidence from a large number of other studies dealing with individual reactions to comparable danger situations. The major psychodynamic hypotheses that emerge will be summarized in Chapter 17.

Further material pertinent to the psychodynamic hypotheses, including new evidence and additional theoretical elaborations, will be presented in Part II, which is comprised of Chapters 18 through 26. This material is based on behavioral studies, using two different observational approaches. One approach consists of case studies of a series of surgical patients who were intensively interviewed and observed on a hospital ward both before and after undergoing a major operation. If the psychoanalytic method is equivalent to a microscopic examination, the case studies on the surgical ward permit us to look through a magnifying glass that reveals with great clarity some of the most salient features of adjustment at a time when people encounter stressful events. The results point to a number of situational factors which affect the incidence of postoperative emotional disturbances involving exaggerated fears and excessive or misplaced aggression. Another research approach used to investigate the same psychological phenomena consists of extracting correlational data from a questionnaire survey administered to several hundred male adolescents who had undergone major or minor surgery. The results are used to test some of the main hypotheses suggested by the case studies.

The findings derived from all three approaches converge on a few major propositions concerning situational determinants of different modes of response to stressful life events. The theoretical and practical implications of these general propositions, together with the main facts from the behavioral studies, will be summarized in Chapter 26.

Notes

1. Although the term "psychological stress" is frequently used by psychologists and psychiatrists, there is at present no generally agreed upon definition. (See the various definitions which occur in recent reviews of the literature by Basowitz et al., 1955; Haggard, 1949; Hanfmann, 1950; Himmelweit, 1950; Lazarus

et al., 1952; Withey, 1956.) Several writers (e.g., C. Menninger, 1954a and 1954b; Wolff, 1953) have attempted to define it in terms of "homeostasis," with the intention of using the same vocabulary as that of Selye (1950) and other biological scientists who have developed the concept of "physiological stress." A number of psychologists, however, take the position that the physiological term does not necessarily refer to the same type of phenomena as the psychological one, and that it is premature to attempt to integrate the two concepts. Withey (1956) calls attention to three main obstacles: First, the psychologist has no adequate way of defining the psychological condition that corresponds to the homeostatic steady state. Second, when one tries to set up a definition in terms of the nonsatisfaction of needs, it may be quite easy to specify the tolerance limits for healthy and efficient functioning at the physiological level, but "in psychology this degree of precision has not yet been reached." Third, in physiological models of stress, "the *structure* and *organization* of the organism determine the 'selection' and sequence of adaptive or defense processes," whereas in psychological studies of stress, "it seems necessary to include the higher mental processes involving learned behaviors, intelligence level and other complicating factors."

Among those writers whose research deals with behavioral phenomena, there seems to be a fairly high degree of consensus as to the domain of behavioral events to which the term "psychological stress" refers, even though their definitions are formulated in different ways. For most writers, the term is used as a construct which designates a broad class of events involving interaction between extreme environmental stimuli and the adjustive capabilities of the organism. An excellent discussion of the methodological problems entailed by this interactional concept is presented by Basowitz et al. (1955, p. 7):

". . . any stimulus may in principle arouse an anxiety response because of the particular meaning of threat it may have acquired for the particular individual. However, we distinguish a class of stimuli which are *more likely* to produce disturbance in most individuals. The term *stress* has been applied to this class of conditions. Thus we can conceive a continuum of stimuli differing in meaning to the organism and in their anxiety-producing consequences. At one end are such stimuli or cues, often highly symbolic, which have meaning only to single or limited numbers of persons and which to the observer may appear as innocuous or trivial. At the other end are such stimuli, here called stress, which by their explicit threat to vital functioning and their intensity are likely to overload the capacity of most organisms' coping mechanisms."

". . . Ultimately we can truly speak of a *stress situation* only when a given response occurs, but for schematic purposes as well as consistency with common usage, we may use the term stress to designate certain kinds of stimulating conditions without regard for response. Such stimuli are called stress because of their assumed or potential effect, although we well know that in any given case the organisms' adaptive capacity, threshold, or previous learning may preclude any disturbance of behavior."

These authors propose that the term "stress" should be used to refer to the stimulus condition likely to arouse the affective response of *anxiety*. This particular definition seems too narrowly restricted because a given noxious stimulus may arouse anxiety in one person, shame in a second person, and anger in a third; sometimes the same person will display a sequence of different emotional responses or an undifferentiated affective state that cannot be appropriately labeled as "anxiety." It seems preferable to replace "anxiety" by a more generic term—"emotional tension"—which includes anxiety as well as any other form of emotional disturbance. Thus, the events referred to by the term "psychological stress" would be those changes in the environment which typically—i.e., in the average person—induce a high degree of emotional tension and interfere with normal patterns of response. As Scott (1949, p. 61) puts it, "a stress situation . . . may be defined as one in which adjustment is difficult or impossible but in which motivation is very strong."

Although the concept is not rigorously defined, it serves as a useful label for referring to a broad class of psychological phenomena which are likely to have something in common with respect to antecedent causal factors and consequent changes in behavior. In order to avoid some of the confusion that is bound to arise from employing a loosely defined interactional concept, the term "stress" will be used in this book mainly as an adjective to characterize either the disruptive stimuli (e.g., "stress situation") or the changes in overt behavior, affect, or attitude that are evoked by the disruptive stimuli (e.g., "stress reactions").

Following a suggestion made by Withey (1956), the term "threat" will be used when cues heralding oncoming danger occur without any noxious stimuli being actually present. But, as Withey points out, the difference between apprehension concerning anticipated danger and emotional reactions to actual stress stimuli may be purely quantitative.

Three general classes of stress situations have been delineated by Schwab and Pritchard (1949):

(a) *Mild* stresses, the effects of which last from seconds to hours: e.g., annoying insects, public appearances before a large audience, missing a train, and other such minor occurrences in daily life;

(b) *Moderate* stresses, the effects of which last from hours to days: e.g., a period of overwork, a gastric upset, a visit of an unwelcome guest, the temporary absence of a loved person;

(c) *Severe* stresses, the effects of which last for weeks, months, or even years: e.g., prolonged separation from one's family, death of a loved one, drastic financial losses, illnesses, and surgical operations.

It is primarily the third type to which the general hypotheses and theoretical analyses in the present book are intended to apply. In fact, most of the hypotheses refer specifically to "physical dangers," which constitute an important subclass of severe stress situations (see pp. 195–197). But it may turn out, of course, that some of the tentative conclusions drawn from studying surgical patients will prove to be valid generalizations of much wider scope, applying not only to the entire class of severe stresses but to the moderate and mild types as well.

2.

Values and limitations of psychoanalytic research

Up to the present time, the contributions to psychological theory made by psychoanalytic case research have been concentrated mainly in two central areas: (1) The development of the human personality from infancy through adolescence and (2) the dynamics of unconscious motives, defenses, and conflicts underlying the neuroses and other personality disorders. In recent years psychoanalytic interview observations have been restricted almost exclusively to problems of psychopathology and therapy. From the standpoint of developing general psychological principles, the primary value of this research is that it furnishes data which help to account for *developmental sequences and individual differences* in personality characteristics and adjustive or maladjustive behavior. Psychoanalytic case studies have revealed a great deal about the structure and genesis of *personality predispositions* (e.g., deeply ingrained emotional habits derived from childhood experiences) which incline a person to have high or low tolerance for specific types of frustrations, which make for high or low ability to cope with the usual demands of the adult social world, and which make for psychological symptoms that are amenable or unamenable to psychological treatment. In the context of studying how chronic predispositions are developed, much attention continues to be devoted to situational events in childhood, notably traumatic experiences and recurring crises, which appear to play a significant formative role in neurotic personalities. But *situational events* in adult life are rarely investigated by psychoanalysts except in so far as the events function as "precipitating" or "contributing" factors in the onset of symptoms among pathologically predisposed personalities.[1]

Expanding the Scope of Psychoanalytic Research

A large number of important scientific problems outside the field of psychopathology remain to be investigated by the psychoanalytic method. Social scientists in many different fields of research have repeatedly suggested that the scope of psychoanalytic inquiry could be fruitfully broadened to include relatively neglected aspects of interpersonal relations, creativity, and normal emotional reactions in which unconscious factors may play just as important a role as in neurosis (Dollard, 1938; Kluckhohn, 1949; Lasswell, 1948; Leites, 1948). Within the psychoanalytic movement itself, there seems to be a growing recognition of the need to broaden the scope of psychoanalytic case studies, especially in connection with the problems of elucidating the "conflict-free functions of the ego" and the role of successful "sublimations" in coping with restrictions of the social environment (Hartmann, 1951). Specialists in psychoanalysis as well as in bordering disciplines are beginning to devote more attention to intensive case study materials bearing on the environmental conditions of adult life which affect stress tolerance and the "creative" and "healthy" features of normal adjustment. (Erickson, 1950, and White, 1952.)

A few pioneering psychoanalytic studies concerning the effects of environmental stress have appeared so far. For example, Sterba (1946, 1947) has described the way his patients reacted to two outstanding news events: the Detroit race riots in 1943 and the death of President Roosevelt in 1945. Glover (1942) has summarized the comments obtained from a group of British analysts concerning how their patients reacted to the Munich war scare crisis in 1938 and to the air blitz of 1941; M. Schmideberg (1942) has described her patients' reactions to the evacuation of London and to the dangers of the air blitz; H. Deutsch (1942) has discussed her patients' reactions to surgical operations. Many valuable hypotheses concerning unconscious and preconscious aspects of normal reactions to environmental events are contained in these reports, but the pertinent case material is generally compressed into a few summarizing statements or given only in the form of illustrative anecdotes.

At the present time, it seems warranted to repeat once again the suggestion that detailed case reports should be devoted to a broader scope of inquiry in the field of human behavior. Probably the most useful material will come from studies which focus on those environmental variables known from other fields of research to have significant psychological or social effects. In the current life situation of persons undergoing analysis, important events occur from time to time which may provide unique opportunities for studying variables of general scientific interest, even though the occurrences may have relatively little connection with the patient's neurosis or with his therapeutic progress. It seems by no means improbable that, in the long run, psychoanalytic research contributions to the general problems of explaining how adults normally react to environmental changes will prove to be of even greater value for the human sciences than those limited to strictly clinical problems of psychopathology.

Of course, when an important event occurs in the life of a patient, the analyst often does not obtain any clear indication of how the patient's daily activities have been affected and, in the absence of information from outside sources, he can only guess at how the patient's overt behavior has changed in relation to other people. The analyst would, therefore, have to confine his case studies on the effects of environmental variables largely to the changes in emotional reactions, attitudes, fantasies, and other such aspects of behavior directly observable during psychoanalytic sessions. And, the opportunity to obtain case study data of general scientific interest cannot be expected to arise in the treatment of every psychoanalytic patient. Moreover, the practical demands and therapeutic objectives of professional clinical work might sometimes prevent the analyst from obtaining systematic interview records of even those rare sessions which contain important data pertinent to understanding the psychological impact of a current environmental event. Nevertheless, it is likely that many more case study contributions in this field would be forthcoming if the majority of practicing analysts (irrespective of whether or not they are affiliated with a research-oriented clinic or university department) were to become more aware of the potential research value of their daily interview sessions.

Because the potential research contribution of clinical practitioners is becoming increasingly recognized by postgraduate medical schools and psychiatric institutes, excellent instruction in research methods is now becoming available for many psychiatric trainees, some of whom will subsequently go on to receive psychoanalytic training. Moreover, some of the major psychoanalytic institutes have begun admitting "research candidates" into their regular curriculum for medically qualified psychiatrists, thus providing a small number of research psychologists, social scientists, and biological scientists with the opportunity to obtain a didactic personal analysis, to participate in case seminars, and, in some instances, to conduct psychoanalytic treatment of control cases under the supervision of a training analyst.[2] Thus, in the near future there may be a substantial increase in the number of well-trained investigators who will be adequately equipped to conduct psychoanalytic case research.

The suggestion that the psychoanalytic case method should be used to study the effects of situational events in adult life is based on the simple assumption that such events can play a more or less important role, in interaction with predispositional variables, as determinants of changes in adult attitudes and behavior. This suggestion does not carry any implications with respect to the debatable issues raised by K. Horney (1937), K. Lewin (1935), and numerous anti-Freudian critics concerning the relative causal importance of *current* reality factors as compared with predispositional factors which are the product of *past* experiences. Studies of the impact of current events do not necessarily minimize the importance of past experiences. On the contrary, researches concerning the sustained effects of exposure to wartime dangers and to many other types of adult experiences often highlight the crucial importance of latent reaction tendencies which are the residues of childhood experiences. (This is what turned out to be the case in the psychoanalytic study of surgery reported in the present volume, as can be seen by glancing at the summary in Chapter 17.)

In the following chapters, pertinent material will be encountered from which the reader can make his own judgment about the potential value of using depth interview data from psychoanalytic sessions for the purpose of studying nonpathological aspects of an adult's reactions to stressful environmental conditions. There are many other aspects of normal behavior, in addition to those involving psychological stress, which also could be profitably investigated by using such data (Escalona, 1952; Janis, 1956).

The reactions noted in one particular case may, of course, be uniquely determined by the individual's specific combination of social skills, group affiliations, ideological preferences, and personality predispositions. But at least a few of the individual's psychological changes are apt to be generalizable in the sense that they might prove to be typical of a delimited group of persons sharing a common social background or possessing a specifiable constellation of personality characteristics. Some of the individual's reactions might even prove to have such a high degree of generality that the psychoanalytic data on the impact of a given external event could help to predict and explain what will happen to the vast majority of people in modern society as a consequence of being exposed to the same type of event.

If a sizeable number of analysts were to investigate the effects of environmental changes among their patients, it might be possible to discover and test a number of significant hypotheses about regularities in the impact of the changes on certain types of personalities, on the average individual in a given subculture, and perhaps even on the average individual in western civilization. The section which follows will discuss the possibilities of building up large samples of psychoanalytic cases and of replicating case study findings with objectively reported data obtained from psychoanalytic patients in various social strata in different countries.

Improving the Case Method

In recent years, a number of psychoanalysts have begun to examine critically the techniques and traditions of psychoanalytic case studies from the standpoint of improving their methods and increasing the scientific status of their findings. For example, Kubie (1947, 1952) has constructively examined some major methodological deficiencies in psychoanalytic case reports, calling attention especially to the consequences of failing to keep adequate records of interview sessions.

> Because there are no precise records, we have no objective evaluation of the relative efficacy of different concepts, different theories, different technical procedures, different ways of handling the transference situation. For the same reason, we lack any detailed studies of psychoanalytic failures, that necessary equivalent of the post-mortem of internal medicine. And for the same reason also, we lack reports from psychiatrists, analyst or otherwise, who have treated ten consecutive cases of hysterical aphonia, ten consecutive cases of agoraphobia, and other conditions. Instead we have theories and more theories, and ever new and redundant and overlapping terms. Whenever we of the psychoanalytic profession experience frustration, whenever we bump against a difficult problem, we comfort ourselves with a new theory or a new name. This was true of Freud; but let us not forget that it is even more true of the many modern messiahs. All that it is fair to say in criticism of Freud is that in this respect he set us an unfortunate example.
>
> Here again it should be clear that this was an inevitable consequence of the fact that psychoanalysis had to begin as a form of private medical practice. This limited the opportunity for those controlled and recorded obser-

vations which constitute the core of clinical research. Clinical theorizing, however brilliant, does not become clinical research until it is buttressed by precise, repeatable observations, accurately recorded. (Kubie, 1947.)

Benjamin (1950) has also discussed numerous methodological problems in the validation of psychoanalytic theory and has concluded that the psychoanalytic case method is "more *subjective than it need be.*" He points out that there are some obvious limitations which should be taken into account, such as the fact that the interplay between the analyst's interpretations and the patient's associations introduces an effect of the observer upon the observed. For the purpose of increasing the objectivity of the case method, he offers two main suggestions: (1) "that better protocols of psychoanalytic interviews than are now available would strengthen both the heuristic and the verificatory aspects of the . . . method" and (2) that "the method itself be carefully examined for possible techniques which could increase its relative objectivity and accessibility to critical scrutiny without sacrificing its unique heuristic qualities." (Benjamin, 1950.)

In line with the above comments, it could be said that there are additional methodological shortcomings, repeatedly emphasized by some of Freud's scientific critics, which also make psychoanalytic research findings more questionable than they need be. Some of the important difficulties center on the problem of obtaining adequate samples for psychoanalytic investigations. Not only are the available samples usually limited to one or a handful of cases but the entire series of research studies bearing on any given psychological problem are apt to be limited to persons representing only a very small substratum of the total urban population. It is a well-known fact that during the 1950's the vast majority of psychoanalytic patients in the United States have been well-educated neurotics who can afford to pay an analyst at least $15 or $20 per session, four or five times every week, for two or more years.

There is an obvious need for deliberate and concerted effort to replicate the initial findings of each psychoanalytic investigation with a wide variety of additional cases from different social strata. The feasibility of such replication seems to have increased during the past decade. At present there are thousands of neurotic patients undergoing treatment with well-trained analysts. Despite the high concentration on upper income levels, the total population of analysands includes several hundred low income level patients, many being charged minimal fees at psychoanalytic clinics. And there are also hundreds of relatively "normal" persons, who, as psychiatric candidates, are undergoing psychoanalysis for training purposes (Knight, 1953).[3]

Since most psychoanalytic practitioners are affiliated with national or international professional organizations, it should not prove to be extraordinarily difficult to mobilize the research potential of those psychoanalytic observers who have the requisite methodological training. In the future, as research training becomes more extensive, it should be possible to alert those psychoanalysts with research interests to the need for objective replication as well as discovery, thus motivating them to keep systematic records and to pool their data occasionally; then at least a few research studies may have the benefit of the collaboration of several analysts who are separately making comparable interview observations, using mutually agreed upon criteria for investigating the same clinical or theoretical problem. For the long run, then, it seems realistic to expect that repeated observations can be made, providing replications of observations bearing on the causes and consequences of unconscious conflicts, motives, memories, and fantasies. Although large and representative samples may be unobtainable, it should be possible to have crucial replications carried out, more or less independently, by numerous trained psychoanalytic observers in many different parts of the world, with samples including persons of different cultural and ethnic backgrounds from diverse socio-economic strata.

In addition to the difficulties of gathering reliable facts from adequate samples, there are several special problems of case reporting. Some of these have been alluded to in Kubie's and Benjamin's general comments about the need for greater objectivity and are of central importance for attaining what Kris (1947) has referred to as "semantic clarification." Among the most crucial problems are those of giving accurate and unambiguous summaries of the extensive interview data on which the psychoanalytic case findings are based.[4]

The general scientific status of psychoanalytic findings undoubtedly would be quite different today if, after the first few decades of major discoveries, participants in the psychoanalytic movement had paid more attention to legitimate scientific criticisms concerning problems of sampling, replication, and accurate reporting. After all, during the many years since Freud made his last case study, there must have been tens of thousands of persons all over the world who have had psychoanalytic treatment, from whom the data could have been obtained that is needed for testing and developing Freud's verifiable hypotheses. Perhaps the next few decades will bring much greater research productivity along with the growing realization that the mere reinforcement of an esoteric oral tradition, however valuable for purposes of clinical training, nevertheless contributes little in the direction of achieving the major scientific goals toward which Freud directed his entire lifework.

Value of Psychoanalysis for Studying Mediating Processes

In terms of the stimulus-response vocabulary frequently used in current behavioral research, the most general explanatory propositions concerning the dynamics of environmentally induced behavior can be schematized as taking the following form: For all human organisms (*O*) or for some general class of predisposed people (*Op*), the occurrence of a given stimulus situation or event (*S*) will tend to evoke temporary or sustained changes in internal processes (*x*)—including changes in attitudes, fantasies, and other response-produced stimuli (*r-s*)—which mediate a delimited class of observable reactions (*R*). For convenience, such explanatory propositions can be represented by the following symbols: For *Op*, $S \rightarrow x \rightarrow R$. These symbols are introduced because they provide a useful terminology for referring to different classes of antecedents and consequences which enter into general psychological propositions about stressful events.

A significant example of the type of proposition under discussion is the general conclusion which emerged from research studies concerning "near-miss experiences" among people in communities hit by wartime or peacetime disasters (Janis, 1951; MacCurdy, 1943; M. Wolfenstein, 1957). The term "near-miss experiences" refers to a class of environmental stimulus events (*S*) which have been found to produce various overt behavioral disturbances forming a single general class of manifest symptoms, designated as "acute anxiety reactions" (*R*). This relationship has been regularly observed among relatively large numbers of soldiers and civilians of different nationalities—American, English, German, Japanese, etc. What the findings indicate is that for a very broad class of *Op* (e.g., any psychologically intact human being), the probability of *R* (acute anxiety symptoms) will be markedly increased if *S* occurs (e.g., exposure to the sights and sounds of the sudden collapse of surrounding buildings). Given the extensive research data which support the *S-R* correlation, theoretical questions arise as to what mediating processes can account for the effects of the given class of stimuli.

A tentative answer was povided in reports about a relatively small number of cases by psychoanalysts in Britain during the air blitz (Glover, 1941; M. Schmideberg, 1942). The outstanding mediating factors noted in these case studies involved a marked change in the individual's self-attitudes, a loss of the previously effective self-reassuring convictions which had bolstered the individual's sense of personal invulnerability. Once this type of mediating reaction (*x*) was inferred from the additional class of observable responses (*Rx*) provided by the depth-interview data, it became possible to give a more precise specification of the crucial conditions under which anxiety symptoms are provoked. For instance, it directed attention to clinical data showing that the class of effective stimulus events includes, in addition to experiences of pain and injury, instances where the individual remains untouched by the physical impact of a disaster but witnesses its direct effects on other people (see Bond, 1952; Garner, 1945; Grinker and J. Spiegel, 1945a). Moreover, the formulations of the mediating factor led some investigators to design large-scale studies that could provide objective correlational data pertinent to testing the explanatory hypothesis ($S \rightarrow x \rightarrow R$). Thus, for example, some confirmatory evidence was obtained from a study of several hundred U. S. air crew returnees shortly after they had completed their combat duty, comparing high- and low-anxiety cases with respect to conscious beliefs about their personal vulnerability (Grinker et al., 1946).

In general, by carrying out research oriented toward formulating and testing hypotheses about mediating variables, the likelihood is increased that the data will contribute to more precise propositions specifying the observable factors (environmental stimuli and indicators of personal dispositions) which are necessary conditions for the occurrence of a given type of observable behavior. (See the discussions of mediating variables and constructs in the writings of Brunswick, 1952; Hempel, 1952; Spence, 1948; and Tolman, 1949.)

In conducting research on common *S-R* relationships which occur in situations of stress, the mediating symbolic or affective responses are sometimes available to consciousness and, hence, may be investigated by a variety of standard research techniques, including focalized interviews and attitude questionnaires. But when attempting to study some of the more subtle aspects of stress behavior, one must expect to find that the mediating internal responses will prove to be partially or wholly unconscious.

The main advantage of psychoanalytic observations, as compared with other observational methods, is that during the interviews a variety of verbal associations, affective changes, and other behavioral manifestations can be observed (*Rx*) which facilitate inferences about unconscious emotional impulses, attitudes, anticipations, fantasies, and other mediating symbolic responses not ordinarily available to consciousness. After all, few psychologists would claim that objective personality tests, projective techniques, or any other observational device currently available can be compared with the intensive procedures of psychoanalysis as a method for investigating the deepest layers of the human personality and for obtaining detailed personal information concerning the impact of past and present events on the inner life of the individual. Although many observational techniques can be used to study the same basic *S-R* relationships, they do not afford as great an opportunity for microscopic study of unconscious and preconscious processes (Hilgard, 1952).

More specifically, psychoanalytic case research has the following main assets: The technique of free association elicits observable verbal responses in which fantasies, wishes, and conflicts are expressed that are not subject to reliable self-observation and that are ordinarily withheld from the observation of others. Both the form and content of each patient's verbal responses can be investigated in the light of empirical generalizations and theoretical assumptions based on prior psychoanalytic observations of other cases. Furthermore, the observations of each analysand are made during hundreds of sessions, so that, if a given emotional or symbolic response appears to be a reaction to a given inner or outer stimulus, the relationship can be checked by obtaining comparable observations from many sessions with the same subject. In the course of two or more years of psychoanalytic sessions, the observer becomes thoroughly familiar with the personality of the subject, which facilitates discriminating those reactions which are highly dependent upon the occurrences of external stimuli from those that are not. As S. Isaacs (1939) has pointed out, "In no other field of science is the study of one organism, one mind, carried on for such a long period and in such an exhaustive manner."

It is the combination of these particular features that gives the psychoanalytic case method its unique status in the human sciences. With regard to studying the impact of environmental events, the essential point is that the analyst is sometimes in a position to observe repeated instances where: (*a*) the given patient is currently exposed to a specified type of impressive situational event (*S*); (*b*) the patient gives clear-cut indications (which meet the minimal criteria for accepting retrospective verbal reports) that in his daily life he is displaying manifest attitudes and actions which are overt reactions (*R*) to the event; and (*c*) while talking about the event the patient also displays various affective responses and sequences of verbal associations (*Rx*) which are indicators of internal mediating processes (*x*). Thus, a large sample of behavioral instances may be obtained from which to infer a causal sequence ($S \rightarrow x \rightarrow R$) for the particular individual.

An obvious weakness of a single case study, which has already been mentioned, is that it can provide no indication as to whether the relationship applies to all other, many other, a few other, or no other human beings. Thus, even when a causal sequence is repeatedly found in a given person, the investigator cannot be sure that his finding can be generalized to any broad class of persons (*Op*) because the relationship may occur only in an unspecifiable, restricted class of persons sharing a unique constellation of complex predispositional attributes. [To put the matter in more technical language, whenever consistent relationships between independent (stimulus) variables and dependent (response) variables are observed in a case study of one individual, a major limitation of the findings is that there are zero degrees of freedom with respect to individual differences, even though each finding may be based on hundreds of degrees of freedom with respect to the samples of the subject's behavior that enter into the correlation between the independent and dependent variables.]

The huge question mark concerning *Op* that one must attach to generalizations about any antecedent-consequent relationships discovered in individual case studies seems to be generally recognized by most research workers in the behavioral and biological sciences. (See the discussion of methodological problems by Whiting and Child, 1953, pp. 4–15.) In the absence of replications from a large series of comparable case studies, the investigator usually makes "cross inductions," taking into account what is already known from prior research concerning the way in which the stimuli and responses he is investigating are linked with predispositional variables. For example, if a case study were to deal with reactions to an environmental situation in which people encounter marked interference with their daily routines (e.g., during military training), the investigator would undoubtedly take account of the fact that his subject had previously displayed chronic obsessional neurotic tendencies, and, therefore, he would be likely to formulate the tentative hypotheses derived from his findings as applying only to the limited class of persons who have such predispositional tendencies. But, if the same investigator were to study intense emotional reactions evoked by painful physical injury in the same patient, he might decide that existing knowledge warrants formulating his tentative hypotheses as applying to a much broader population (e.g., all persons in western society). Thus, judgments about the generality of case study findings are usually made by evaluating the variables in the light of existing facts and theories. In this way, certain case findings are promptly discarded as being idiosyncratic to the individual observed, whereas other findings may be singled out as potential generalizations which warrant systematic testing.

Although every scientific investigator knows that ultimately his conclusions will be accepted, rejected, or modified by the findings from subsequent research, the value of his case studies will be very slight indeed if none of the general hypotheses suggested or implied by his findings turn out to be confirmed. In order to maximize the chances of arriving at valid generalizations, the case investigator, from the very outset, can take account of prior research findings concerning the psychological consequences of the antecedent variable he is investigating, selecting for intensive study those examples of manifest reactions which have already been found to occur with a sizeable incidence among a specifiable class of persons or among representative samples of a large population. Intensive studies of one or a few individuals probably will have the greatest chance of arriving at valid general laws concerning the impact of environmental events if such studies are confined mainly to ferreting out the mediating psychological processes which can account for the occurrence of widely observed overt reactions.

The proposed selective procedure does not involve the obviously erroneous assumption that phenomenologically similar behaviors always follow from the same psychological causes; rather the assumption is that among all the various reactions elicited in different people by a common environmental stimulus, those reactions which are phenomenologically similar have a somewhat higher probability of being mediated by the same internal (symbolic and emotional) responses than those which are phenomenologically dissimilar. If the latter assumption is correct, it follows that the case investigator should attempt to separate the manifest reactions of his subject which appear to be *uniquely idiosyncratic* from those known to be *typical*, in the sense that they characterize the manifest behavior of at least a sizeable percentage of other persons who had been previously observed in the given type of stimulus situation. The investigator can then concentrate his research efforts on investigating the psychological factors which enter into the typical relationships rather than the idiosyncratic ones. He may thereby maximize his chances of arriving at a causal sequence ($S \rightarrow x \rightarrow R$) which will constitute a *prototype* for many other cases.

Outline of Part I

In the chapters of Part I which follow, psychoanalytic interview data are used for the purpose of investigating the internal processes which mediate a patient's overt reactions to the external dangers posed by a surgical operation. An attempt is made to orient the investigation toward understanding "typical" stress reactions displayed by the patient and to exclude those behavioral manifestations which were idiosyncratic or of unknown generality. Many different types of comparative data on the way people react to the danger of injury or death were used in order to select typical reactions. The specific procedures will be described in the next chapter, which also includes a brief summary of the patient's social background and life history up to the time of the surgical experience.

Taking account of the need to separate psychoanalytic observations from inferences, the chapters dealing with the psychoanalytic research are organized in the following way: One chapter will be devoted to describing in narrative form what went on in the psychoanalytic sessions during the initial premonitory phase of the surgical experience. This chapter will be followed by a purely theoretical one, in which the implications of the observations are discussed in relation to the findings from other studies of stress behavior for the purpose of formulating general hypotheses about mediating processes. The same alternating pattern will be followed with respect to each of the successive phases of the stress episode, i.e., a descriptive chapter on the psychoanalytic observations will always be presented separately and will then be followed by one or more theoretical chapters. (Case observations are given in Chapters 4, 6, 9, 11 and 14; hypotheses on the dynamics of stress behavior are presented and discussed in Chapters 5, 7, 8, 10, 12, 13, 15, and 16.)

For convenience in cross-referencing, the major hypotheses are numbered and italicized in the text. These are the hypotheses which are most definitely supported by evidence from the psychoanalytic case study and which, in the light of evidence from other sources, appear most likely to be generally applicable to large numbers of persons in similar stress situations. The author has not hesitated, however, to present some additional psychoanalytic hypotheses (stated without being numbered or italicized) for which the evidence is less substantial in that: (*a*) the pertinent psychoanalytic data are incomplete or (*b*) other studies of stress behavior do not provide any clear-cut indications as to the generality of the overt stress reactions in question. All of the hypotheses, whether numbered or unnumbered, are put forth as tentative generalizations which, in the author's judgment, may ultimately prove to be confirmed and for which the currently available evidence provides more or less preliminary substantiation. The main psychodynamic hypotheses will be re-examined in Part II, in the light of the behavioral research findings based on the author's intensive interviews of a small sample of hospitalized surgical patients and the survey data from a fairly large sample of adolescents who reported on their surgical experiences.

Notes

1. Freud's earliest work was not so sharply restricted to investigating predispositional aspects of abnormal behavior. Many of his researches were directed toward understanding various types of reactions to environmental situations which he selected for investigation because of their general psychological interest, quite aside from any connection with psychopathology. Included in his studies on the psychology of dreams, for instance, were inquiries concerning the normal changes in fantasy activity which take place under conditions of sleep, from which he inferred mediating processes involving a reduction in internal censorship (S. Freud, 1904, 1905b, and 1930). Similarly, normal psychological reactions evoked by various classes of social stimuli occupied Freud's attention in his studies of grief (1917), humor (1916), idealization of leaders, social conformity, and related topics (1921). In his monograph on *Wit and the Unconscious* (1916), for example, Freud was attempting to discern a mediating psychological process that occurs in all normal adults—in this instance, one that could account for the pleasure produced by certain types of interpersonal communications (jokes, wit, the comic). However, on the negative side, it must be said that Freud frequently failed to give an adequate account of the psychoanalytic interview evidence which he presumably used to evaluate his insightful hypotheses. Except for his detailed monograph on the psychology of dreams (1930), in which he draws upon interview material from his clinical practice, Freud's writings on normal processes rarely refer to any specific evidence from psychoanalytic investigations of his patients. In his contributions on humor, group behavior, and other normal aspects of adult life, he rarely cites anything more than some anecdotal examples from his own pioneering efforts at self-analysis or from his incidental nonpsychoanalytic observations of friends and acquaintances in daily life. Other psychoanalysts who discuss these same psychological problems seem to follow Freud's example with respect to omitting any detailed presentation of pertinent case study data from their patients. Only very fragmentary material bearing on such problems can be found in those reports which attempt to describe or summarize the data obtained from psychoanalytic interviews.

In published case reports, detailed accounts are sometimes given of current situational factors in relation to the patient's nonpathological fantasy productions (e.g., hypnagogic reveries) and parapraxes (e.g., slips of speech and forgetting of names). But here again, the central interest is much the same as in studies concerning the role of the current reality situation in the production of abnormal symptoms: most carefully examined is the case material on the "psychopathology of everyday life," which helps to illuminate the pathological processes involved in neuroses, character disorders, or psychoses. The only other situational stimuli of adult life that have been extensively discussed in psychoanalytic case reports are those pertaining to the interaction between analyst and patient (problems of effective therapeutic technique and the psychology of transference and countertransference). Even in this limited area, much of the interest has been centered on understanding the relationship between interview stimuli and changes in neurotic attitudes and symptoms. Thus, psychoanalytic interview data continue to be reported almost exclusively for the purpose of increasing knowledge about psychopathology or about ways of modifying the personality predispositions which give rise to psychopathological disorders.

2. Because of the lack of opportunity to obtain training in psychoanalytic techniques, few psychologists or social scientists are equipped at present to conduct psychoanalytic case research. During the last two decades, many quasi-legal and professional obstacles have been set up by the "official" psychoanalytic organizations in the United States with the intent of restricting the practice of psychoanalytic therapy to the medical profession. Since it is impossible for anyone without an M.D. degree to become a member of the American Psychoanalytic Association, all lay analysts, including many prominent clinicians trained in European institutes, are generally regarded as "illicit" practitioners. This situation has influenced American universities to avoid giving trainees in clinical psychology any courses on the application of psychoanalytic techniques to the treatment of emotional disorders. Such a policy gives rise to an anomalous unfamiliarity with the psychoanalytic case study method among research workers in psychology and the social sciences. As Benjamin, Grinker, Kubie, and other analysts have repeatedly pointed out, much misdirected time and energy are devoted to studying, developing, and evaluating all sorts of laboratory techniques and standardized tests that are intended to investigate "unconscious" processes by research workers who know hardly anything at all about the prime methods from which most present-day knowledge of psychodynamics is derived.

Fortunately, the lack of sophistication concerning the technical aspects of psychoanalysis is beginning to be corrected by the efforts of a few leading training analysts who are aware of the need to provide adequate psychoanalytic instruction for experimentally oriented psychologists and for other research specialists in the human sciences. As a participant in a training program for research candidates at the New York Psychoanalytic Institute, the author became acutely aware of the differences between the training in psychoanalysis available to university graduate students and that offered to professional psychoanalytic trainees.

3. Professional census statistics, presented by Knight in his Presidential Address to the American Psychoanalytic Association at the end of 1952, indicate that during that year there were 996 postdoctoral students affiliated with eleven "official" psychoanalytic institutes in the United States. The current crop of students, according to Knight, differs from those of the 1920's and 1930's— ". . . perhaps the majority of students of the past decade or so have been 'normal' characters . . . not so introspective, inclined to read only the literature that is assigned in institute courses . . . [with] interests [that] are primarily clinical rather than research and theoretical. Their motivation for being analyzed is more to get through this requirement of training rather than to overcome neurotic suffering in themselves or to explore introspectively and with curiosity their own inner selves." (Knight, 1953.)

4. In order to test certain of the most complicated psychoanalytic propositions, it will undoubtedly be necessary to develop reliable quantitative techniques of semantical content analysis that can be applied systematically to interview protocols (Auld and Murray, 1955; Dollard and Auld, 1955; Janis, 1943; Lasswell, 1938.)

Before such an enterprise can lead to successful means for testing significant hypotheses, however, a great many major obstacles must be overcome, the most important of which involve the problems of translating major psychoanalytic constructs into objective terms that are unambiguously connected with the raw data of psychoanalytic observations. To begin with, the most feasible content analysis procedures probably will be those which enable the analytic investigator to test *short-term predictions* concerning his patient's verbal behavior. For example, many hypotheses concerning the differential effects of a given type of analytic intervention on transference attitudes, fantasies, and defenses can be tested by: (*a*) systematically studying the content of the patient's associations in the two or three sessions following each instance when the given type of intervention was used, and (*b*) comparing the content analysis results with those obtained in similar sessions following comparable instances when other types of intervention were used. After content analysis techniques have been developed for the study of short-term changes in behavior, it will probably be much easier to work out appropriate modifications to apply to longer series of sessions and thus to extend the systematic investigations to *long-term changes*.

Even when the observer is merely trying to summarize some of the most elementary data concerning unconscious phenomena obtained from psychoanalytic interviews, a number of special requirements should be regarded as essential for indicating the status of the evidence. In continuous case seminars conducted at psychoanalytic institutes, sharp disagreements sometimes occur among experienced analysts, as well as among the trainees, regarding such questions as the following: What evidence, if any, shows the analyst to be correct in surmising that a patient's politely worded complaints about him at the beginning of the session are indicative of unconscious hostility? Can a patient's fragmentary recollections of a childhood sexual experience in the associations given to a dream be regarded as a genuine memory? Intense debates are occasionally provoked if a reporting analyst happens to make grossly incomplete observational statements which refer more or less vaguely to only a fragment of the evidence from which he has made his inferences. His judgment is likely be questioned, for example, if he makes the mistake of confining his remarks to such generalizations as "The patient was outwardly friendly and deferential but made criticisms of the analyst which reflect latent negative transference," or "His associations led to the recovery of a memory of childhood masturbation." In the course of a seminar dispute, the reporting analyst usually amplifies his remarks by citing a great many detailed observations, and sometimes his evidence is sufficiently clear-cut to convince everyone present that he had, in fact, encountered a genuine instance of negative transference or that his patient was recalling an actual childhood event.

Despite exposure to numerous seminar experiences of this kind, however, most psychoanalytic writers continue to fill their published case reports with vague and ambiguous statements, taking no cognizance of the need to describe what was actually observed with sufficient clarity and in sufficient detail to convey the status of their case evidence to fellow analysts (even omitting from consideration the problems of communicating the positive and negative features of the evidence to a more general audience of students of psychology, psychiatry, and the social sciences).

Perhaps the simplest way to illustrate the gross ambiguities that occur in psychoanalytic case studies is to consider a typical statement concerning the "reconstruction" of a childhood memory. An analyst may assert, for instance, that his psychoanalytic investigation indicates that the patient had undergone a specific type of traumatic experience at a certain period of childhood. In making such an assertion, the analyst may mean any of at least six different things so far as the nature of his evidence is concerned:

(*a*) The patient *spontaneously recalled* the specific event during one or more psychoanalytic sessions, and, in addition to displaying *behavioral and verbal consistency,* the patient also produced or described *independent external evidence* (e.g., a contemporary newspaper clipping, or a family letter) to verify the event. (See M. Bonaparte's, 1945, famous example of the use of independent evidence in verifying a primal scene memory.)

(*b*) No external verification was available but the patient *spontaneously recalled* the event during one or more analytic sessions while displaying consistent *behavioral signs* of genuine recollection, and, at other times in the analysis, gave numerous associations which were *internally consistent* with respect to the specific content of the "memory." (See the comments about laughter, blushing, transitory somatic symptoms, and signs of internal consistency with respect to the patient's productions during psychoanalytic sessions in the discussion by Ferenczi, 1912.)

(*c*) No external verification of the event was available and the patient did not spontaneously recall it but gave *confirmatory postintervention associations,* such as the recollection of "new memories which complete and extend the construction" after the analyst had communicated his conjectures about the event on the basis of the patient's (preintervention) associations. (See S. Freud's, 1932, account of the criteria for confirmatory associations in judging the validity of psychoanalytic interpretations.)

(*d*) No external verification of the event was available, the patient did not spontaneously recall it, and after the analyst had communicated a reconstruction of the memory, the patient's (postintervention) associations were too ambiguous to be regarded as confirmatory; nevertheless, there were numerous *specific "derivatives" in the preintervention associations,* from which the analyst inferred that the patient actually had undergone and retained the experience, even though it remained inaccessible to awareness. By "derivatives" is meant verbalizations derived from repressed memories and impulses, symbolically expressed by means of "associatively connected ideas that are less objectionable to the conscious ego" (Fenichel, 1945, p. 17). (See also S. Freud's, 1918, illustrations of the way free associations are used to infer those crucial childhood events which "are as a rule not reproduced as recollections, but have to be divined—constructed—gradually and laboriously from an aggregate of indications.")

(*e*) No positive evidence was obtained with respect to any of the various criteria referred to in (*d*); nevertheless, after a careful retrospective examination of his detailed case notes, the analyst judged—on the basis of his knowledge derived from the psychoanalytic literature and from his own experience with similar cases—that it was plausible to postulate the given traumatic experience (as a hypothetical "construction") because it appeared not only to account for otherwise unexplained psychoanalytic observations but also *fits in consistently with all the known facts about the patient's life history and personality development.* (See the comments by S. Isaacs, 1939, concerning the way analysts attempt to confirm or modify their conclusions about the meaning of a patient's story concerning past events by observing the consistencies and variations in the patient's repetitions of the story during successive phases of the analysis.)

(*f*) No evidence at all can be cited, but when he thought retrospectively about the treatment of the patient, the analyst had a *general clinical hunch or impression* which inclined him to postulate the particular childhood memory; although the analyst made no attempt to examine the case notes in detail (or had not recorded any), he had a general sense that the postulated memory fit in well with his global recollections of the psychoanalytic case material. (See the discussions by Brierley, 1951, and Reik, 1949, on the importance of "empathy" and "intuitive" processes.)

The above six categories are not exhaustive but merely represent some typical combinations of the *eight criteria* which appear to be the main ones used to evaluate any psychoanalytic hypothesis asserting that a patient has experienced a given childhood event: (1) spontaneous recall of the event during one or more analytic sessions; (2) independent external evidence of the event; (3) consistent behavioral signs of the genuineness of the recollections bearing on the event; (4) internal consistency of the recollections bearing on the event; (5) specific (symbolic) "derivatives" of the event in preintervention associations; (6) confirmatory associations after the analyst's intervention focused attention on the inferred event; (7) over-all consistency of the inferred event with respect to the entire set of case history data; and (8) the observer's global clinical impression of the plausibility of the inferred event. The eight criteria can occur, of course, in many other combinations in addition to those described in the six categories. The latter were selected so as to highlight one simple fact about psychoanalytic findings, which is sometimes difficult to grasp from reading psychoanalytic reports, namely, that *the supporting evidence can range from being very substantial to very flimsy.* The first category (p. 30), for example, comes close to meeting the criteria of reliability and validity that most legal experts and historians require for deciding that an alleged event probably had occurred. At the other end of the scale, however, the last category would be evaluated by most analysts (as well as by most research workers in other fields) as important for arriving at new hypotheses about a patient's unconscious processes, but of such questionable reliability and validity as to offer very little empirical weight to the analyst's conjectural reconstruction. In other words, an analyst's over-all recollections and impressions of his unrecorded psychoanalytic observations would be regarded, at best, as increasing the empirical probability of the reconstruction by a barely noticeable difference over what it would be had the analyst merely indulged in crude armchair speculation based solely on the obvious clinical diagnostic facts regarding the onset and development of the patient's emotional disorder, without taking any account whatsoever of the patient's free associations. Expressing a point of view that is beginning to be shared by many research-minded psychoanalysts, Kubie has emphasized that as long as analysts rely on unrecorded impressions or memories, their case reports are of little value as evidence: "After a time, the observer can no longer differentiate clearly and surely what the patient has said from what he himself has said . . ." (Kubie, 1952, p. 117).

The criteria discussed above are formulated with reference to the problem of reconstructing childhood memories; but similar criteria (with some modifications in wording, especially concerning the nature of external verification) would apply to other major types of constructions inferred from psychoanalytic data, e.g., unconscious fantasies, the latent content of dreams, and the infantile impulses and defenses that enter into "transference" symptoms.

One of the main values of discussing such criteria is that merely to designate them can help to provide at least a rough answer to the question that so often besets the psychoanalyst who is trying to condense or summarize in a reasonable amount of space the voluminous interview data accumulated from hundreds of hourly sessions: How much information should be included? Obviously, as a bare minimum, the report should at least give sufficient information to indicate for each reconstruction the type of evidence on which the main inferences are based. (In Chapters 4 to 16 the author has attempted to adhere to this minimal standard, at the obvious cost of some apparently tedious elaborations of observational details.)

Ultimately, along with other improvements in the methods of psychoanalytic case study research, more refined categories for specifying the status of the evidence will undoubtedly be developed to take into account differential degrees of reliability and validity.

3.

The psychoanalytic study of surgery

The opportunity to obtain depth interview observations bearing on the emotional impact of surgery arose unexpectedly in the course of conducting a lengthy psychoanalysis with a psychoneurotic patient. The psychoanalytic treatment was conducted by the author according to standard Freudian principles. It was done under the auspices of a research project that had been set up in collaboration with medical colleagues in the Department of Psychiatry at Yale University (including a training analyst who was available for supervision of the treatment).

Research Procedures

Descriptive records were routinely kept of the psychoanalytic sessions which took place before, during, and after the stressful period, and these were sufficiently detailed to permit a precise assessment of the psychological changes evoked by the surgical experience. Taking account of the problems of extracting potentially valid generalizations from a single case study, the author concentrated his research efforts on discerning unconscious factors that enter into *typical* reactions to external stress stimuli.

The psychoanalytic treatment had been going on for about two years when the patient (a middle-class woman in her late thirties) began to fill her sessions with associations in which she expressed thoughts, feelings, and fantasies concerning an impending surgical operation on her leg. Then, a few weeks after the operation had been performed, when the patient resumed psychoanalytic treatment, her sessions were again filled with salient details about the surgical experience. At the time, the author was routinely keeping detailed notes on each session, not because he had expected to make a special study of the data bearing on surgery but because the psychoanalytic observations of this particular patient were being used in a longitudinal study of attitude changes in relation to personality needs. Subsequently, when the patient recovered from an acute postoperative depression, the author began to realize that he had learned a great deal about the emotional changes induced by the surgery and that he had the opportunity of studying his records for further information concerning the unconscious motives and defense mechanisms that came into play when the patient was coping with external threats to body integrity. In contrast to the usual psychoanalytic case study, however, the author's inquiry was directed entirely toward understanding the effects of external situational events, including such problems as the following:

1. Why did certain irrelevant events (e.g., a quarrel with a co-worker) have the effect of stimulating acute fear concerning the dangers of surgical mutilation?
2. How did the patient's autistic fantasies and anticipations change when she received realistic information from the surgeon and from others concerning the dangers associated with the surgery?
3. Which types of interpersonal relationships had a reassuring effect or had some influence on the patient's modes of psychological defense in the face of the impending danger?
4. In what way was the patient disappointed by the behavior of other people during the stress episode and how did she attempt to deal with the disappointments?
5. How did external events occurring during the stress episode contribute to the drastic changes observed in the patient's manifest attitude and mood, such as the following: (*a*) during the preoperative period, shifting from complete unconcern about the impending threats to ap-

prehensive overconcern; (*b*) during the postoperative period, shifting from expansive elation to acute depression?

In seeking to discover the causes and consequences of the patient's inner adjustment to the stress situation, the author attempted to take account of the various methodological problems discussed in the preceding chapter. The following procedures were used in an effort to insure a high degree of accuracy and objectivity with respect to each of the three main steps in this study: (*a*) Reporting the psychoanalytic observations; (*b*) drawing conclusions about the patient's stress behavior; and (*c*) deducing tentative hypotheses concerning the determinants of stress reactions that are likely to occur among large numbers of people.

1. *Case notes were recorded immediately after each psychoanalytic session, giving a full account of what the patient said and what the analyst said.* The main goal was to record the *substance* of each participant's statements. A special effort was made to reproduce the expressive quality of the patient's verbalizations so as to retain something of the personal flavor of her speech at times when she was revealing her inner feelings. Somewhat less care was expended in attempting to set down the exact phrasing of the analyst's comments, except for his main interpretations; but an effort was always made to record the gist of every analytic intervention.

There is at least one type of distortion which should be kept in mind when reading the numerous quotations from the analytic sessions in subsequent chapters, and especially when examining the complete record of an entire preoperative session in Chapter 6. Except when a slip of speech occurred or an unconventional phrase was used, the patient's prose was apt to be condensed and smoothed out. Since the records were intended to preserve the substantive content of what was said, they do not include many instances of redundant phrasings, false starts, dangling sentences, or the usual varieties of incidental hemming and hawing that always characterize natural speech. Repetitive phrases and incomplete sentences tended to become consolidated into single statements, and faulty sentence constructions were likely to be improved. Of course, the smoothing-out process applied to the analyst's statements as well as to the patient's, and, consequently, quotations from the protocols might convey a somewhat exaggerated impression of the over-all efficiency with which the two people communicated with each other.

If phonographic or tape recording equipment had been used, a more complete verbatim record obviously could have been obtained. But, since the nature of the research required only a careful summary of the content of each session, the possible gains from using a mechanical recording device did not appear to warrant the potential risk that the presence of a microphone might, to some extent, disrupt the analysis of this particular patient (a woman with strong obsessional tendencies and with an unusually high degree of conflict over exhibitionistic impulses). Taking cognizance of the fact that the records could not be as complete as a tape recording, the analyst made every effort to avoid major omissions or changes in wording that might alter the meaning of the content.

Despite all precautions, any note-taking procedure which requires the analyst to prepare his summaries of the voluminous verbal data obtained from each 50-minute session suffers from the disadvantage of presenting an opportunity for unintentional biases and distortions to enter into the records. The author's working assumption, however, was that, even without the use of a recording machine, the probability of gross errors would tend to be quite low if an experienced research worker took rough notes during the interview itself and then completed his observational report immediately thereafter, without permitting any substantial time lapse in which memory distortions could easily develop. Moreover, some of the sources of "contamination" and bias were probably minimized because at the time the analyst recorded his notes, he did not have in mind studying the patient's reactions to surgery; he did not formulate the main psychodynamic hypotheses until *after* he had recorded and examined *all* of his case notes.

2. *The psychological effects attributable to the external threats, dangers, and deprivations imposed by the surgery were ascertained by means of longitudinal intrapersonal comparisons.* Specifically, the patient's reactions observed in psychoanalytic interviews during the two months comprising the surgery episode were compared with the reactions she had displayed during the preceding two years and during the succeeding year and one-half of her analysis. Detailed records were available for approximately 600 ("nonsurgical" control) sessions in addition to 12 preoperative sessions and 8 postoperative sessions in which the surgical operation was more or less in the focus of attention. In deriving hypotheses concerning reactions to external stress situations, the 20 "surgery" sessions were carefully examined for any unusual responses—affective outbursts, impulsive actions, fantasies, preoccupying thoughts, defensive maneuvers, etc.,—which appeared to be linked with the patient's awareness of the threatening aspects of the surgery and *which she did not ordinarily display at times when no such external*

threats were present. It was possible, therefore, to select potential instances of stress reactions in such a way as to exclude the patient's habitual modes of responding to the ordinary mild stresses of daily life and other such chronic personality manifestations. Thus, the longitudinal data available for lengthy time samples preceding and following the critical period of stress were used to establish a norm or base line for the given patient so as to be able to isolate the unique behavioral fluctuations evoked by the unique environmental stimuli present during the surgical episode.

3. *In order to select prototypic reactions, the patient's stress reactions were compared with those of other persons who had been observed in similar stress situations.* An attempt was made to orient the investigation of mediating psychological processes toward understanding "typical" stress reactions and to exclude those behavioral manifestations which were either idiosyncratic or of unknown generality. Five different types of comparative data were used, all of which pertain to *the way people react when exposed to external situations involving the danger of body damage or death.*

(*a*) *Studies of surgical cases.* The existing psychological and psychiatric literature is relatively sparse on this topic, but a few important observations have been made by various clinical investigators. Although largely impressionistic in character, some interesting and insightful case discussions were found, especially in the clinical reports by Bernstein and Small (1951), H. Deutsch (1942), Fessler (1931), Levy (1945a and 1945b), Lindemann (1944), and Rosen (1950, 1952). As an additional source of observational data for assessing the typicality of the psychoanalytic patient's overt behavior, the author made use of his own research studies (described in Chapters 18 to 26). The data were obtained from intensive case studies of 30 surgical patients and from a survey of 220 male adolescents who reported on their reactions to major and minor surgery. Most of these phenomenological data had already been analyzed and were, therefore, taken into account at the time when the psychoanalytic case material was examined.

(*b*) *Studies of nonsurgical cases hospitalized because of incapacitating illnesses or injuries.* Among the few outstanding psychological studies in this category are those by Hamburg (1953) on victims of mutilating accidents and deforming diseases, Ruesch and Bowman (1948) on chronic illnesses, and Wittkower (1949) on tuberculosis patients undergoing sanatarium treatment.

(*c*) *Studies of persons exposed to peacetime disasters.* Since the time of Prince's (1920) classical study of how people behaved during the Halifax explosion in 1918, there has been a growing body of descriptive literature on the psychological aspects of community catastrophes. Especially valuable for present purposes were the numerous reports prepared in recent years under the sponsorship of the Committee on Disaster Studies of the National Research Council. (As a member of this Committee from the time of its inception in 1951, the author has had access to large numbers of interview protocols of disaster survivors as well as mimeographed research reports on disaster behavior, many of which have not yet been published; see the list of reports in Fritz and Williams, 1957, and M. Wolfenstein, 1957.)

(*d*) *Studies of civilians exposed to wartime bombing attacks.* In a volume on *Air War and Emotional Stress* (1951), the author has previously presented a comprehensive survey and analysis of the available scientific literature concerning the psychological effects of air attacks on the British, German, and Japanese populations in World War II. The generalizations drawn from this analysis provided the initial framework of facts and theories concerning stress reactions with which the author commenced the present series of psychological investigations of surgery. Danger situations of wartime have been much more carefully and extensively studied by psychiatrists, psychologists, and sociologists than those of peacetime and, consequently, this category, together with the next one, constitute the main sources of detailed empirical information concerning typical reactions to environmental stress.

(*e*) *Studies of military personnel exposed to the hazards of combat.* The reactions of combat ground troops and combat air crews have been widely studied by a variety of observational methods, ranging from psychiatric interviews to large-scale questionnaire surveys. Useful reports concerning typical stress reactions of military personnel were found in the comprehensive monographs by Kardiner and H. Spiegel (1947), W. Menninger (1948), Grinker and J. Spiegel (1945a, 1945b), and Stouffer et al. (1949).

Since all five of the above sources of information pertain to human reactions in situations where serious physical dangers are anticipated and actually experienced, they were used conjointly to help identify those manifest reactions of the psychoanalytic patient which could be regarded as typical instances of overt stress behavior. Certain of the patient's overt reactions were judged to be atypical or of unknown generality because they were found rarely or not at all in the numerous observational reports on how people behave under conditions of stress. Many of the patient's behavioral manifestations, on the other hand, appeared to be representative instances of common reactions to stress situations—reactions that were known to occur regularly in a sizeable percentage of exposed people, irrespective of obvious differences in personality characteristics, socio-economic background, or nationality. The latter were selected as "typical" stress reactions and were given the highest priority in the psychoanalytic inquiry, the primary goal being the discovery of the mediating psychological determinants.[1]

Description of the Patient

In view of the limitations of a single case study, discussed in the preceding chapter, it is important that every psychoanalytic case study provide detailed background material in order to take account of possible sources of individual differences in behavior. As psychoanalytic data on stress behavior begin to accumulate, subsequent investigators will need to know the social and personality characteristics of each subject in order to explain the different ways individuals react to the same circumstances of stress. Moreover, even when examining only one psychoanalytic case study, information about the patient's neurotic disturbances, his social class origin, his present family situation, his occupation, and his daily activities furnish part of the essential context necessary for the most elementary understanding of why he thinks, feels, or acts one way rather than another. Accordingly, the remainder of this chapter will be devoted to giving a brief account of the patient's background, with which the reader should become familiar before proceeding to the psychoanalytic observations of the patient's reactions to the threat of surgery. (Additional information on the personality of the patient will be presented in Chapter 10, when discussing specific hypotheses concerning predispositional determinants of stress reactions.)

The patient, whom we shall call Mrs. Blake,[2] had been referred for psychoanalysis by a psychiatrist after he had been treating her once a week in psychotherapy for over a year. Since Mrs. Blake was unable to afford the standard fees for psychoanalysis, the psychiatrist explained to her that the author could take a case at a minimal fee. The opportunity to do so arose because the author was engaged in a psychoanalytic research project (under joint sponsorship of the Departments of Psychiatry and Psychology) at the Institute of Human Relations, Yale University.

At the time of the initial interview the patient was 39 years old, and had been married for 17 years. She lived with her husband and three children in a middle-class apartment house located fairly close to the downtown area of New Haven. Her eldest child, a boy of 15, was followed by a girl of 13 and a boy of 9. When her youngest child started public school, she took a full-time job as salesclerk, and, subsequently, became the assistant manager in a sales section of a large department store. Her husband was steadily employed as a postal inspector. Without the supplementation of Mrs. Blake's earnings, his income would not have enabled the family to buy a new car, to take an annual vacation trip, to pay the orthodontist to straighten their daughter's teeth, or to purchase various pieces of household equipment that are a standard part of most American middle-class homes.

Mrs. Blake was a well-groomed, middle-aged woman, unostentatiously dressed, usually in a well-tailored suit. Despite her fairly athletic build, her short stature, wide hips, and somewhat plump extremities gave an over-all impression of her being rather overweight. Her face, however, was not plump, and, in fact, the taut skin and drawn mouth gave her almost a gaunt, haggard look.

Mrs. Blake's language and manners were typical of a college-bred American woman. A slight British inflection in her speech, which was predominantly Bostonian, reflected the fact that she had spent the first years of her childhood in England before her family had migrated to Massachusetts. Mrs. Blake's father had been a highly respected but financially unsuccessful pharmacist in a small town near Boston. Evidently he was less interested in his business than in the duties connected with the local chapter of a religious fraternal organization in which he was an officer. Throughout her childhood, the patient was aware of the fact that her father was continually in debt.

According to Mrs. Blake's impression, her mother "slaved" from early morning until late at night, never relaxing. Part of the time her mother had worked in the pharmacy, taking charge of all the business accounts. The rest of her time had been devoted to taking care of the family and performing the usual household duties in addition to making all the clothes for her five children.

By dint of extremely rigid budgeting, the parents managed to save enough money to send three of the children to college. The patient spent three years at a small denominational college for women. The parents chose the college in accordance with their conviction, as fervently religious Protestants, that thorough religious instruction should be provided at every stage of a child's education, even through the college level. Not sharing this attitude of her parents, the patient was often in trouble with the college authorities because of her failure to attend religious services regularly. She sometimes violated the rigid rules governing the students' social life, and was once caught with a small group of her classmates attending a dance at a nearby coeducational college. As a result, she and the other girls were expelled. The reaction of her parents surprised her. They did not reproach her but dismissed the whole matter with the attitude, "Oh, well, Dorothy always has been the black sheep of the family!"

The parents displayed the same resigned attitude a year later when she decided to marry Joe Blake, a young man from the west coast who, although quite acceptable to the parents in all other respects, had been married before and had a child. After the divorce, his first wife had married a wealthy California business man and kept the custody of the child; Mr. Blake was required to pay only a very small stipend for its support. Since they lived 3,000 miles apart, the second Mrs. Blake never encountered the first, nor did the husband maintain any contact with his former wife and child.

After the first year of marriage, the patient felt that she had made a mistake, and that she had never really been in love with her husband. The marriage was punctuated with intense quarrels, separations, and extramarital affairs on the part of both husband and wife.

At the beginning of the first interview, Mrs. Blake asserted that the unsatisfactory marriage was the main source of her unhappiness. She said that she wanted psychoanalytic treatment in order to fulfill two main objectives: The first was "to have enough courage to be able to leave my husband." She described Mr. Blake as a superficially attractive man who was really a self-centered baby, sexually passive, almost impotent, and more interested in men than in women, except on rare occasions when he would be violently jealous of her. The second goal was to become more independent and successful as a career woman; she wished to overcome certain personal handicaps in order to work more efficiently and to advance more rapidly to an executive position at a higher level.

In response to questions about the nature of her personal handicaps, Mrs. Blake described a variety of neurotic symptoms which interfered with her job: chronic constipation together with toilet ceremonials which made it necessary to spend an inordinate amount of time in the lavatory every day; frequent headaches, although a neurologist's examination had failed to discover any organic basis for them; phobic avoidances which sometimes prevented her from performing her job duties because she could not enter certain sections of the department store where she worked. She also described severe anxiety attacks which occasionally occurred when she was alone, especially on nights when her husband was away. These attacks reminded her of a male cousin who became insane and had committed suicide; sometimes she could not dispel the disturbing thought that she was destined sooner or later to meet the same fate.

Another complaint was that she behaved in such a way as to antagonize her children and other people with whom she was in daily contact: "I am so fussy, and overbearing; I'm afraid that no one likes me because I've become so completely domineering and aggressive, like my mother." Nevertheless, in describing her social life, she asserted that she was well liked, and even admired, by many friends, and that at social gatherings she and her husband were regarded as the "life of the party." Similarly, despite the numerous neurotic disturbances she had described, she gave a picture of herself as being a fairly competent worker on the job.

During the two years of psychoanalysis which preceded the unexpected occurrence of the surgical operation, the dominant unconscious themes in her free associations concerned infantile ambivalent longings toward her weakly passive father and her oppressively autocratic mother. (See pages 111–114, for details concerning the underlying structure of the patient's neurotic conflicts.) The operation came at a time when her chronic ambivalence toward love objects was focused sharply on two persons, her father and her daughter. Ruminations about them had been stimulated by two recent events; one was the death of her father, which had occurred five months earlier. Although she had felt somewhat depressed and suicidal during her father's terminal illness, Mrs. Blake had completely evaded the psychological work of mourning. At the funeral, she had felt "glad of his death," because she thought it would enable her to develop a more friendly relationship with her mother. She persistently maintained that she now felt completely indifferent about her father. Much of the analyst's activity during this period consisted in calling the patient's attention to the various ways in which she managed to isolate her feelings from her intellectual awareness of the magnitude of the loss.

Against this background, a second, less important event was shaping up, and this had the effect of arousing latent ambivalent tendencies toward the patient's daughter, an eighth-grade student at the time. As a result of inattentiveness and misbehavior, the girl had received failing grades in two courses. Although it was almost time for graduation from grammar school, the home room teacher adamantly maintained that the girl should not graduate and should be required to repeat the two courses during the next school year, an action which would prevent her from starting high school in the fall. Although aware of the fact that this action would be a black mark on her daughter's record and might even disrupt the girl's entire educational career, Mrs. Blake felt reluctant to confer with the teacher and was completely inhibited with respect to taking any steps toward mitigating her daughter's punishment. Earlier in her psychoanalysis, Mrs. Blake had begun to realize that when she treated her daughter with excessive indifference or harshness she was expressing the same sort of detached punitive attitude that she felt her mother had directed toward her. The patient's associations to the current problem led to various childhood experiences and certain transference reactions which appeared to be causally related to her inability to come to the aid of her daughter. These constituted the central topics of the analytic sessions immediately preceding the ones in which the necessity of undergoing a surgical operation became the main focus of attention.

Notes

1. From the discussion of "typical" stress reactions, it is apparent that the term is used to refer to *S-R* relationships which can be expected to occur fairly universally among all types of people. Thus, the psychoanalytic findings which reveal internal responses that may mediate such typical reactions are tentatively formulated as universal reaction tendencies (*Op* = every intact human adult in modern society). Most of the hypotheses derived from the psychoanalytic study fall into this category. In addition, there are a few hypotheses (see pp. 111 ff.) which attempt to describe personality predispositions underlying the readiness to develop exaggerated fear reactions in response to threat stimuli; in these hypotheses, *Op* is explicitly restricted to a class of persons who share a specified constellation of personality characteristics.

The procedure of selecting typical stress reactions was used because it was assumed to be a useful means for increasing the chances of arriving at hypotheses that will prove to have some degree of generality. But the procedure is not regarded as a rigid methodological requirement that must be applied to every psychoanalytic finding, and, in one outstanding instance, the author did not follow the procedure. The exceptional instance was an unexpected finding concerning "unrepression" which strongly suggested the occurrence of an involuntary reaction to stress and which, if confirmed, might lead to the discovery of a hitherto unobserved *S-R* correlation (see Hypothesis 14, p. 188).

2. In order to preserve the anonymity of the patient, all names of persons and places have been altered. For the same reason, various minor circumstantial details, which are not relevant for understanding the psychoanalytic observations, have been replaced by equivalent details.

4.

The patient's premonitions

The interviews to be described in this chapter cover a two-week period during which the patient became aware of her organic disability, obtained the advice of her physicians, and made the decision to submit to surgery. Mrs. Blake had suffered intermittently from acute leg pains for almost a week before she consulted a physician. In the analytic sessions during this particular week, it became apparent that the delay was partly due to her fear of being told that she needed a surgical operation. Although she had been given considerable medical information by a physician, who had treated the same ailment in the past, her expectations concerning the threat of surgery began to be interwoven with fantasies of being mutilated. The repeated autistic themes in her daydreams, together with the associations to a night dream which occurred shortly after she had decided to see a physician, provide a unique opportunity to discern some of the unconscious sources of a psychoneurotic patient's fear of surgery.

SESSIONS 1–4: INITIAL PREOPERATIVE REACTIONS

The first reactions directly stimulated by the impending operation were observed in an analytic session three and one-half weeks before the surgery was actually performed. For convenience in referring to the various analytic sessions that are reported below, the initial session relating to the surgical operation will be called "Session 1" and the subsequent ones will be numbered consecutively in chronological order. Session 1 occurred after the patient had been in psychoanalytic treatment for approximately two years. It followed a weekend during which Mrs. Blake had experienced a considerable amount of pain in her right thigh. During this session, Mrs. Blake said she was afraid that something might be seriously wrong. When the analyst asked if she had considered going to a physician to have her leg examined she responded that she was "too scared" to go because she might need an operation.

Several years earlier she had had similar pains and the physician had told her that, if there were a recurrence, surgery would be necessary. Now, she claimed, her main fear was that the operation would create an ugly scar which would permanently ruin the appearance of her leg. But her associations soon led to daydreams expressing a much more profound concern about body mutilation: she imagined that the operation would turn out to be an amputation of her entire leg.

During the same analytic session in which she first spoke about the danger of a mutilating operation, Mrs. Blake displayed three other reactions which appeared to be closely linked with her fear of body damage.

The first was unusually intense guilt feelings accompanied by explicit expectations of being punished or destroyed for her own misbehavior. The particular event upon which this exaggerated sense of guilt was centered seemed to be a minor aggressive action directed against one of her subordinates. She described how, on that very morning, she had set up a new rule concerning the working hours of the four saleswomen under her supervision. The purpose of the rule was to deprive one of the older employees, toward whom she felt both attracted and repelled, of the opportunity to rearrange her days off to suit her own convenience. During the past two years Mrs. Blake had used her authority on numerous occasions to inflict similar restrictions upon the same woman; but she had not felt so guilty about it before. In a manner that almost directly exemplifies the "talion" principle described by Freud (1910, 1913), Mrs. Blake expressed the fear that her own fate would be to suffer severe bodily loss because "what I did to that woman was like cutting some vital organ out of her body."

The second main reaction during Session 1 was the recollection of a vague childhood memory which she said was "upsetting." She remembered that once when her mother took her to visit at her aunt's house, she had been horrified at her aunt's behavior. Part of the horror was aroused by seeing the aunt lift up her skirt and wash her genitalia, the appearance of which impressed the little girl as being ugly and dirty. Even more horrifying were the "spooky" things the aunt had said, none of which Mrs. Blake could remember during this particular session. (As will be seen in Chapter 9, what her aunt had said was recalled in a later session, on an occasion when Mrs. Blake's fear of the impending operation was even more intense, viz., in the very last analytic hour before going to the hospital.)

The third reaction was of quite a different character. In contrast to the guilt and anxiety involved in the first two reactions, a positive affective state was manifested. Immediately after speaking about the shocking episode of seeing her aunt's vulva, Mrs. Blake asserted that there was something attractive about the idea of becoming a cripple. She went on to explain that the loss of one or both of her legs could result in greater happiness because then she would be comforted and treated more warmly by other people. While speaking about this positive anticipation, she remembered an episode which had already been recalled several times earlier in the analysis. At the age of eight she had been taken on a train by her father to visit friends in the country for several days because her mother was about to give birth to another baby. While looking out the window at one of the stations where the train stopped, she saw a little crippled boy in a wheel chair. It seemed to her that the boy was being lavished with affection by the two women accompanying him. She recollected that at the time she felt very envious and began to daydream about being just like him, with the conscious expectation that as a boy she would be more highly valued by her parents and, as a cripple, she could never again be sent away from home.

During the next three analytic hours (Session 2–4), Mrs. Blake continued to complain about the pains in her leg. But she gave no further associations to the topic, even though the analyst mentioned it several times.

SESSIONS 5 AND 6: ANALYSIS OF A PREOPERATIVE DREAM

Further material bearing on the nature of the three reactions noted in Session 1 occurred a week later, shortly after Mrs. Blake had decided to be examined by a physician. At the beginning of Session 5, she again asserted that the physician would probably recommend an operation, and she expressed concern about being left with a visible scar. This possibility immediately called to her mind a dream that had occurred on the preceding night. Since the prospective operation was the topic initially associated with the content of this dream, it seemed quite probable that Mrs. Blake's anticipated examination by the physician and her fearful attitude toward the contemplated surgery formed a significant part of the day's residue that entered into the formation of her dream:

> I was looking at my face in a mirror and noticed that there was a large pimple on my cheek. I pressed it and was surprised to see a long bony thing come out that looked like spaghetti. As I pressed it, more and more came out. It was very rigid, going straight up from out of my face. I had a great feeling of satisfaction as I pressed it. I felt proud and pleased that I was able to produce this thing even though I knew it was abnormal. I thought to myself that mother will be delighted.

The pimple in the dream constituted the specific element to which Mrs. Blake associated the ugly scar on her leg that might be caused by the operation. After recounting the dream, she spontaneously produced four additional associations to the dream:

1. Pressing the pimple was similar to the way her pimples used to be squeezed by her mother. She remembered that her mother used to become quite exhilarated by this activity and would often exclaim, "Now just look at that nasty little worm!"
2. The bony, rigid object that came out of the pimple called to mind a long, erect penis. This penislike appendage sticking out of her face reminded her of the way she used to play at being a boy when she was about six years old. A favorite game at that time was to place a stick inside her panties as a make-believe penis and then to squat down to pretend to urinate into a pot, in the way she had once seen her father relieve himself when she slept in her parents' room at a summer cottage.
3. The reference to mother in the dream was linked not only with memories of the squeezing of her pimples but also with the recollection that she used to be afraid of being caught playing with the make-believe penis. She had thought that, if she were discovered at this secret activity, father would only be embarrassed, whereas mother would become enraged and would punish her severely.
4. Without mentioning any specific element of the dream, she reported the following transference fantasy shortly after having referred to the dream: The analyst had not been dangerous as long as she had nothing that could be taken away, but now he has become dangerous because she has regrown something; she did not know what it could be, but whatever it was, she had recently recaptured it and wanted to avoid losing it again.

The analyst's interpretations during the two sessions when the patient gave the above associations to the dream were confined entirely to the patient's mixed feelings toward the analyst, the nature of which may be surmised from the last association. No attempt was made at this particular time to give Mrs. Blake an over-all interpretation of the unconscious tendencies suggested by the dream material. In later sessions, however, the analyst took account of the latent content of this dream, as revealed by the above associations, in attempting to understand and to interpret to the patient some of the unconscious determinants of her emotional reactions to the operation.

As the patient associated to the dream, the author gradually became aware of the parallels between the dream material and the content of the earlier analytic session in which Mrs. Blake had spoken for the first time about her premonitions concerning the impending operation. The three main emotional reactions which she had displayed at that time—and which she continued to display intermittently throughout the entire preoperative period—seemed to have their counterparts in the dream material.

First, a major reaction in the earlier session had consisted of feelings of guilt along with the anticipation that the surgery would be a punishment for past and present moral offenses. This type of reaction seems to be directly reflected in her associations to her own actions in the dream, which apparently symbolized an act of masturbation. She remembered being involved in forbidden sex play and being afraid that mother would catch and punish her.

Secondly, there had been the reaction of ill-defined horror, connected with the recollection of having become profoundly upset by the sight of her aunt's genitals. Without necessarily assuming *a priori* that this was to be understood as an expression of "female castration anxiety," the analyst was left with the marked impression that the way she originally related these feelings of horror was very similar to the way she related her last associations to the dream—the associations which had to do with her vague sense of danger concerning the potential loss of some unspecified part of her body at the hands of the therapist.

Thirdly, there had been the contrasting theme of gaining various gratifications, especially maternal care and affection, by becoming a cripple. Very similar in content is the dream association of eliciting mother's warmth and enthusiasm by submitting to the pimple-squeezing operation.

Taking account of the various overlapping memory fragments and the current expectations expressed in the patient's associations to the dream, the analyst surmised that the latent content involved a wish to attain forgiveness and love from a punitive maternal figure (mother, surgeon, analyst). There are also some indications in the dream material that the patient was attempting to reassure herself that she would be able to gain pleasure from manipulating her body and that she would not lose anything (e.g., the protrusion which she produces remains attached to her body). From the standpoint of understanding the latent fears implied by this preoperative dream, there seem to be three central themes that can be summarized as follows: (*a*) I am guilty of having indulged in sexual acts that mother has forbidden; (*b*) my punishment might be to undergo (once again) the horror of losing part of my body (perhaps a repetition of the earlier fantasied loss of the offending genital organ); and (*c*) by submitting to this horrible punishment I will be forgiven and can regain the sort of love my mother used to give me. (See the pertinent life history data on pages 111–114 and 128.

SESSIONS 7 AND 8: INDIFFERENCE VERSUS AGITATION

The day after reporting the preoperative dream, Mrs. Blake phoned for an appointment with her family physician. During the following weekend she was examined by the physician and was referred to a surgeon, who, after further consultation, informed her that an operation would be the best form of treatment. She accepted his recommendation and agreed to enter the hospital a week later. In Session 7, which followed this eventful weekend, Mrs. Blake said nothing at all about it. Instead, she spoke almost exclusively about a topic which had occupied her thoughts in Sessions 2, 3, and 4 during the preceding week, namely, her worries concerning the school problem which affected her daughter (see page 42). She ruminated at great length about her desire to "thrash the whole thing out" with the home room teacher or to "go over her head" to the school principal; but she felt unable to do so because of her uneasiness and uncertainty about the consequences of handling the situation in an aggressive way.

The next day, in a casual, bland manner, she mentioned: "Incidentally, I am going to have an operation next week and so I won't be able to come for analysis for two weeks after that." When the analyst called attention to the contrast between her present casual manner and her anxieties about the operation during the preceding week, she explained that the operation was not at all serious and that she was looking forward to a very pleasurable vacation in the hospital. She expected not only to escape from all the responsibilities of daily life but also to get lots of attention and solicitous care from everybody. She recalled having been worried about the disfigurement of her leg last week, but felt no concern now because the surgeon told her that the scar would gradually fade away and eventually become so faint as to be barely noticeable. She went on to express a mild feeling of disappointment that her surgeon was not going to perform the operation at the University hospital, which was located across the street from the analyst's office. Instead, she would have to go to an affiliated hospital about two miles away. The latter hospital had the advantage that it was only a few blocks away from her home but, still, she wished that the consolidation of the two hospitals—which the newspapers said was scheduled to take place within a few months—had already occurred because then she would be hospitalized in the building close to the analyst's office.

It now occurred to her that she had meant to tell the analyst about the operation during yesterday's hour but had forgotten all about it. In fact, the operation had been hardly on her mind at all yesterday; it had seemed very unimportant compared with the serious problem of having to deal with Mrs. Lucas, her daughter's home room teacher. Last night she had been very agitated about this school problem as well as about something the analyst had said. It was something that had had no effect on her at first but, in the evening, had caused a violent headache, from which she had been suffering ever since. The offending remark was actually a question the analyst had asked when she had been trying to explain her feeling of being unable to offer any opposition to Mrs. Lucas' harsh method of handling the child's problems. (Following up certain of her remarks, the analyst had asked if she felt that Mrs. Lucas belonged to the upper-class social set of the town.) This question, which she had answered affirmatively, was the cause of her emotional agitation. Although it had made no impression at the time, the analyst's question had suddenly seemed like an accusation that she was socially inferior to the teacher. The more she had thought about this possible accusation, the more upset she had become, until finally, it was as though the analyst had "stabbed me right in the head." She claimed to have been deeply "injured" by it, just as when, a few months earlier, her mother had made a matter of fact comment about their financial insecurity and had offered to lend her and Mr. Blake some savings. The "accusations" by her mother and the analyst were true, she asserted, but terribly damaging because they put her into the category of a crude, lower-class person. That was the "real" reason she felt unable to oppose Mrs. Lucas' will—"I'd rather do nothing about it, just let her push me around."

At this point in Session 8, Mrs. Blake began to display slightly agitated movements, shifting her position on the couch several times, placing the pillow over her face, and finally sitting bolt upright on the couch. Suddenly she burst out weeping: "I wish I didn't have the responsibility for straightening things out at the school—I wish I could love my daughter more—I feel like an awful heel—I ought to tear that school apart and force Mrs. Lucas to do the right thing!"

After this outburst, the analyst remarked on the fact that she was obviously feeling very upset and had been struggling to hold very strong feelings in check, as shown by her agitated behavior during this hour as well as during the preceding night. He referred to the impending surgery, reminded her that she had forgotten to mention it in yesterday's session, and asked whether her concern about the operation might be one of the main reasons for this agitation. Instead of answering this question, Mrs. Blake announced that she had just thought of something that would explain why she was so upset about Mrs. Lucas: The woman reminded her of a lady from New York who once visited at her parents' home. The lady was very flirtatious and seemed to be trying to seduce her prim father by using all sorts of coy tricks. During the remaining few minutes of the session, Mrs. Blake continued to speak about how ineffectual she felt in the presence of women like the New York lady and Mrs. Lucas. Thus, she managed to ignore the analyst's first attempt to show a connection between her emotional agitation and the decision she had just made to submit herself to surgery.

5.

Superego mechanisms

The hypotheses to be discussed in this chapter deal with reactions observed in the analytic sessions which were described in the preceding chapter. We have seen that when the patient became aware of the objective threat she initially displayed three main reactions: (1) intensification of *guilt* feelings; (2) exacerbation of *neurotic anxiety* symptoms; and (3) development of *optimistic fantasies* about compensatory satisfactions. These appear to be typical stress reactions, inasmuch as all three have been observed in many persons who face similar external crises, such as major surgical operations, the prospect of prolonged illness, the threat of peacetime disasters, and wartime dangers.[1] It seems reasonable to expect that the underlying dynamics revealed by the psychoanalytic method might help to illuminate the nature of guilt, anxiety, and fantasy reactions in persons facing similar external dangers. The psychodynamic hypotheses to be presented, although not necessarily intended to be applied universally, are offered as plausible theoretical propositions which may help to explain certain of the emotional and behavioral reactions to stress found among a sizeable percentage—and possibly even the majority—of persons in modern society.

All of the hypotheses deal with *unconscious* factors that may be determinants of the observable behavior produced by objective threats to body integrity. In deriving hypotheses from the available psychoanalytic evidence, the author has repeatedly relied upon one of Freud's basic theoretical assumptions, namely, that powerful external forces can penetrate to the deepest layers of the human personality, arousing the weak and helpless child that is normally submerged under the external mask of conventional adult behavior (S. Freud, 1920).

Thus, a general assumption running through all the theoretical discussions in this book is that stress experiences tend to arouse apparently outgrown modes of response to childhood dangers. The primitive affects, fantasies, and defenses that had become habitual ways of adjusting to external threats during the early years of a person's life, although partially superseded by new habits, remain as latent reaction tendencies in the adult personality. These latent tendencies will be called forth once again whenever powerful threat stimuli are encountered.

Guilt Reactions

An outstanding feature of the patient's guilt feelings is that they are centered almost exclusively upon her own aggressive wishes and actions. For instance, she expects to suffer some violent form of retribution for a new administrative ruling which she has devised deliberately to restrict the freedom of one particular female employee. Many times in the past the patient had used this same (motherlike) woman as a target for her hostility, but rarely had she consciously felt guilty about doing so.

There is additional evidence which also indicates a lowering of the patient's threshold for guilt in response to her own aggressive impulses. In trying to handle her daughter's school problem, she was extraordinarily inhibited in asserting her own views to the teacher or the principal. The inhibition was linked with a momentary conception of herself as a rather shabby, inarticulate inferior who has no right to make any demands. This self-derogatory attitude was at variance with the patient's ordinary conception of herself as a socially competent, energetic "go-getter," who can easily manipulate others through the use of her superior intelligence and verbal skills. That the patient was temporarily experiencing an acute impairment in self-esteem is further suggested by the particular way in which she distorted the meaning of the analyst's question concerning the social status of the home room teacher. In her bedtime ruminations, she became convinced that the question must have been intended as an invidious reference to her own inferior social status.

There are several indications that the patient was by no means unaware of the covert aggression involved in her acquiescence to the teacher's plan, the net effect of which would be to impose a severe penalty on her daughter. At the moment when her guilt feelings burst forth in the form of agitated weeping and explicit self-accusations ("I am an awful heel"), she was acutely conscious of the fact that in failing to oppose the teacher she was failing to protect the child.

In effect, the patient expressed an unusual degree of guilt with respect to her dealings with the teacher, with the elderly employee under her supervision, and with her second oldest child, toward each of whom she had previously expressed openly ambivalent attitudes. On the basis of what was learned about the nature of her guilt feelings, the following hypothesis is suggested with the expectation that it may provide a part of the explanation for the remarkable increase in guilt reactions so frequently noted in a wide range of personalities under conditions of impending deprivation or danger.

Hypothesis 1A. *Exposure to a threat of body damage (as in the case of an impending surgical operation) tends to sensitize the individual to unacceptable hostile and destructive tendencies in his own aggressive behavior, so that even relatively minor aggressive actions, which are normally tolerated without affective involvement, are consciously or unconsciously felt to be violations of inner superego standards.*

An equivalent way of formulating the hypothesis would be to say that threat situations induce a more or less temporary change in a person's superego functioning in the direction of more rigorous self-scrutiny and harsher self-criticism of his own aggressive behavior. This hypothesis provides, at best, only a partial explanation of the rise in guilt feelings that accompanies awareness of impending danger. Even if fully confirmed by subsequent psychodynamic research, the hypothesis is limited in that it specifies only one preceding link in the causal chain which leads up to the guilt reactions—the excitatory cause of guilt, so to speak.

The hypothesis leaves open the following questions: Why does anticipated danger mobilize a greater need for inner vigilance with respect to aggressive behavior? A possible answer to this question might be derived from the commonly held assumption that any threat of body damage mobilizes aggressive impulses. Taking account of the savage violence that sometimes breaks out among endangered animals (as well as among people), a number of theorists have postulated that dangers which threaten the survival of an organism will arouse emotional excitement which can develop into either fear or aggression, instigating either flight or fight (Hebb, 1949; Murray, 1938; Rado, 1942; Saul, 1947; Simmel, 1944). The heightening of the aggression drive presumably increases the organism's readiness to attack any perceived obstacle to goal attainment; in humans, this tendency can be regarded as a primitive mode of defense, either an innate biogenic mechanism or the product of quasi-universal frustration experiences whereby the infant learns to eliminate various types of noxious stimuli by discharging its excitement in violent movements. In any case, if the strong arousal of the aggression drive inclines the adult individual to attack indiscriminately, in ways that violate social norms, an intense inner conflict will be generated. The superego component of the conflict is aroused, of course, as a consequence of parental training and other socialization experiences involving the internalization of cultural taboos which require one to curb aggression and to confine its discharge within the acceptable channels of one's society. An external threat situation is capable of arousing a powerful aggression drive to such a degree that a person may find it difficult to control his inclination to release unacceptable impulses (H. Deutsch, 1942; Grinker and Spiegel, 1945a; Wittkower, 1951). When this occurs, the internal conflict may be partly resolved by means of greater self-scrutiny and vigilance, as specified by Hypothesis 1A. Thus, the intensification of guilt feelings and of superego restraints evoked by external threats could perhaps be explained as an effort to cope with such a marked increase in aggression that the person feels himself to be in danger of losing control over unacceptable hostile impulses.

Such an explanation, however, still remains incomplete because it hinges on the assumption that the aggressive tendencies mobilized by an external threat of body damage will necessarily be *unacceptable* to the personality, requiring inner surveillance to ward off anticipatory guilt reactions. Moreover, the actual occurrence of overt violence or antisocial action appears to be quite rare among people facing physical dangers (Glover, 1942; Janis, 1951; USSBS Report, 1947a and 1947b). In times of crisis, aggressive behavior typically takes the form either of energetic protective action or of purely verbal "griping" that is socially harmless. Consequently, if endangered people feel afraid of releasing damaging aggressive impulses, they are displaying an unrealistic fear that might be considered as irrational or neurotic.

Why, then, should the arousal of easily controllable aggressive tendencies create internal disturbances of the type that would ordinarily be expected to occur only when aggression threatens to become uncontrollable? Undoubtedly there are some persons suffering from neurotic character disorders for whom any increase in aggressive impulses will be felt as a superego violation. But it seems improbable that this type of neurotic disturbance characterizes the large numbers of persons who have been observed to display guilt and ascetic behavior in times of impending danger (see pp. 61–62).

In the case of the psychoanalytic patient, the same problem arises: Why are the aggressive impulses aroused by the threat of external danger felt to be so dangerous and unacceptable? Under ordinary circumstances she reacts to external provocations with defiance or anger but without any remarkable increase in guilt feelings. Why does the aggression activated by the threat of surgery produce intense guilt whereas other provocations to aggression generally do not?

An important clue to the underlying dynamics of the patient's guilt reactions emerges in her associations to the preoperative dream. The latent content, it will be recalled, involved an intense preoccupation with retribution and parental punishment. A very similar theme runs through the patient's transference reactions during all the preoperative sessions. In Session 6, she explicitly reported feeling afraid of the analyst and had the accompanying fantasy that he would punish her for some undefined misbehavior by taking away a precious part of her body. From the dream associations and the transference reactions we can infer an unconscious equating of the new threat posed by the surgical operation with old childhood threats of parental punishment. The emotional reactions and defenses of the patient, with their obvious flavor of intimidation, suggest that the objective danger is felt to be a highly personalized one. It is as though instead of an impersonal surgeon having recommended a standard surgical operation as the best solution for her medical problem, an angry parent had threatened to thrash her for being a "bad" girl; she must try to mitigate the assault by acknowledging her faults, by inhibiting any incipient impulse to struggle or to retaliate, and by trying to behave like a very "good" girl.

This particular form of mitigation attempt—trying to be on one's best behavior—is likely to be learned by the average child in our culture as a product of repeated bitter experiences at the hands of an angered parent. Probably by the age of five, the average child already knows that if father or mother becomes so strongly aroused as to threaten a violent beating—or whatever is the most damaging punishment the parent is thought to be capable of executing—he had better be careful to avoid expressing resentment or doing anything that might provoke the full fury of the attack. The patient's temporary inhibitions with respect to aggression could be accounted for by assuming a transfer of childhood feelings of intimidation (originally produced by real or fantasied threats of physical assault from a parent) to the new objective threat of physical assault from the surgeon.

Hypothesis 1B. *Any objective threat of body damage, even though consciously appraised as an event that cannot be influenced by one's own behavior, will tend to be unconsciously assimilated to childhood threats of parental punishment for bad behavior: The individual will strive to mitigate his fate in the same way that, as a child, he succeeded in mitigating the parent's punishment—primarily by controlling his aggression and by making sure that he gives no cause for provoking the maximum penalty.*

The intimidation pattern to which the above hypothesis refers has been discussed elsewhere by the author as a probable explanation for the increased adherence to conventional moral standards and the formation of new taboos among urban populations at times when they were subjected to wartime threats of bombing attacks.

> In London, numerous individuals appeared to adhere obsessively to certain self-imposed formulae: "If I do this (or refrain from doing that) there will be a raid." A wide variety of verbal taboos was also observed. In target cities, some people would not permit certain ideas to be expressed, such as "there has not been a warning tonight," on the grounds that it would tempt Providence. In unbombed towns, there was a similar taboo against making any comments about the air blitz elsewhere for fear that talking about what happened to other cities might bring it to them too.
>
> . . . From her psychoanalytic practice, M. Schmideberg [1942] noted an increased tendency to deny pleasures to oneself as an attempt to propitiate fate: the raids would come as punishment if one engaged in "bad" behavior or if one indulged in highly pleasurable activities. . . . Many of the rituals and avoidances which occurred among the British seem to be attempts to deal with the threat of external danger as if it were a threat of punishment for wrongdoing.
>
> People who are facing the prospect of illness, unemployment, or any extreme form of deprivation will often attempt to ward off the danger by making sure that they do not deserve to be punished. Evidently, this was one of the dominant types of reaction among the bombed population of Britain. Stringent self-control and efforts to live up to purified moral standards seem to have submerged incipient hedonistic strivings. (Janis, 1951, pp. 168–169.)

On the basis of the present psychoanalytic observations, the tentative explanation can be carried one step further. According to Hypothesis 1B, childhood anticipations concerning the intentions of an angry father or angry mother are transferred more or less intact to impersonal danger events in adult life. It is these unconscious anticipations which are now singled out as the critical factor in the heightening of superego vigilance under conditions of external threat; they could give rise to the same propitiation responses that had been learned early in life as a means of coping with the parents' threats of severe punishment.

Compensatory Fantasies

Closely linked with the patient's guilt and childlike concern about being punished were her morbid fears of being mutilated by the surgeon. Time and again the patient put forth the wholly unfounded notion that the operation would turn out to be not the surgical repair of blood vessels, which is what the surgeon had told her it would be, but, rather, an *amputation* of her entire leg. Coupled with this exaggerated expectation of mutilation was a change in the transference relationship, which also involved unrealistic fears of body damage. Although continuing to rely on the analyst for affection and reassurance, the patient nevertheless began to experience a sense of unknown danger while lying on the couch. She was unable to dismiss the anxiety-laden fantasy that the analyst threatened to deprive her of some precious bodily possession.

It seems probable that all these morbid fantasies were manifestations of neurotic anxiety produced by the arousal of repressed psychosexual conflicts. Particularly suggestive in this connection were the recollections of the horror she had experienced as a young child upon unexpectedly seeing her aunt's genitals and hearing an adult conversation about something "spooky" which, as was learned in a later session, referred to a mutilating disease (see Chapter 9). The unconscious significance of these memories could not be ascertained with any degree of certainty until the very last preoperative session (12), at which time the patient not only managed to recall what the spooky conversation was about but also produced a long series of associations in which she ventilated a variety of infantile "castration" fears stimulated by the imminent surgery. Accordingly, further discussion of the nature of the inner dangers underlying her morbid fantasies will be deferred until a later chapter (see pp. 108 ff.).

For the present it is sufficient to note that the patient was attempting to ward off intense neurotic anxiety, as well as guilt, stimulated by the realization that she must soon submit her body to the surgeon's knife. Because of the high degree of emotional tension, she was strongly motivated to erect and maintain a variety of psychological defenses, most of which were only hinted at in the sessions described so far. One particular mode of defense, however, had already emerged very clearly and, in fact, became quite apparent in Session 1 when the possibility of surgery was first mentioned—reliance upon fantasies of compensatory gratifications. Such fantasies appear to be fairly typical among people who face extreme threat situations. Bettelheim (1943), for example, has described the compensatory daydreams and irrational expectations about the future that characterized the mental activity of political prisoners in Nazi concentration camps. Grinker and Spiegel (1945a) state that in the thoughts and daydreams of men in combat:

> . . . home assumes the characteristics of a magical fairyland. All the faults and difficulties in the economic and social structure of the individual's home environment seem to fade away. The people at home become endowed with unrealistic attributes of beauty, kindness, generosity, and are considered to have the soldier's return home as their only desire. Mothers become the most loving and kind individuals, wives assume a beauty and character far from real, and children are model and have no faults. To a lesser extent this rosy hue surrounds the figure of the father or the brothers. For a time at least, there is an attempt to envisage their fathers without the role of authority, fantasying them as equals or pals. They think of going on fishing or hunting trips or sitting in "bull sessions" with them. All in all, anticipation of the return home is extremely unrealistic since the returnee expects the perfection of paradise in the "new life." Actually the return home to a "brave new world" is fantasied as a rebirth.

Among surgical patients, the dominant compensatory fantasies are apt to be based on the more or less realistic hope of being cured of the distressing illness or relieved of the painful disability that makes it necessary to have the operation (S. Blanton and V. Kirk, 1947; Kennedy, 1953; Titchener et al., 1956). But in our patient it is apparent that over and above any such reality-oriented aspirations, there were other satisfactions of an infantile character which she hoped to obtain from the surgical experience. By examining the regressive nature of this patient's fantasies, some insight may be gained concerning the *sources* of the compensatory anticipations that occur among people exposed to comparable threat situations.

In the midst of telling about her dire forebodings of terrible loss, the patient summoned up the childhood memory of seeing a crippled boy from a train window. She then revived the daydream of becoming a cripple, by which she had sought to overcome the profoundly disturbing sense of desertion engendered by the forcible separation from her mother at the time of the birth of her younger sister. It will be recalled that the central theme of the daydream was that through losing part of her body she could gain mother's loving care and prevent any further separations (see p. 46).

The same theme is embedded in the preoperative dream material in which she equated the anticipated experience of undergoing an operation with that of allowing mother to squeeze her pimples. From the entire set of associations, it appeared that the wish-fulfilling tendency of the dream hinged precisely upon the remembrance of earlier episodes in which she had achieved some momentary satisfaction of her longings for maternal affection. Evidently she was falling back on reassuring memories of times when she had gained close contact with her mother and simultaneously had experienced an abatement of superego tensions as a consequence of submitting her body to maternal manipulation. The same compensatory notion can be discerned in what she said in Session 8 about why she was looking forward to the impending operation: she expected to receive attentive care (maternal affection) and to feel free from responsibilities (decreased guilt).

The following hypothesis is suggested on the basis of the psychoanalytic data indicating that the patient's current anticipations were linked with the compensatory themes that characterized her thoughts and fantasies in comparable threat situations in the past.

Hypothesis 2. *When a person faces an objective threat of body damage, he will spontaneously attempt to alleviate guilt and anxiety by thinking of compensatory gains, the content of which derives from fantasies which functioned as effective reassurances in childhood threat situations.*

This hypothesis is predicated on the assumption that early in life every individual goes through a learning process of developing fantasies which will function as reassurances with which to meet recurrent threats. The content of such fantasies is probably derived partly from unintentional training experiences, as, for instance, when parents try to sooth a sick or frightened child by allowing it to have special compensatory indulgences or by promising special gratifications after the suffering is over. Later on, when the child has become more independent of the parents, it may spontaneously make promises of the same kind to itself, some of which probably have to do with anticipated relief from chronic feelings of guilt and anxiety. Whatever the source of a compensatory fantasy, as long as it succeeds in markedly lowering emotional tension when the child is highly anxious or upset, it will tend to become fixated as a habitual means of gaining relief in similar emotional crises. (See Dollard and Miller 1950; English and Pearson, 1945; Erikson, 1950; Murray, 1938.) According to this theory, the compensatory fantasies that are most frequently and most powerfully reinforced by the reduction of emotional tension during childhood are the ones that will be most likely to survive into adulthood. One would expect such fantasies to be called forth as an habitual internal response whenever the person faces a danger situation that is perceived as similar to the childhood situation in which the fantasy had succeeded in producing emotional relief.

It will be noted that the ascetic tendencies specified by Hypothesis 1B refer to *actions*, whereas the self-indulgent tendencies specified by Hypothesis 2 refer solely to *fantasies*. The use of compensatory fantasies to gain reassurance concerning anticipated stress experiences does not necessarily imply a strong desire for immediate gratifications or a tendency to engage in acts of self-indulgence. During periods of impending danger, in wartime for example, there are often unique opportunities for obtaining forbidden gratifications because of the temporary relaxation of coercive forces within the community; but people rarely take advantage of such opportunities until *after* the danger has terminated. (H. Deutsch, 1942; Glover, 1942; Janis, 1951; J. Spiegel, 1953; M. Wolfenstein, 1957.)

The inhibition of self-indulgent activity implied by Hypothesis 1B would presumably not occur if the punishment were no longer perceived to be a threat. Especially after having undergone actual suffering, most people may be inclined to try to obtain the compensatory rewards which they had previously promised to themselves (see pp. 141–148). During the preoperative period, indulging in fantasies of compensatory gratifications appears to be wholly compatible with the heightened superego pressure toward avoiding "bad" behavior. In fact, the compensatory fantasies in the case of our patient seem to have had the effect of helping her to be a "good" girl, to do what the doctors said she ought to do. Her fantasies about what she would gain from the operation helped to bolster her decision to follow the advice of the medical authorities rather than to run away from the frightening surgery. Perhaps one reason for this had to do with the *transformation of passivity into activity* implied by her conception of the operation as a desirable means for attaining what she wanted. The compensatory fantasies may have enabled her to feel that to some extent the imposed operation was entirely of her own choosing—a decision to gain various anticipated rewards—rather than a threat situation toward which she was passively being pushed by pressure from others.

When people use compensatory fantasies to bolster their decisions to submit to threatening ordeals, they do not necessarily refuse to admit the fact that deprivation and suffering may be entailed along with the anticipated rewards. In the present case, however, the patient's emphasis on compensatory gratifications seemed to be closely linked with denial mechanisms that operated in the direction of shunting off any awareness of the unpleasant aspects of the operation. In the next two chapters, further insight into the nature of the compensatory fantasies will be sought by examining the context of the precarious denial defenses in which they were embedded.

Notes

1. Many observational reports and reviews of the literature on psychological stress describe the intensification of guilt feelings and the arousal of neurotic anxiety symptoms which occur when people are facing imminent threats of physical danger. Among the major references which describe these reactions are the following.

(*a*) Among patients facing the threats of surgery: Bernstein and Small, 1951; Blanton and Kirk, 1947; H. Deutsch, 1942; Fessler, 1931; Hill and Silver, 1950; Kirk, 1949; E. Klatskin, 1952; Levy, 1945a; Michaels, 1943; Mittelman, et al., 1945; Nunberg, 1949; Ochsner, 1950; Pearson, 1941; Prugh et al., 1953; Rosen, 1950 and 1952; Schilder, 1942; Sutherland et al., 1952; Sutherland and Orbach, 1953; Titchener et al., 1956.

(*b*) Among patients with serious or chronic illnesses: Bernstein and Small, 1951; Brody, 1956; B. Cobb et al., 1954; Hammerschlag, 1952; Kaplan, 1956; Muncie, 1934; Robinson et al., 1956; Schilder, 1938; Seidenfeld, 1949; Sutherland and Orbach, 1953; Wittkower, 1952.

(*c*) Among pregnant women facing childbirth: Caplan, 1951; H. Deutsch, 1945; S. Haas, 1952.

(*d*) Among civilians facing peacetime or wartime dangers: Burgum, 1944; Glover, 1941 and 1942; Janis, 1951; Rickman, 1938; M. Schmideberg, 1942; J. Spiegel, 1953; Vernon, 1941; Withey, 1956; M. Wolfenstein, 1957.

(*e*) Among men in the armed forces facing the threats of combat: Bychowski, 1944; Garner, 1945; Glass, 1953; Grinker and J. Spiegel, 1945a and 1945b; Hadfield, 1940; Hastings et al., 1944; Kardiner and H. Spiegel, 1947; Mira, 1943; Saul, 1947, Stengel, 1944; Stouffer et al., 1949.

The following are some of the main references which suggest that optimistic fantasies about compensatory gratifications may occur frequently under circumstances where people realize they might be injured or killed: Flugel, 1945; Greenson, 1949; Maskin and Altman, 1943; K. Menninger, 1934; Rosen, 1952; Schilder, 1938 and 1942, M. Wolfenstein, 1957.

6.

A crucial preoperative session

This chapter will be devoted to a single psychoanalytic hour (Session 9). At the beginning of the session, the analyst was struck by the extreme degree to which Mrs. Blake was defending herself against anticipatory fear, exaggerating the pleasant features of the operation and avoiding any thoughts about the unpleasant aspects. Throughout the session, one of the main activities of the analyst was to raise doubts in the patient's mind as to whether the excessive optimism she expressed represented the whole truth about her attitude toward the operation. At first it seemed as though the analyst's comments were having little effect but, toward the end of the hour, the patient had an outburst of extraordinarily intense emotion. The remarkable transformation in Mrs. Blake's behavior during this session was, without doubt, the most dramatic occurrence in her entire psychoanalysis. At the moment when she could no longer maintain her denial defenses, her state of acute agitation was the most extreme instance of uncontrolled emotion that she ever displayed on the analytic couch.

Because the drastic changes in the patient's emotional behavior reveal so much about her struggle against anticipatory fear, it seems desirable to present a full account of the verbal associations which occurred during the session. The record of this particular session contains many significant details concerning the way in which the patient's unconscious conflicts and mechanisms of defense were manifested during the period when she was reacting to the external threat posed by the impending operation. Accordingly, the complete protocol will be given which contains in condensed form a record of practically everything that the patient and analyst said during the entire psychoanalytic session. (See the methodological discussion on pp. 35 ff., which describes how the verbatim notes were recorded.)

Readers familiar with the technical aspects of psychoanalytic practice will recognize that the analyst's interventions during this session represent an attempt to adhere to the standard technique of consistently analyzing the "ego defenses" (Fenichel, 1941; S. Freud, 1933, 1936). Throughout the session, priority was given to two outstanding problems. One involved negative transference, obvious signs of which had been appearing in the analytic sessions during the preceding week. These signs again became apparent at the beginning of Session 9, not only in the patient's free associations but also in her overt social behavior (coming late and not apologizing). In view of these manifestations, the analyst felt that until the negative transference reactions were explicitly dealt with no lasting effects could be achieved from interpreting other motives underlying the childhood fantasies and attitudes expressed in this session. For the same reason, no attempt was made at this particular time to reconstruct the repressed portions of the early memories recalled during this hour.

The second problem, by no means unrelated to the first, was a central one discussed in the preceding chapter—the marked distortion of reality in the patient's conception of the surgical operation, which was now only four days off. At the outset of the session, the analyst was cued to the likelihood that the patient was actively struggling against latent fears of being killed because her opening remarks, in which she manifestly denied feeling afraid, contained a suggestive allusion to the threat of surgery: "It would kill me if I had to give up those things." In dealing with this problem as well as with the negative transference reactions, the analyst's goal was to help the patient overcome her automatic, inefficient defenses so that, eventually, she would be able to develop more successful means of coping with her emotional problems.

It must be emphasized that this particular session was somewhat atypical in one important respect: the analyst intervened much more frequently and talked at much greater length than usual. For several preceding sessions the analyst had been quite inactive, listening carefully to the patient's associations in an attempt to understand why she could not admit to herself that she was apprehensive. By the end of Session 8, the analyst felt he understood fairly well what it was that the patient was trying to deny, and he felt the time was ripe to interpret her strenuous effort to ward off anticipatory fear and to call attention to certain transference reactions which appeared to be closely linked with her fantasies about the impending operation. Perhaps the analyst's spontaneous tendency to be very active during this session was also influenced by his realization that there were only a few days left before the patient was to undergo the operation, for which she appeared to be psychologically unprepared because of her extreme efforts to maintain an unperturbed attitude.

Taking account of the technical principles pertaining to the analysis of ego defenses, the analyst directed his interpretive remarks primarily toward showing the patient that she was defending herself against painful feelings before trying to point out exactly what outer and inner dangers were disturbing her and why she was so strongly motivated to ward them off.

One needs no special knowledge of psychoanalytic technique, however, to discern how a few relatively simple questions and comments by the analyst were sufficient to release the powerful emotions she had been struggling to hold in check. Nor does one need any special background in psychology to be able to appreciate the intense emotional turmoil that must have been going on internally before it erupted on the surface during this session.

SESSION 9: EMOTIONAL CRISIS

Patient arrives five minutes late. Walks slowly to the couch, speaking without looking at the analyst.

PATIENT: I know that I am late and I ought to apologize but I can't. I really don't want to. (Lies down on couch. Pauses for several seconds before speaking.) Actually I'm feeling quite good today. I'm glad the surgeon said I won't have to give up smoking or wearing high-heel shoes. Those were the only two things that I was scared of. It would kill me if I had to give up those things. But now I know that I don't need to worry about those things any more. I can see that it really is better to face the facts than to keep on feeling afraid, like I felt before I went to the surgeon.

ANALYST: But I wonder if you really are facing the facts. You say that you were afraid only of those two things: having to give up smoking and wearing high heels. Last week, before you saw the surgeon, those certainly weren't the main things that you feared. The main fear you expressed was that he might tell you that you need an operation. And you were afraid that an operation might somehow lead to you losing your leg. Actually, it turns out that one of your fears has come true: your fear that you would need an operation was borne out by what the surgeon said.

PATIENT: Last week I did feel afraid of having an operation, but I don't feel that way any more. I'm looking forward to it. I think that I'm going to enjoy being in the hospital. They treat you like a baby, a dear little baby. That's what this operation means to me now. I know that I had been worried about my leg getting worse and having to be amputated. But now I know there's no danger of that at all. The operation is very simple and I'm going to have a really nice rest. Everyone will give me lots of affection. The whole thing will be a nice experience.

ANALYST: Do you really think that's true? Aren't you leaving out the unpleasant aspects of the operation?

PATIENT: Well, I know there will be some pain, of course, but I don't care about that. It won't be so bad, and everyone will feel sorry for me and treat me affectionately. I remember one of my neighbors went to the hospital for something or other, and when she came home she told me that she loved being in the hospital. She said she felt lonely at home alone all day all the time and she loved the attention she got at the hospital. I feel exactly the same way about it only I wouldn't admit it to anyone but you. I was surprised she admitted it to me. I'd hate to admit that I'm so lonely that I'd welcome an operation just to have contacts with people, but that is the way I feel. That's why I'm looking forward to it. I don't get enough satisfactions in other ways. I've told you all about that before.

ANALYST: Yes, and usually when you say that you don't get enough satisfactions it turns out to be a complaint directed against me and against this treatment.

PATIENT: I think I lose satisfactions rather than gain them from this treatment. It makes me more aware of how remote I am from everyone I know. I suppose I have gained a little from it. I can get a little closer to my children at times, and to Joe. And I've lost some of my fears. Yesterday we had a big group of visiting firemen from out of town who came to our section to get a briefing, and the boss asked me to give a little talk to them about the system we use. Before, I would have been scared to death to stand up in front of them, really panic-stricken. But, yesterday, I just felt a little keyed up. Once I got talking, I was completely confident. I was surprised to hear myself saying some of the damndest things! But I didn't care. I could see that I had the audience with me every minute of the way so I just spoke right up. I think I was very persuasive and I felt real proud of myself. So you have helped me in some ways. To be a better worker, that is. If I keep it up, I'll turn out to be a real good worker. That seems to be what you're trying to accomplish with me. If I keep it up, I'll end up being a person who will just be satisfied to work all the time, to take on more and more responsibility, just to plug away at it during every waking minute. A real drone. You don't give me any sexual satisfaction. That's what I really need. You are the only one who could give it to me and you won't have an affair with me. That's why I have to look around for substitutes for sex. I'm afraid I'll get to be just as bad as

Miss Quincey. She's an old maid and has nothing to live for except her work. She doesn't even want to take her vacations or weekends off because she prefers to work. That's the worst fate of all, to have nothing but work. I would rather be dead than to be like that. I want to feel that I belong to someone, that there is someone who likes me, not just for what I do, but for myself. And there is nobody who does.

ANALYST: During the last week you have said many things which indicate that you want to have me treat you affectionately, to give you some tangible sign that I like you for yourself, not just for the things you do to try to please me. Probably that's one of the main motives behind your desire to have a sexual relationship with me at the present time. And this same motive seems to affect your relationship with other people too. Yesterday you told about some similar feelings toward your husband. And for the past week you have been very disturbed about your inability to deal with the teacher at your daughter's school. After all, you gave in to her plan, even though you objected strongly to it. The main reason you gave was that you felt self-conscious and couldn't bear the idea that she might have a bad opinion of you. You wanted her to like you, and you were disturbed at the thought that she might not.

PATIENT: Why do I want a woman like her to like me? Is it because she has a New York accent like the woman who stayed at our house? The one father flirted with when I was a little girl? (Long pause.) I can see myself as a little girl—sort of a visual image—standing between father and mother. I am thinking "which one will like me?" Mother is looking at father, very upset; she's all taken up with his flirtation. Father is looking away, watching the New York girl sitting on the beach. This whole thing is at the beach, the same beach where I played in the sand when mother almost drowned. Father and mother are both completely taken up and neither notices me. That whole thing is so vivid that I can see it, but I don't know if it's a real memory. I think I just concocted it out of different scraps of memory. The New York woman is like a snake in the garden of Eden. If I attract her and make her like me, that would make me feel satisfied. Father would be real mad and mother would too. You know, while I'm telling you this, I can actually see it going on, sort of like a movie; I can actually see my mother's face getting angrier and angrier. The reason why mother gets so angry about it is that if I take the New York woman away from father, he will come back to mother and become more threatening to her. He will do something terrible to mother if I take mother's rival away. I never thought of that before. I wonder if that has something to do with my sex problem. When I saw the surgeon he wanted me to go to the hospital for the operation right away but I wanted to postpone it for a week because I wanted to try to solve my sex problem with Joe first. When I'm in the hospital I want to have the feeling that Joe is home waiting for me, and that he's concerned whether I'll pull through it or not, whether I live or die. I want to be sure that he's completely tied down and under my thumb. I know now that I can't get that done. Tomorrow is my last hour here before the operation and I won't be any further along than I was last week. But my plan was to spend this whole week working on my sex problem so that Joe and I could have very good sex relations all this week and then he would be disarmed. I should have worked more on my fear of sex instead of all those things, so I could disarm him.

ANALYST: What are your associations to the idea of disarming your husband?

PATIENT: I wanted to seduce him, to make him weak. To disarm him would be to de-leg him, to make him helpless. Isn't that what seduction amounts to? A seduced person will give up all will to resist, become completely helpless, like putty, so that from then on the other person can do anything at all without any opposition.

ANALYST: You know, those are the very same words you have used to describe your fear of this treatment. You've said many times that you are afraid that I will seduce you into becoming helpless, like putty, and that I will mold you into whatever I want and that you would be unable to resist.

PATIENT: Yes, I know it.—No I don't! I don't know what you mean. You just seduced me into saying "Yes!"

ANALYST: And so, right at this very moment, you are afraid of being seduced and you feel that you must resist the danger.

PATIENT: You are dangerous! But still I want you to help me. I'm not getting any place on my sex problem. I don't really want Joe; it's just that he's all I've got. He's like Sam, my first boyfriend, when I was fourteen. I always felt he was my "inferior" boyfriend and I really didn't care for him very much, but he was the only one I had. So I let him kiss me and do almost anything he wanted to. Like that time we were lying down on the floor in the library after the building had been closed. The 'phone was ringing—just like it did here just now—and the more it rang the more scared I got. I don't know why I let Sam make love to me, he was such an inferior person. I had the same feeling about father too. I felt he was such a weak and incompetent and inferior man.

ANALYST: And evidently you have the same feeling toward me today, too.

PATIENT: Yes, I can admit that all right! I can't admit that I'm attracted to you, but I can admit *that*.

ANALYST: When you referred to my 'phone ringing just now, you showed that you feel that this situation of lying on the couch right here is like the time you were with Sam, when you were lying on the floor. You let him seduce you to some extent, but you felt all the while that he was inferior. Your feelings about me today must be much the same. You say that you wanted to have my help this week, but, still, today when you arrived late you said you couldn't apologize. Didn't that express the same attitude: that there is no need to apologize if you don't feel like it, because I am an inferior person?

PATIENT: (smiles) I did have that feeling as I was walking in your office. I noticed that your walls need painting, and I remembered that when I had that thought here once before I was really criticizing you and feeling that you are inferior. You must despise me! I wouldn't blame you if you just threw me out. I told my father once that I felt contemptuous. He gave a speech once at a big picnic of his fraternal order and, I didn't say it right out, but I told him that I thought the speech was sort of silly. He was very hurt and he just looked at me with a hurt expression and said: "You say the most cutting things! Some day someone will cut you down. Someone will take you down a peg or two." You must feel the same way about me. Why don't you do it? Why don't you cut me down?

ANALYST: You seem to be trying to provoke some sort of punishment from me. Your behavior reminds me of the way a child will try to provoke punishment from a parent, as a way of testing to see what the parent will do about it.

PATIENT: It's sort of like a game. Kind of flirting around but escaping just before the spanking. Or then there is a spanking, and the baby screams but then it is cuddled and there is a reconciliation. Like father always did if he spanked me. He would kiss and make up right afterward. Then I would wonder if that proved that father was stronger, because I would be sort of humble and let him kiss me and make up.

ANALYST: It seems quite clear that you are trying to provoke me right now in the same way as when you were a little girl, when you would sometimes try to provoke your father to spank you and make up. The reason for this must have something to do with your wanting some signs of affection from me.

PATIENT: If I got a spanking it would wash away all my sins. It would make me clean again. Like an enema, it would clean out all the bad.

ANALYST: Many times in your analysis we have seen what enemas mean to you: complete loss of control. It isn't simply a punishment you seem to be thinking about but . . . (Patient interrupts before analyst has completed his statement.)

PATIENT: You mean the enemas my mother gave me when I was little? I resented them and sometimes I wouldn't let them work. I'd hold the stuff in for hours. An operation involves enemas too. I've heard they always give an enema beforehand to clean you out so you won't soil on the operating table. Like when a person dies, he lets out all his secretions. Isn't that a horrible thing? I know that I won't let go when they give me an enema before my operation. If I don't let go, though, I'm liable to let go on the operating table. I'll be unconscious so I won't know about it, but still I'll be embarrassed to have that happen. I'm sort of worried about being embarrassed that way because I know that I won't let go when they give me the enema. (Patient begins to show much more agitation in motor movements than usual, rapidly twisting the ring on her finger, crossing and uncrossing legs, frequently shifting position on couch.)

ANALYST: That's the first time you've mentioned being worried about the operation since the time the surgeon told you that you would need to have it. But you seem to have picked a rather unusual thing to be worried about. As you said, you wouldn't be likely to be actually embarrassed on the operating table especially because you would be under an anesthetic. I wonder if there isn't something else about being on the operating table that is the thing you are really more worried about?

PATIENT: Before you go under from the anesthetic, do you tell things? Do the people in the operating room listen to what you say and gossip about the things you have told? That would be awful! That would really worry me to death!

ANALYST: Still, it's doubtful that this is the main thing you fear about the operation. After all, suppose you did talk freely while going under the anesthetic. Do you really believe that the things you might reveal would be so unusual that the people in the operating room would pay that much attention to them?

PATIENT: You're right, I guess. I don't really dread that. If I did say anything embarrassing when they give me the anesthetic, it would just make me more human, that's all. It would just make me more like other human beings.

ANALYST: Our time is almost up today but, before you go, I think it's important for you to realize that there is a particular kind of fear concerning your operation which you have been expressing in a number of different ways. Are you aware of what it is?

PATIENT: I don't feel any particular fear of the operation. I'm really looking forward to it. I think it's going to be enjoyable being in the hospital.

ANALYST: But you have been expressing a fear that you might die. For instance, you said that you want your husband to be concerned about whether you will live or die. And just a few minutes ago you said that the loss of secretions produced by an enema is like the loss of secretions that occurs when a person dies. Then you said that you would resist an enema, that you wouldn't allow yourself to lose secretions that way. In other words, the idea of losing control over your bowels disturbs you very much, partly because it means becoming like a dying person. So when you say that you look forward to the operation and that nothing particularly worries you, I wonder if that isn't just a facade, a way of deceiving yourself, a way of escaping from the fear of death.

PATIENT: My God! (Sits up on couch and cries loudly for several minutes.) My God, my God! I can't stop crying. (Lies down but continues to cry. Clutches at the pillow, holds it over her face, then lifts it up.) I'm scared to death. Oh God, I'm afraid I'll never come out of the anesthesia. I'll die! Or else I'll have an embolism and they will have to cut off my leg. Embolisms can go to the brain and kill you. It's supposed to be such a simple operation, but I know that an embolism can occur and that makes it terribly dangerous. Why do you make me think of that? I don't want to think of it. What good does it do? It won't help me. Do you think it does you good to think of how frightened you are?

ANALYST: What is your answer to that question?

PATIENT: I suppose if a person is going to die he ought to prepare himself for death.

ANALYST: You speak as though you expect to die from the operation. Now we can understand why you set up this unrealistic belief that the operation was going to be an enjoyable picnic. You weren't able to allow yourself to think about the dangerous aspects of the operation for the simple reason that you have a very exaggerated fear of it. Your surgeon has made it very clear to you that the operation is a minor one. You know that while there may be some very unpleasant things connected with it, it isn't the sort of operation that anyone is likely to die from. Still the fantasy you just expressed is that the operation is somehow going to kill you. In your fantasy either you don't come out of the anesthesia or you develop an embolism. This exaggerated idea frightens you so much that you haven't allowed yourself to think about it at all, to face that fact that the operation will be no picnic. You haven't been able to look at the operation realistically, to accept the fact that the operation will be neither a picnic nor a funeral.

Patient remains silent, shows a decrease in agitated motor movements. Analyst announces, "Our time is up today." Patient remains on couch for a half-minute, then slowly rises, walks to table, takes handkerchief out of handbag, and dabs at her eyes. Faintly murmurs "goodbye" and walks slowly out of the room.

7.

Causes and consequences of intellectual denial

In the foregoing session, the main mechanisms used by the patient to control her intense preoperative fears can be seen quite clearly. This chapter will examine further the powerful emotions underlying the patient's pseudo-optimistic attitude, which she consciously maintained throughout most of the session, even though it was belied by numerous involuntary signs of agitation and by her final emotional outburst.

There is a marked contrast between the manifest content of the first part of the session, with its repeated emphasis on compensatory gratifications, and the earlier sessions (1–6), in which the patient had freely admitted feeling afraid of various realistic and unrealistic dangers. Such admissions abruptly ceased as soon as the operation was no longer merely a remote possibility. When the operation became a concrete reality, scheduled only a few days off, the patient disclaimed her fears and tried to persuade both herself and the analyst that there was no danger at all. Thus she maintained a facade of optimism, bolstered by the belief that the operation would be a wholly rewarding experience.

Minimization of Personal Vulnerability

The change in the patient's manifest attitude seems to be similar to certain emotional phenomena noted in related kinds of threat situations. Grinker and Spiegel (1945a and 1945b) report that ruminations about injury and death, characteristic of certain phases of precombat training (e.g., "gangplank fever"), were surprisingly absent among army troops and combat flyers on the first occasions when they actually entered the dangerous combat zone.

. . . the primary reaction to combat is usually detachment and objective interest. The anti-aircraft fire may look like a spectacular but harmless Fourth of July celebration, entertaining but not dangerous.

. . . many men have this feeling [that although others may die, "it can't happen to me"] at the beginning of a combat tour and in most of them it appears to be based largely on good previous experiences with reality. Their past has been so secure or any insecurities have been so well mastered that they enter combat with a large reserve of confidence and cockiness. However, as they lose friends in combat and have narrow escapes of their own, they usually become less convinced of their own invulnerability and this type of protection against anxiety is not very reliable." (Grinker and Spiegel, 1945a, pp. 127 and 130.)

Similar phenomena have been observed in tornadoes, floods, and other peacetime disasters (Committee on Disaster Studies, 1955; Diggory, 1956; M. Wolfenstein, 1957) as well as in civilian wartime disasters (Glover, 1942; Janis, 1951; MacCurdy, 1943; M. Schmideberg, 1942).

The patient's behavior can be viewed as an instance of the paradoxical decrease in fear that sometimes occurs when awareness of danger increases (Kris, 1941 and 1944). Such a paradox can be accounted for by the following generalization suggested by the present psychoanalytic data.

Hypothesis 3A. *The closer an anticipated threat of body damage is perceived to be (in space or time), the greater will be the individual's motivation to ward off anticipatory fears by minimizing the potential danger or by intellectually denying that he will be seriously affected by it.*

According to this hypothesis, any external sign that increases a person's awareness of the proximity of a threat will tend to elicit an increase in denial tendencies. Such tendencies are manifested by overoptimistic expectations which (1) minimize the probability that the potential danger will actually materialize; (2) minimize the magnitude of the potential danger; (3) maximize the person's ability to cope with the danger; (4) maximize the person's chances of receiving adequate help from others to mitigate the danger; or (5) maximize the gains or gratifications to be derived from the potential danger situation. All five types are illustrated in the patient's responses during Session 9.

That the minimizations observed in Session 9 were motivated by an effort to ward off disturbing affect is indicated by the intense emotional outburst elicited when the analyst's comments prevented the patient from remaining convinced of her own optimistic statements. By calling attention to the illusory character of the patient's expectations, the analyst prevented the minimizations from operating effectively as a means of avoiding uncomfortable thoughts about the threatening aspects of the operation. But as long as intellectural denial was maintained, overt fear reactions evidently were successfully inhibited.

Even without the intervention of an analyst, of course, attempts at denial may fail to reduce fear. Sometimes overoptimistic and minimizing beliefs about an impending danger situation will be broken down by impressive communications from an authoritative figure (Hovland et al., 1953, pp. 56–96) or by the skeptical comments of relatives and friends, or even by the remarks of a stranger who describes his own harrowing experiences in the same kind of danger situation (Barker et al., 1946; Bernstein and Small, 1951; Wittkower, 1952). Hence, it does not follow from the foregoing hypothesis that the heightening of denial tendencies elicited by perceptions of increased proximity to a danger situation will necessarily have any effect on *overt manifestations of fear*. That is to say, the hypothesis does *not* predict that, as the threat is perceived coming closer, the person's bodily or verbal expressions of fear will necessarily decrease. What the hypothesis *does* predict for such a situation is only that there will be more vigorous efforts at minimizing or ignoring the impending danger. Such efforts might succeed, at least for a short time, in actually reducing the level of overt fear. But, when there are inescapable signs that great danger is actually at hand, the person's attempt to deny the threat may fail completely and the individual may then experience an attack of acute fear.

In the case of our patient, efforts to minimize the danger seemed to show a steady increase as the time for the operation came closer and closer. But her overt expressions of fear showed a curvilinear relationship: (*a*) Before she saw her physician (e.g., Session 1), she had freely indulged in apprehensive fantasies of a masochistic character and her level of overt fear was fairly high; (*b*) in Sessions 7 and 8, after having made all the arrangements for the operation, she expressed very little fear; (*c*) during most of Session 9, she continued to show only rather subtle manifestations of fear until the analyst's interventions became effective, at which time her level of overt fear rose again to a new peak; and (*d*) as the time for the operation drew closer, the level of overt fear rose even higher (see pp. 101–106).

Thus, despite her vigorous and persistent efforts, the patient's attempts at minimization functioned only as a temporary stopgap. Perhaps they cut down somewhat on the frequency with which she experienced affective disturbance, but they certainly did not succeed in eliminating her fears. In fact, the emotional outbursts which occurred after repeated denial efforts—as in the case of the analytic session reported in the preceding chapter—were even more intense than those which had occurred before the patient became stimulated to engage in intellectual denial.

From the above clinical observations, one is led to infer the following supplementary proposition:

Hypothesis 3B. *When a person attempts to minimize the danger after becoming aware of a potential threat, fear reactions are not extinguished but, rather, are temporarily held in check only so long as no clear-cut signs of danger are brought to his focus of attention.*

The predisposition to react with overt fear in response to signs of impending danger evidently is not removed even when the person consciously feels convinced that the threat is unimportant or that he will easily manage to avert the danger. Any time the person encounters impressive evidence or authoritative assertions which induce him to reconsider his optimistic assumptions, he is likely to display in full strength the fear reactions which he had temporarily managed to inhibit.

Defensive Processes in Intellectual Denial

The temporary character of the fear-reducing effects achieved by intellectual denial raises a question as to the nature of the defensive processes involved. In many standard textbooks on personality dynamics, denial is described as an important mechanism, coordinate with repression, projection, isolation, compensation, and other such defenses. However, there seems to be little agreement as to the relationship that denial bears to the other defense mechanisms, and there is a great deal of inconsistency regarding the pathological implications of denial. Some authorities say that denial is essentially a psychotic or borderline psychotic defense (e.g., A. Freud, 1936, p. 97), whereas others use the same term to refer to relatively normal processes (e.g., Federn, 1952, pp. 263–264, and Kris, 1952, p. 42). Much of the ambiguity stems from the fact that the term is used to cover widely different aspects of psychotic, neurotic, and normal thought processes which have only one main feature in common; namely, that the individual manages to ward off unpleasant affect by failing to appraise correctly some undesirable aspect of a past, present, or future predicament.

Perhaps some misunderstandings can be cleared up by distinguishing between those instances where a person ignores *ambiguous signs* of threat from those where he disregards *clear-cut evidence* of loss or danger. The latter, which will be referred to as "pathological denial," includes all instances where a person rejects a painful fact about his present environment even though it can be clearly perceived and is generally regarded by others in his community as unquestionable. Typical instances of pathological denial have been described in the literature on the delusions and morbid elations of the chronically ill and the bereaved (Barker et al., 1946; Bellak, 1950; B. Cobb et al., 1954; Fahrenkamp, 1931; B. Lewin, 1950; Lindemann, 1944; Rosen, 1950; Schilder, 1938, 1942; Strecker et al., 1938; Weinstein and Kahn, 1955, and Wittkower, 1949 and 1952). Thus, for example, a patient who is suffering from tuberculosis might deny being ill and refuse to stay in a hospital; a widow might deny that her husband is dead after attending his funeral.

At the other extreme are those highly ambiguous situations of potential adversity where the probabilities of loss or danger cannot be accurately ascertained at the moment but must await further developments. Intellectual denial of any such potential danger will be referred to as "minimization" of the threat. Typical examples of minimization are to be found in any hospital ward where patients are waiting to be taken to the operating room (H. Deutsch 1942; Hamburg, 1953; A. Kennedy, 1953; Rosen, 1952; Titchener, et al., 1956).

Probably we should think of the two types of situations as extremes on a continuum of ambiguity-clarity. The necessity of taking account of the degree of ambiguity arises when one attempts to assess the psychological significance of any given instance of intellectual denial. Does the denial imply a high degree of personality disorganization? Will the person be unresponsive to factual clues and impressive communications which are intended to correct his misinterpretation of "reality"? Will he persistently fail to take precautionary action despite being exposed to authoritative advice and other persuasive influences? Answers to such questions would depend partly on the characteristics of the reality signs that are being ignored (where on the continuum of ambiguity-clarity is the denied evidence located?). The closer it is to the ambiguous end of the continuum, the less pathological the denial attempt.

Many normal persons characteristically fail to take advantage of opportunities to learn about future dangers that might someday materialize. When unavoidably exposed to warnings or other clues pertaining to such dangers, they tend to ignore the ominous significance of those unfavorable signs which lend themselves to alternative interpretations; or they selectively recall and give most weight to those favorable signs which permit them to maintain a relatively unperturbed attitude about what the future holds in store for them.

Only when a situation approaches that of clear and present danger does denial behavior become a serious deviation in the sense that it is essentially delusional in character and suggestive of a psychotic break with reality.[1]

Still another factor should also be taken into account when one is attempting to draw psychodiagnostic inferences from a person's use of a denial defense: Does the person categorically deny the possibility of danger, refusing to give any consideration whatsoever to perceptible threat cues; or does he, rather, simply minimize the probability of danger, admitting some qualifications that take perceptible threat cues into account? In the face of signs of impending danger, *the more unqualified the denial, the greater the deviation from normal reality-testing behavior.*

In the light of the above considerations, it is important to call attention to the fact that the denial reactions encountered in the present psychoanalytic case study—and, as a matter of fact, throughout this entire book—do *not* include any instances of the pathological type of reaction. Rather, the responses with which we are concerned consist of anticipations and judgments which minimize *potential* dangers in the *future.* In all such instances, there are definite signs of threat which inform the person that some form of danger or deprivation is *likely* to occur, but there is no conclusive evidence that the danger has actually materialized. Moreover, the examples of intellectual denial observed in the psychoanalytic patient (and in the surgical cases to be discussed later [pp. 251–273]) are essentially of the *qualified* species; the individual distorts but does not completely disregard those aspects of reality which point to the likelihood of personal involvement in danger. Our theoretical assumptions and hypotheses concerning denial tendencies are, therefore, to be understood as applying primarily to "minimizations," the relatively nonpathological variants of intellectual denial.

Returning now to the case material, we note that the patient's denial of the potential dangers that might be entailed by the impending surgery takes numerous different forms. The psychoanalytic data are sufficiently detailed to warrant an attempt at a hypothetical reconstruction of the psychological processes underlying the defensive components in the patient's overoptimistic attitude toward the impending operation. The following generalization is suggested by the observations from Sessions 1 through 9 concerning the mechanisms involved when a person indulges in intellectual denial: Judgments and expectations which tend to minimize potential dangers in the future appear to be the joint product of suppression, repression, and related adjustment mechanisms which operate together to create and maintain pseudo-optimistic attitudes. A number of such mechanisms, will be examined in order to see how they contribute to intellectual denial.

1. Suppression of Unpleasant Thoughts

As already noted, one of the most frequent manifestations of denial tendencies takes the form of minimizing the chances of being seriously affected by potential dangers or deprivations. Such beliefs began to be verbalized by the patient on the first occasion when she informed the analyst of her decision to have the operation (Session 8, pages 49 ff.). She said that the operation was not at all serious and her stay at the hospital would amount to nothing more than a pleasant vacation. These optimistic judgments were reiterated and amplified in Session 9. From the material which emerged during the latter session, it appears that such judgments were partly the result of *suppression* of certain thoughts which would ordinarily lead to a more objective view of the probabilities of danger. The one-sided way the patient discussed her anticipations of what the operation experience would be like, and especially the way she responded to the analyst's questions about the other side of the issue, suggests that the patient's mental set was such that she would allow herself to focus only on the pros and avoid thinking about the cons. Thus, when the analyst induced her to consider the unpleasant aspects of the operation, she briefly mentioned the fact that there would be some postoperative pain, but very promptly changed the subject back to the compensating gratifications which would make her welcome the operation (see p. 66). At the very end of the session, after the analyst's interventions had finally broken down her minimizations, the patient, in a state of acute agitation, frankly admitted her intention to suppress fearful anticipations: "Why do you make me think of that? I don't want to think of it."

2. Isolation and Repression

Coupled with the suppression of unwelcome ideas were avoidance responses which cannot ordinarily be controlled by purely voluntary efforts and which appear to be *unconsciously* determined. At times the patient showed a remarkable degree of isolation of affect from mental content, as when she blandly announced in Session 8 that she would soon be going to the hospital to have the operation. In Session 9, at the moment when she acknowledged that the operation would cause some pain, she spoke in a completely unperturbed manner, maintaining a cheerful, almost euphoric exterior.

The isolation seems to have been partly facilitated by her deliberate set to suppress unpleasant trains of thought. Thus, her fears were not apt to become strongly aroused so long as she continued to avoid thinking about what the painful experiences would really be like; unpleasant affect would not be likely to mount as long as she could merely allude to the unpleasant details in passing, at a time when she was having many vivid fantasies about the affectionate pampering she would receive. But her emotional indifference was probably the consequence of *repression* as well as suppression. At several different points during Session 9, as well as during the two preceding sessions, the patient showed temporary memory gaps combined with retrospective distortions of recent events and other parapraxes which involved a failure to recall information pertinent to the impending surgical experience. When these memory disturbances occurred, the patient's free associations contained numerous displacements, symbolizations, and other "primary process" signs which are indications of repression.

The memory lapses began in Session 7, when the patient forgot to tell the analyst about the scheduled operation after the crucial weekend during which she had been examined by two surgeons and had accepted their joint recommendation. When she did think of the operation in the next session, her comments indicated that the act of forgetting was not a matter of conscious suppression but an unintentional slip (see pp. 49–50). Then came the memory distortions in connection with her recollections of what she had feared during the preceding week. In Session 8 she recalled only that she had been worried about being disfigured by the incision scars; in Session 9 she thought that the loss of smoking and high heels were the only things about which she had felt really concerned. Thus, she selectively recalled precisely those former sources of worry which, in the light of new information and assurances obtained from the surgeon, were no longer felt to be serious threats.

The patient's failure to remember the content of her recently verbalized fears was subsidiary to the repression of something else of far greater significance. The major repression, partially uncovered during Session 9, was the patient's unverbalized fantasy of being mutilated or killed while lying helplessly anesthetized on the operating table. In her free associations to many diverse topics, this particular fantasy was indirectly expressed, through metaphorical or symbolic references.

The same kind of unconscious defense which psychoanalysts frequently observe when someone is struggling to ward off neurotic anxiety stemming from past traumas of childhood seems to have been used by this patient, as a means of warding off the fears generated by an external threat.[2]

3. Rationalization and Displacement

Despite her extensive use of unintentional as well as intentional devices to ward off disturbing affect, the patient did not wholly succeed in remaining emotionally calm. We have seen that she experienced intense outbursts of emotional agitation not only while on the analytic couch but also while at home. Nevertheless, she still attempted to deny that her agitated state was in any way connected with the dangers posed by the impending operation.

Here again, we find that the denial involves an isolation of affect from the affect-arousing thoughts. In the example of isolation discussed earlier, we saw that the patient denied feeling upset at the moment when she was acknowledging that the operation would cause pain and suffering. What we must now add to this observation is the fact that, at times when undeniable emotional upset occurred, she displayed the converse type of isolation; i.e., she invented *rationalizations* to explain her emotional state in such a way as to continue to deny that she was experiencing any anticipatory fear of body damage. Such rationalizations have been observed in other types of physical danger situations (Hastings et al., 1944; Wittkower, 1952; Wolfenstein, 1957). In describing some typical examples, B. Lewin (1950, p. 54) refers to the phenomenon as "denial of the emotional impact of reality" in contrast to denial of external danger. Thus, for instance, a person might admit a serious injury or the death of a loved one but believe "that it did not matter."

Fear-denying rationalizations sometimes involve a combination of two types of *displacement:* (*a*) misidentifying the external source or thought stimulus which evokes the fear reaction; and (*b*) mislabeling the fear reaction as some other, more or less irrelevant, affect. In Session 8, we had a prime example of denial involving both types of displacement. The day after deciding to undergo the operation, the patient developed a state of emotional tension which became increasingly acute during the evening and continued throughout the night. She acknowledged having been emotionally upset but asserted that it was really a delayed reaction to something the analyst had implied the previous day concerning her social status. Instead of fear, the affect was supposedly shame or humiliation.

In a less obvious way, the same type of displacement appears in the patient's rationalizations of her emotional tension during Session 9. While talking about enemas and other matters pertinent to the impending surgery, she showed increasing motor agitation as well as verbal signs of increasing emotional tension. When it finally reached a level where she could no longer maintain that she felt completely unemotional, she attributed her concern exclusively to the danger of disgracing herself (by revealing confidences or by soiling herself while under the influence of the anesthetic). Thus, she continued to deny her fears of the surgical procedure itself and again described her present worries as though she merely felt anticipatory shame or embarrassment. The patient's rationalizations, of course, may have contained a large grain of truth in that they represented some of the many dangers which worried her. But the denial defense broke down precisely at the point where she was shown that she had been describing her affect incorrectly and that her concern about being embarrassed was far from the whole story. When her dysphoric feelings could no longer be blamed on other matters, the patient was flooded with affect and suddenly began to ventilate her overwhelming fears of being exposed to surgical assault.

From the above observations it appears that rationalizations involving the displacement of affect may play an important supplementary role in the maintenance of denial attitudes. As is implied by Hypothesis 3B, one cannot expect suppression and repression to be one hundred percent efficient in eliminating a person's emotional tension at a time when he knows that a potential danger situation will soon be at hand. Once he becomes aware of his own uneasiness he is apt to start thinking about what it is that arouses these feelings ("why am I so upset?"). This, in turn, would lead the person to become more aware of the disturbing implications of the situation he is about to enter. The rationalization defense, therefore, may be conceived as a means of escape from thinking about the causes of current emotional tension to prevent fear reactions from snowballing. By giving himself convincing reasons as to why he is feeling somewhat upset, a person can avoid certain of the most disturbing inner cues, viz., thoughts or images which explicitly and vividly represent the most dreaded possibilities of suffering and loss. The latter are apt to be replaced by other thought sequences which the person has learned from prior experiences do not create such painful feelings. The substitution of one thought sequence for another enables the person to prevent his fears from building up.

The important psychological function of displacement rationalizations, as seen in the light of the psychoanalytic evidence, suggests the following general hypothesis, which might be regarded as a corollary to Hypothesis 3B.

Hypothesis 4. *Under conditions where a person is strongly motivated to deny an impending danger, he will tend to rationalize his self-perceptions of residual emotional tension by mislabeling his affective state and attributing it to other, less fear-arousing, circumstances.*

4. Defensive Dominance and Negativism

Closely related to the patient's fears of being damaged or killed while under the anesthetic was a specific internal source of conflict activated by the patient's realization that she would soon have to submit her body to surgery. In her free associations, one can observe multiple indications of a combined longing for and fear of being infantalized, particularly with respect to losing control over what might happen to her body.

In Session 9, her statements about enemas and involuntary release of body secretions point directly to the activation of an acute conflict between passive submissiveness and stubborn defiance—a conflict that probably originated in the childhood struggle against parental interferences with excretory functions and related bodily processes.

In this connection it should be recalled that a major theme in the latent content of the preoperative dream of pimple squeezing (pp. 47–49) involved willing submission to parental punishment. We have also noticed several other signs indicating that a major source of preoperative anxiety in this patient is the inner danger of giving in to masochistic tendencies. This brings us to one of the outstanding features of Session 9: the patient's efforts to deny that she is or will be in a submissive state of helplessness. No single piece of crucial evidence can be cited to demonstrate that the patient was defensively warding off awareness of the dangers of passive compliance. Nevertheless, one can discern repeated manifestations of an energetic struggle against passivity which is symbolically conveyed by her words and even "acted out" during Session 9. These manifestations, which mainly take the form of aggressive expressions of dominance and negativism, will be briefly reviewed for the purpose of attempting to draw some inferences as to the specific defensive processes involved. Such inferences, however, must be regarded as much more conjectural and tentative than those pertaining to the other mechanisms which have already been discussed, and for which the analytic evidence is much more clear-cut.

An outstanding manifestation of negativism in Session 9 is the patient's announcement that she "won't let go" when the time comes to have the enema which she knew would be routinely administered as part of the standard medical preparation for the operation. It is noteworthy that this forecast turned out to be a self-fulfilled prophecy: according to her subsequent postoperative account (in Session 13), she felt willing to take the enema on the night before the operation was scheduled but, without consciously intending to do so, retained the fluid. (To the "amazement" of the ward nurses, she absorbed the entire enema and had no bowel movement whatsoever.) In making the forecast (and subsequently, when involuntarily confirming it), the patient probably was unconsciously expressing her refusal to be submissive. The refusal pertains to a sphere of action that constitutes one of the earliest modes of infantile resistance against parental interference—retention of faeces. In the primitive language of the body, the patient seems to be asserting her protest: "I won't give in to their demands, I won't let them take anything out of my body!" [3]

A second clue to the patient's ambivalence and defensiveness toward demands for passive compliance in the hospital is to be found in her repeated assertions about "being treated like a baby." Here she seemingly acknowledges that the hospital experience will entail some degree of infantalization. Presumably, she realizes that she will have to allow the doctors and the nurses to handle her body, to take care of intimate physical matters. But from her comments it is obvious that she is not taking account of the main implications of the childlike status of a hospitalized patient, which were as well known to her as to anyone living in a middle-class urban community. She takes no cognizance of the fact that she will be required to put up with all sorts of regulations of daily habits that are normally assumed to be an inviolate part of an adult's autonomy and that she will be expected to "be a good girl" with respect to accepting whatever distressing manipulations, intrusions, or treatments the medical staff may decide to inflict upon her. Indeed, the patient's notion of being treated like a baby does not seem to include any component of helplessness or dependency; she claims that she will take advantage of the opportunity to be pampered by exploiting the situation to elicit a maximum of solicitous care and affection. Thus she avoids acknowledging that there will be strong external pressures for passive compliance by repeatedly assuring herself that she will take command and will make everyone give her what she wants. Her regressive fantasy of hospitalization seems to be that of becoming an omnipotent child who can control the parental figures administering to her bodily needs instead of being under their domination.

Another important indication of the patient's defensive struggle against passive submissiveness comes from the transference reactions manifested in the patient's free associations and in her behavior toward the analyst. In an earlier session (5), we saw that her associations equated the danger of being mutilated by the surgeon with the danger of being deprived of important body functions by the analyst. Moreover, the associations to the preoperative dream (Sessions 5 and 6) also contained signs of an unconscious equation between the operating table and the analytic couch. In Session 9, the dangers of the anesthesia are described in terms that apply directly to the free-association technique: one is induced to talk freely, to reveal too much, and to lose control over primitive impulses. During this session the patient also accuses the analyst of being "dangerous"—a "seducer" with whom she "flirts around," provoking him to attack and punish her, but "escaping just before the spanking." In her struggle against the analyst's power, the patient's defensive strivings for dominance become apparent in the associations she "acts out" as well as in the content of her verbalizations: (*a*) she arrives five minutes late for the session; (*b*) she announces that she refuses to apologize for being late; (*c*) after complaining that she gets very little out of the analysis, she aggressively demands that the analyst give her sexual gratification; (*d*) she vehemently accuses the analyst of "seducing" her into accepting a statement that she asserts is not true (the content of the statement being that she is afraid the analytic treatment will make her helpless and unable to resist the analyst's influence); (*e*) she readily admits feeling that the analyst, like her father and her husband, is a weak, incompetent, and generally inferior man; (*f*) when she realizes the extent to which she has been derogating the analyst, she momentarily expresses fear of retaliation and then tries to provoke the punishment: "Why don't you cut me down?" What the patient is saying in all this dominating, provocative, and negativistic behavior seems to boil down to this: "No matter what happens here, even if you throw me out, I must be the one who remains in control and who determines everything that goes on."

Finally, we come to the patient's peculiar expressions of dominance and hostility toward her husband. She begins by saying that, before going off to the hospital, she would like to overcome her sex problem (frigidity and related inhibitions which she had frequently described in earlier sessions as resulting from an ill-defined fear of being damaged in intercourse). But she wants to accomplish this for the special purpose of tying down, dominating, and disarming her husband. Her associations then lead to the somewhat bizarre notion of "de-legging" him, which she equates with seducing him into a completely helpless state such that "the other person can do anything at all without any opposition." A major element in this fantasy seems to be a reversal of sex roles: she becomes the active attacker instead of the passive victim. (It should be noted at this point that the patient often daydreamed about having one or another masculine attribute, but she rarely produced fantasies with openly castrative or sadistic content; during the preceding two years of analysis, there was certainly no other instance in which the manifest content had to do with mutilating her husband.)

The specific body zone which is the target of her fantasied attack against the husband provides a clue as to why she produces such a fantasy at the present time. The wish to be the dominant person rather than the submissive one evidently applies not only to the sexual sphere but also to the impending surgical experience. Perhaps she is falling back on a sexual fantasy of long standing ("I am the attacker and he is the victim,"), as a means of coping with the new source of anxiety posed by the anticipated surgery. In Session 1 we saw that the patient's anxiety was explicitly centered on the danger that her leg would be amputated; in her fantasy, she denies this danger by assigning to her husband the role of passive victim and by identifying herself with the surgeon.

This fantasy is probably best understood as a manifestation of the well-known mechanism of *identification with the aggressor* (A. Freud, 1936, pp. 117 ff.). Originally described as a defense used by children to cope with overwhelming fears of a powerful parent, this mechanism has also been observed in adults who are under the realistic threat of severe punishment from powerful authority figures—for example, among German concentration camp prisoners (Bettelheim, 1943) and among U. S. Army recruits in a basic training camp (Janis, 1945). In the present case, the fantasied identification appeared to be closely linked with her striving to transform the image of herself as a passive victim into one in which she retained complete control.[4]

All of the patient's defensive maneuvers, which involved so many different levels of regression, were probably used to enhance her sense of power and mastery, so as to ward off a very specific source of intense anxiety stemming from an unresolved psychosexual conflict. In later chapters, when additional material is presented concerning the patient's exaggerated fear of surgery, it will be seen that she was afraid of being overwhelmed by feelings of helplessness partly because of an irresistible impulse to submit her body to be mutilated by the powerful man with the knife.

Notes

1. The occurrence of *unambiguous reality clues to oncoming danger* is a necessary, but not a sufficient condition for pathological denial. At the time when a disaster strikes, and sometimes just beforehand, many people fail to appreciate the magnitude of the disaster and remain inordinately calm (M. Wolfenstein, 1957). Under these conditions, intellectual denial may have a markedly benign effect, enabling the person to plan his protective actions or to carry out the emergency orders he is given without his efficiency being seriously impaired by emotional agitation. Thus there are some extreme instances of denial that cannot be regarded as pathological even though clear-cut signs of danger are misinterpreted or ignored.

There are also other instances of nonpathological denial which occur in persons who temporarily develop symptoms of apathy or depersonalization at a time when they are confronted with an extraordinarily serious threat such that no protective action or escape appears to be possible (Greenson, 1949; Schilder, 1938). Probably when the threat involves being utterly helpless to ward off grave danger, even the most healthy persons cannot "take it" without resorting to an extreme form of denial defense. In all such instances, however, the impairment in reality testing seems to be of very short duration.

From what has just been said, it appears that a precise differentiation between pathological and nonpathological denial may require some specifications in addition to the clarity of the reality signs that are misinterpreted, e.g., the duration of the period during which the misintepretations occur, and the nature of the objective threat that would be anticipated if the reality signs were correctly interpreted. Thus, for example, a denial reaction would not be considered as "pathological" if clear-cut danger clues had not been repeatedly ignored over a long period of time or if the situation implied by the perceptible clues was an apparently inescapable threat of total annihilation.

Additional factors may need to be specified, of course, in order to improve the utility of classifying denial reactions into the two categories, "pathological" and "nonpathological."

The distinction between these two categories is important in so far as it enables correct predictions to be made about the personality characteristics of anyone who is displaying one or another form of denial. When a person's denial reaction is diagnosed as "pathological," the term carries the implication that he will prove to have an abnormally low degree of stress tolerance in general and that he can be expected to display other grossly pathological symptoms of severe neurosis or psychosis.

2. The recurrent themes and vivid imagery in the patient's numerous incidental references to her body bear many of the telltale signs which analysts use to identify the derivatives of unconscious processes (see the statement of the main themes in the interpretation given toward the end of Session 9, pp. 70–71, and also the summary of the patient's manifestations of an unconscious conflict involving passive submissive tendencies, pp. 82–85). The psychoanalytic evidence leads to the inference that an intensive intrapsychic struggle was going on directed against inner dangers which had been mobilized by the external threat of body damage—a struggle of the kind that is apt to be implicated whenever a repressive mechanism is actively at work. Some clues as to the nature of the inner dangers against which the patient was defending herself were described earlier in the discussion of Hypothesis 1 (pp. 56–57), particularly those pointing to the unconscious significance of the operation as a mutilating punishment for past misbehavior connected with the patient's guilt-laden hostility toward her mother. But until additional preoperative observations are presented in the next chapter, it is premature to consider the reasons why this patient reacted to the threat of surgery with so much alteration in her normal ego functions. For the present, it will merely be noted that from the evidence presented so far we are not yet justified in concluding that the patient's memory disturbances pertaining to the operation are necessarily signs of a deeply repressed conflict of the sort which, in Freud's theory of mental organization, is assigned to the "system unconscious" (S. Freud, 1930, pp. 610–621). In terms of Freud's constructs, the main examples of forgetting which we have been examining might be regarded as belonging to the "preconscious system," inasmuch as the patient, with relatively little aid from the analyst, was able to become aware of what she had temporarily forgotten. Nevertheless, it is useful to designate the temporary lack of awareness and the memory lapses pertaining to the anticipated surgical experience as instances of "repression" because this designation highlights the fact that, over and above any manifestations of *intentional* turning away from disturbing thoughts, there were also various indications that the patient was *unconsciously curtailing her own thought processes.*

3. The patient's concentration of interest on the enema probably was the consequence of a regressive maneuver to which she resorted as a "last ditch" defense against the anxieties generated by the threat of surgery. As the patient's denial efforts began to break down, her fantasies became increasingly infantile in character; she conceived of herself first as actively and aggressively mastering the danger situation and then as achieving a passive-receptive form of mastery. It is this regressive type of defensive striving that furnishes the context for understanding why the patient's (phallic) fear of being mutilated by an amputation was replaced by the (anal) fear of being overwhelmed and annihilated by an enema.

4. In addition to satisfying defensive needs and regressive sado-masochistic motives, the patient's fantasy of de-legging her husband might also have an additional defensive function. As a consequence of unconsciously equating the surgical operation with parental punishment (Hypothesis 1B), she may be offering up her husband as a substitute victim. The latent attitude expressed in the fantasy might

be to the effect that "somebody has to suffer—let it be him rather than me." The fear-reducing value of a "scapegoat" attitude of this kind might stem from ubiquitous childhood experiences in which severe punishment is sometimes averted because a parent's anger is deflected away from oneself onto the other parent or sibling. Despite the fact that the victim is a love object, the child may, in a moment of danger, welcome the fact that the full brunt of the attack is being borne by someone else. The same infantile attitude sometimes occurs in the external danger situations of adult life and seems to play an important role in generating postdisaster guilt and suicidal depression especially if a close friend or relative is injured or killed. (Garner, 1945; Grinker, 1944; Grinker and J. Spiegel, 1945a and 1945b; Kardiner and H. Spiegel, 1947; M. Schmideberg, 1942.) In such cases the underlying dynamics of the depression seem to involve the attitude that "I don't deserve to live because at the time when danger struck I wanted him to be the victim rather than me."

8.

Arousal of affiliative needs

In the preceding chapter, we have seen that much of the patient's aggressiveness was purely defensive in character. Her attitude toward love objects before and during the preoperative period was acutely *ambivalent*, containing strong positive components as well as negative ones. So far, in concentrating on the manifestations of hostility and negativism, we have examined only the negative components. But this leaves us with an incomplete and somewhat distorted picture of the way in which the anticipation of danger affected the patient's interpersonal attitudes and behavior.

To correct our view, we must take cognizance of the signs of a concurrent upsurge of positive feelings—the intensified longing for affection and, as the patient put it, the need "to feel that I belong to someone." Thus, her seemingly cold-blooded statements about wanting to dominate and victimize her husband cannot be taken at face value as being the whole story because she also informs us that her reason for postponing the operation was to bind him to her sexually and affectionately: "I want to have the feeling that Joe is home waiting for me and that he's concerned whether I'll pull through or not. . . ." It will be recalled that the emotional significance of this aspect of her attitude toward her husband was emphasized by the analyst in the final interpretation which evoked the sudden unblocking of her intense affect (pp. 70–71).

There is a similar dual character to the patient's plans for exploiting her status as a hospitalized patient. On the one hand she intends to dominate the nurses, to trick them into treating her in such a way as to make her feel like an omnipotent child. But, on the other hand, what she specifically wants is to be treated as a "dear little baby" so that, like the neighbor who had confided in her, the attentiveness of the hospital staff will help to overcome her intense feelings of loneliness: "I'd hate to admit that I'm so lonely, that I'd welcome an operation just to have contacts with people, but that is the way I feel."

Finally, we must recognize that underneath her surface aggressiveness toward the analyst, there is an undercurrent of frustrated longing for affectionate response. In much of her provocative behavior she is simply falling back on the somewhat masochistic devices she had learned to employ as a child, at times when she felt neglected or unloved—devices which were intended to elicit at least some small degree of parental interest. In subsequent sessions, there is a great deal more evidence of her desire for sympathetic attention from the analyst. For instance, after the operation was over she admitted that the postponement of the operation, about which she spoke during Session 9, was motivated by the wish to establish closer affectionate ties not only with her husband but with the analyst as well. Moreover, the postoperative sessions also reveal that her hunger for reassuring affection remained unabated throughout the entire hospitalization and convalescence period, during which time she attempted to compensate for the lack of contact with the analyst by developing an intense, preoccupying interest in the surgeon. Although sometimes masked by surface eruptions of defensive aggressiveness, the patient's heightened need for interpersonal affiliation and affection seems to be one of the most outstanding motivational changes evoked by the threat of surgery.

In wartime, especially at moments when people are suddenly faced with the imminent danger of being injured or killed, they show a tremendous upsurge of interest in interpersonal contacts oriented toward establishing firm affectionate bonds.[1] A basic psychological need fulfilled by the increase in affiliative behavior may be that of overcoming certain specific fears derived from childhood experiences in which deprivation and suffering came to be associatively linked with signs of losing parental love and being left alone. The following hypothesis, originally suggested on the basis of wartime observations of the fear of social isolation displayed by people under threat of air attack (M. Schmideberg 1942; Janis 1951), may apply equally to the threat situation confronting surgical patients.

Hypothesis 5. *When faced with potential body damage, a person is likely to experience a reactivation of childhood fears of parental abandonment, as a result of which he will have an unusually high need to be reassured that he is affectionately regarded by love objects and by other persons upon whom he is emotionally dependent.*

That the patient was re-experiencing childhood fears of the sort specified in the foregoing hypothesis is suggested by several different aspects of her behavior during Session 9. Perhaps the most direct evidence is contained in her recollections of an episode in which she felt she had been abandoned by both parents. Of special importance in establishing the linkage between the recollected abandonment experience and her present need for affectionate reassurance is the fact that a long-forgotten memory came back to her just at the point where the analyst was commenting on her desire to have some tangible sign of affection from him. The patient had asserted, in a somewhat depressive way, her wish that someone would genuinely love her ("there is nobody who does"), and the analyst had responded by talking about the many different ways in which this longing had recently been expressed toward him and other persons, such as the school teacher. It was then that the patient's associations led her to a childhood scene in which she felt acutely lonely and neglected as a result of her parents' exclusive involvement in the triangle created by a flirtatious female visitor ("Father and mother are both completely taken up and neither notices me . . ."). As she spoke about these childhood events, her sentences were in the present tense and, simultaneously, her affective responses began to approach the intensity of an unassimilated painful event which is being currently relived. While recalling childhood fantasies about breaking up the triangle, she began to visualize her parents' anger with almost hallucinatory clarity ("I can actually see it going on, sort of like a movie. . . ."). Then, immediately after recollecting this emotionally charged memory, her next associations led her to reveal that she had postponed her operation so as to have one more week of analysis, allegedly to make sure her husband would be tied down.

The particular context in which the childhood memory was recollected suggests that the patient's emotional responses to the impending surgery were heavily colored by a revival of childhood fears of being unloved and abandoned. The re-experiencing of these feelings appears to have energized the patient's strong desire to strengthen affectionate bonds with both husband and analyst before beginning the period of separation when she would have to go off to meet whatever fate was awaiting her in the hospital.

The "triangle" situation so vividly recalled in Session 9 might, of course, be a screen memory which represents in more tolerable form a related traumatic experience (see Session 12, page 104). But whether we regard the recalled episode as a screen memory or as the recollection of a genuinely formative experience, the dominant theme of *suffering from loss of parental love* tends to bear out the implications of Hypothesis 5.

The "triangle" episode is not the only childhood memory of being abandoned that the patient brought up in her associations to the anticipated surgery. In Session 1 (pp. 44–46), immediately after speaking about the possibility that the pains in her leg might necessitate a surgical amputation, she recalled an incident from her eighth year which involved feeling envious of a crippled boy seen from a train window at a time when she was being taken away from home because her mother was about to give birth to another child. Her envy of the crippled boy was explicitly focused on the notion that he was being lavished with affection and could never be separated from his parents. In Session 9, the sequence of associations included an additional element which was not so obvious in the earlier session, *viz.*, the memory of the envied crippled boy turned out to be directly linked with the patient's current urge to seek affectionate contact. As will be seen in the next chapter, a similar linkage became apparent in Session 10, during which the patient repeatedly made undisguised attempts to elicit the analyst's sympathy and love: she again focused on the childhood memory of the crippled boy but this time it was immediately after having expressed the fear that, when she left to have the operation, it might be the last time she would ever see the analyst.

Thus, the psychoanalytic evidence points to a direct connection between: (*a*) the strong need for reassuring affection aroused by the threat to body integrity in adulthood and (*b*) the reactivation of childhood fears of parental rejection and abandonment.

Notes

1. A marked tendency toward increased valuation of primary group membership together with greater dependence on love objects, on group leaders, and on anyone else who is capable of functioning as a protective parental figure has been

repeatedly noted in studies of military combat units (Glass, 1953; Grinker and Spiegel, 1945a, 1945b; Haggard, 1949; Shils and Janowitz, 1948; H. Spiegel, 1944; Stouffer et al., 1949b) and of civilian populations exposed to bombing attacks (Glover, 1942; Janis, 1951; Levy, 1945; M. Schmideberg, 1942; Thouless, 1941; Vernon, 1941). A similar increase in dependency and group cohesiveness has been observed among survivors of peacetime disasters (Brownlee, 1931; Committee on Disaster Studies, 1955; Wallace, 1954; M. Wolfenstein, 1957) and also among sick people requiring surgery or suffering from serious illnesses (Barker et al., 1946; Schilder, 1938; Shands, 1955; Finesinger et al., 1951; Sutherland and Orbach, 1953; Wittkower, 1952).

9.

Awaiting the operation

This chapter describes the last three sessions preceding the operation. Session 10 was originally supposed to be the last before the patient left for the hospital. But, as it turned out, the operating-room schedule was so crowded that Mrs. Blake's operation had to be postponed for several days, during which time she came for two additional psychoanalytic sessions (11 and 12). In these preoperative sessions two main tendencies were observed: first, a growing emotional tension which mounted to very high intensity as the impending operation approached; second, a variety of new trial-and-error attempts to develop inner psychological defenses to ward off the mounting anxiety. During this suspenseful period, the most outstanding feature of the analytic sessions was the upsurge into consciousness of primitive fears together with florid neurotic fantasies. The content of the fantasies and the accompanying free associations point to specific childhood conflicts which had never been adequately resolved, and which may account for some important features of the defensive maneuvers used by the patient to cope with the approaching threat of surgical assault.

SESSION 10: VASCILLATION

Probably as a direct consequence of the temporary breakdown of her denial efforts, Mrs. Blake showed a marked increase in overt fear symptoms during the session immediately following the one reported in Chapter 6. She began the hour with speculations about how long she might be away from analysis, wondering if the surgeon had been really telling the whole truth about how serious the operation would be, or if he had perhaps exaggerated the speed with which she would recover. This implicit expression of fear was followed by a lengthy description of the obsessional thoughts with which she had been preoccupied for several hours, ever since receiving a telephone call from one of the nurses at the hospital. Because the operation was an elective one, the nurse asked whether Mrs. Blake would prefer to have it next Tuesday or Thursday. Promptly Mrs. Blake chose Thursday but changed her mind a moment later and asked to have it scheduled for Tuesday instead. Long after the telephone conversation was over, she mulled over the choice. She explained to the analyst that various practical considerations were causing her to vacillate between arranging to get the operation over with at the earliest possible date and waiting until the later date. For instance, if it were to take exactly two weeks to recover, the later date would be preferable because it would give an extra weekend before returning to work; on the other hand, she could not expect to accomplish very much on her job during the two extra days while awaiting the operation.

When the analyst pointed out that in discussing these vacillations she had omitted any direct mention of her inner feelings, Mrs. Blake immediately admitted being somewhat worried about the operation. Then, after a long pause, she said: "I'm wondering if today will be the last session I ever have; maybe I won't ever see you again." This feeling made her think of the time when, as a little girl, her parents had sent her away to camp for an entire summer. She had cried so much beforehand that her parents had almost deceided not to send her. Mrs. Blake recalled that while at the camp she had been continually homesick and had feared that she might never see her parents again. The train trip to the camp also reminded her of the earlier trip during which she had observed from the train window the crippled boy supported by two loving women.

Mrs. Blake's disturbed feelings appeared to subside as she dwelt on the image of the crippled boy toward whom she had consciously felt envious because he could never be neglected by his mother or separated from his family. She then spoke about having recently put something over on the owner of the parking lot where she regularly left her car when coming for the analytic sessions. She told the man that, although she had paid for her parking space for the entire month, she would not be using it for the next few weeks because of the operation. He had sympathetically volunteered to give her a refund for the period she would be away. After telling about this incident, Mrs. Blake's next association was that she might not have the operation after all. The following excerpt shows rather clearly that she was still attempting to maintain, in somewhat modified form, the very same type of intellectual denial as in the preceding session, having not yet adequately "worked through" the analyst's interpretation:

PATIENT: I wonder if I really need the operation. Maybe I should call off the arrangement at the hospital. I haven't had any pain at all in the last few days. I think my leg has cured itself. If I don't have any pain I don't see why I would need to have the operation. Anyhow when I saw the surgeon, I exaggerated the amount of pain I had. That's why he said to have an operation. There's really nothing wrong with my leg.

ANALYST: Do you think that you succeeded in misleading the surgeon so that he made the wrong diagnosis?

PATIENT: No, I know I couldn't mislead him one little bit. Everyone says he's the best man in town when it comes to a condition like the one I have. And he sent me to another diagnostician too, to be absolutely certain. I know that both doctors are topnotch. I don't doubt their judgment. And I know that my leg isn't really right; there is something wrong with it.

ANALYST: Well, then, what you said a moment ago was not something that you really believe.

PATIENT: But I believed it when I said it.

ANALYST: Evidently it was something that at the moment you wanted to believe. It was the same sort of thing you said at the beginning of yesterday's hour—that the operation experience would be entirely pleasurable. By the end of the hour you realized that it wasn't true and you became extremely fearful and upset. Today you have again been trying to control your fear in almost the same way. This time you tried to deny that there is anything really wrong with your leg so that you could feel justified in postponing or calling off the operation.

PATIENT: I was just thinking that the surgeon said I **could** postpone the operation if I wanted to. My leg could be treated by wearing a certain kind of bandage. But I guess that wouldn't be a good idea. He said that sooner or later I would need the operation, and he recommended that I have it now. If it must be done sometime, I want to do it now. It won't be so bad. I still think it will be nice being taken care of in the hospital, with no responsibilities. I wouldn't want to miss all that. That's what I said yesterday, isn't it?

ANALYST: You keep coming back to the idea that the operation is going to be pleasant. You allow yourself to avoid thinking about the unpleasant aspects because there are certain things about the operation that frighten you very much. You keep trying to avoid the upsetting feelings you experienced yesterday by trying to convince yourself that either you don't need it or else that it will be a pleasant experience.

PATIENT: I know it. I know the operation won't be pleasant at all.

This particular portion of the analytic hour seemed to be a repetition of the main trend in the preceding hour, although in a considerably attenuated form. Much more readily than in the previous hour, the patient admitted feeling anxious when the analyst called into question her optimistic statements.

While speaking about being worried, the patient again displayed some overt emotion, but with much less intensity than on the previous occasion. Then she began to ventilate a pessimistic notion to the effect that the operation would ruin her sex life: it would set her back because abstinence from sex relations would be medically prescribed for a long time; moreover, she would lose all interest in sex and would be unable to work on her sexual inhibitions in the analysis. When the analyst said that there was probably also some deeper fear that lay behind her concern about the way the operation would interfere with her sex life, she became somewhat agitated. She asserted that she really thought of the surgical procedure as cutting off her leg, and to lose the leg would mean to lose part of her self. Her next association was that she would lose certain "masculine powers" about which she often daydreamed. "I will lose the secret power of a man that I have always hoped to get; the operation will make me feel more like a woman; I won't be able to imagine myself as a female Jesus or an angel or fairy in disguise."

After elaborating on fearful amputation fantasies, she returned to the theme that had been implied in her associations concerning the memory of the crippled boy seen from the train window: instead of losing power she could exploit her infirmity to gain control over others and to elicit affection. As she continued to reiterate this theme during the remainder of the analytic hour, her anxious feelings subsided.

Throughout Session 10, the analyst received the impression that Mrs. Blake was continuing to strive for a reassuring fantasy that would be more plausible and more effective in alleviating her fears than the earlier attempts. The fantasy of gaining power to elicit affection from others appeared to be essentially another denial of her fearful expectations that she might be overwhelmed by feelings of being helpless and loveless. For the present she was still clinging to the comforting belief that she would be able to capitalize on the operation. Instead of passively experiencing the deprivations that would be imposed on her, she could actively master the situation in such a way as to make the personal gains exceed the losses. Her associations clearly showed that the goal of eliciting sympathy, affection, and special concessions was applied not only to the hospital personnel who would be taking care of her after the operation but also, more immediately at hand, to the analyst. Toward the end of the session, as Mrs. Blake became increasingly aware of the latent content of the fantasy, she felt increasingly self-critical and dissatisfied with it. The change in her attitude is illustrated by the following sequence extracted from the record of the last half of the analytic hour:

> After an operation you are allowed to be like an infant and no one expects anything of you, they just give you things . . . I expect to be changed into a darling, appealing baby . . . but I feel confused about all of this. Aren't you going to tell me what the operation is supposed to transform me into? . . .
>
> I expect more power from the operation. I can use my helplessness to make people show affection . . . I suppose I'm a stinker but I think I will be able to fool people into giving me affection . . . it won't be the real thing of course, but I don't care as long as they do what I want. I could fool everyone. I could fool you and make you do some special things for me. But I'm not so sure of that. I guess that wouldn't really work.
>
> The trouble is the whole thing is a fake because I'd just be forcing affection instead of getting the real thing, just playing on peoples' sympathy. Like father did to get me to submit to whatever he wanted me to do. I expect to do the same thing. The woman I visited in the hospital caught me with my guard down and I started to cry. I can do the same thing to other people. But I'm a real skunk. What's wrong with me? I'm trying to play a game just to elicit sympathy. When I said the operation would make me into an old lady and would make me lose all interest in sex, I just wanted to give you a picture of me that isn't true.

The true picture, according to her final associations, was that she wanted the analyst to feel sorry for her so that he would allow her long-standing wishes concerning the analysis to be realized—namely, that instead of requiring her to give free associations, the analyst would pamper her, make love to her, and protect her from all danger.

SESSION 11: REACTIONS TO POSTPONEMENT

The arrangement made in Session 10 was that Mrs. Blake would telephone the analyst, presumably in about two weeks or so, when she had recovered from the operation sufficiently to resume analysis. On the day when her operation had been scheduled, she called the analyst to let him know what had happened at the hospital that morning. She had been informed that her operation would be postponed for three days because an unexpectedly large number of emergency surgical cases had been given priority. During this telephone conversation the analyst made the remark that a postponement of this kind can be a rather unpleasant experience, especially when one is informed of it only at the last minute. He asked whether she had in mind the possibility of arranging to come for her regular analystic sessions during the interim. She was surprised at this question ("I never thought of that") but promptly gave an enthusiastic affirmative response.

When she came the next day, her first association was to the telephone call. She said her intention in calling had been simply to pay a compliment to the analyst by keeping him informed—"a tribute to your kindness and interest in me." But after hanging up, she realized that the call had been changed into something else and then she began to feel hurt. The analyst should not have expressed sympathy nor reminded her that she could return to analysis if she wanted to. At the last session she had tried to seduce him into expressing sympathy but had she succeeded, she would have felt gratified about his having fallen for her tricks. The telephone call, however, was quite a different matter. When the analyst spoke sympathetically, that ruined everything.

Exactly what was it that the analyst ruined? For several hours before making the call she had been feeling very "high" as a result of the postponement. Early in the morning, as the nurses began to prepare her for the operation, she had been quite upset. Then, when informed that the operation had to be canceled, she momentarily felt bewildered and could not grasp it. Suddenly she was able to snap out of it with the thought, "This is a wonderful opportunity to play a joke on everyone." From that moment on she had felt happy, carefree, and full of energy.

She took a cab from the hospital to her office and arrived in time to attend the last few minutes of the regular meeting held each week for the department store managers and their assistants. Feeling gay and conspicuous, she made a dramatic entrance. Since all of them knew she had been given sick leave to have an operation that day, she had expected the group to become so startled that "they would just about drop dead." Instead, no one seemed the least bit surprised or interested, but merely greeted her with polite "hellos" and went on with the business under discussion. For a moment she felt terribly deflated but then decided "if they don't give a damn about me, I don't give a damn about them."

After the meeting she continued to feel slightly let down until she came to her own office where some of her colleagues really did show the warm, excited greeting she had so keenly anticipated ("Oh, what in the world are you doing here?!") She had been looking forward to producing this sensational effect and, once having succeeded in doing so, her elated mood was fully restored. For several hours she plunged into work, accomplishing "a tremendous lot." She even overcame with ease her usual inhibitions about contacting socially prominent clients with whom she was supposed to discuss certain business matters. When the time of day arrived for the analytic hour she "paid the tribute" of telephoning the analyst. She felt that the analyst threw cold water on her because what he said over the telephone made her realize that the postponement was only a temporary matter and not a real cause for jubilation.

After the letdown of the telephone conversation, Mrs. Blake's elated mood was replaced by a mood of the opposite sort. Now her main feeling was that her case was hopeless. This attitude was not applied to the impending surgical operation, however, but was expressed only with respect to her psychoanalytic treatment. Her feeling was that she really could gain nothing from psychoanalysis, either at present or in the future:

> If I had a disease like cancer, then you could remove it—or if I needed to have my leg amputated, it could be taken away. But mental disease is different. There's nothing to be taken away and that's why I can't get any benefit from coming here. I've been fooling you into thinking that I have something to lose, something that you could take away that would make me better. But there is nothing there for you to take.

The patient was told that her statement sounded like an attempt to cover up her fear that the analyst might want to take away something of great importance to her. Her reaction to this interpretation was to admit that she had been struggling against the danger of feeling too affectionate toward the analyst. (Earlier in the analysis she had achieved some degree of insight into her defensive avoidance of affection and had recalled many vivid episodes of being exploited and disappointed by her mother at times when, as a child, she had wanted to express her love; but she had continued to justify her policy of avoiding affectionate entanglements on the grounds that she must avert the danger of becoming so compliant as to be an easy victim to exploitation at the hands of any person she loved.) Now she felt, allegedly for the first time, that her wariness was not really justified: "I want to let people be nice to me and I want to be able to feel grateful and friendly toward them, not always thinking that they will take something away from me."

SESSION 12: PARADE OF PAST HORRORS

The sense of hopelessness and the somewhat depressive feelings which Mrs. Blake began to express in the session following the postponement were greatly amplified in the next session, which was the last one before the operation actually took place. At the beginning of the hour she retold some of the incidents that had occurred during the brief period when she had felt jubilant about the postponement, except that this time she included some additional material which showed even more clearly how superficial her elation had been. She now reported that while gaily walking down the hospital corridor on her way out of the building, she caught a glimpse of an old man who lay gasping on his bed. The sight of the dying man made her think of her father on his deathbed and for a moment her gaiety vanished; she felt a pang and wanted to cry. But once out of the hospital her elated mood came back and dominated her feelings until it was again momentarily shaken when she walked into the business meeting and received only perfunctory greetings from her business colleagues, from whom she had been hoping for "some sign of real interest and affection." Her next association was that on the day her father died she had experienced no grief whatsoever but, instead, had become unusually carefree and gay.

At this point the analyst told her that it seemed quite clear that she was apt to become unusually gay at times when she wanted to cover up feelings of the opposite kind and that her gaiety after the postponement was apparently an attempt to escape from unpleasant feelings about the impending operation. This comment elicited an admission of intense fear together with further elaborations of the ambiguous notions she had expressed in the preceding hour concerning the reason why she could not be helped by analytic treatment:

> I didn't feel concerned about the operation that day. But now I guess I am getting frightened by it. I am really frightened! (Pause) There's something I thought of yesterday but didn't tell you. It was something in connection with the idea that if I have nothing to be removed from my body you can't cure me. But it seems too ridiculous to mention (Pause) I know I should tell whatever things I think of but—well, the thought was that I don't have a rotting penis that needs to be amputated.

Following this reluctant admission, Mrs. Blake got up from the couch, walked over to the table on which she had placed her handbag, searched for a small packet of tissues, and then returned to the couch. As she resumed her position she remarked that the analyst undoubtedly had the mistaken idea that she took the tissues because she was going to cry, but the real reason was only that she needed to blow her nose. On the basis of Mrs. Blake's facial expression as she made this remark, the analyst responded with the question: "What would be so awful about it if you did start to cry?" Her response was:

> I can't let myself cry. I would dissolve if I cried. Then you'd leave me. If I cried I couldn't pull myself back together.

This explicit statement of her fear of dissolving seemed to unblock the intense emotions she had been struggling to hold in check. During the remainder of the analytic hour, her tone of voice and tense body movements worked up into a crescendo of agitated anxiety as she recounted a series of fantastically gruesome associations which were linked with the notion of dissolving. This series of associations contained ten different fantasies or images, in the following sequence:

1. To dissolve into tears is like being transformed into urine or "BM" or some other *hideous secretions* that would disgust anyone and would especially repel the analyst.

2. Dissolving is like becoming a bloody mess, as in a novel about *genital mutilation.* The novel, called *The Doctors,* was one she had read a few years ago. The story involved a woman with a vagina which was blocked because of scar tissue. Mrs. Blake was shocked by the description of an incident in which the woman's husband became uncontrollably aroused and painfully forced an opening with his erect penis. She felt so terrified, as she read the gory details, that she had almost fainted.

3. Once she actually did faint as she read a gruesome story about a *brutal, mutilating rape.* It was a book called something like *Mother India* which told about a young girl being sexually attacked. In her middle teens, she used to read the book in the bathtub. Once, while lying in the tub, she became panicky as she read a passage that vividly described how a man's penis tore the raw, tender flesh of the young girl. At that time she had fainted and almost drowned. (The analyst commented that these fantasies about mutilation seemed to be connected with her fear of the impending operation.)

4. What she really needs is a very *dangerous hemorrhoid operation.* If she were carefully examined by her surgeon or some other physician, this is what she would be told. Just before the operation was postponed, as she was being sponged around the thighs and buttocks with some sort of antiseptic, the nurse unexpectedly told her that she had hemorrhoids. She ought to tell the surgeon to cancel the leg operation which she doesn't really need since there is no pain any longer. Instead, she should allow him to perform a hemorrhoid operation. But after her last hemorrhoid operation, she had been informed that another such operation probably would be too dangerous to perform because she had developed so much scar tissue. (The analyst called attention to the similarity between this statement and the theme of the novel about the woman with scar tissue in the vagina.)

5. Her *vagina has a hideous infection,* because it gives off a terrible stench and a gruesome secretion. Once she had an infection which a

gynecologist told her had spread to the vagina from the rectum. Now she has a similar infection, only much worse. It started last night and hasn't yet been examined by a physician, but it will certainly prove to be something hideous. Isn't the analyst aware of the awful rotting stench? (The analyst answered that he was very much aware of the similarity between the notion of a rotting stench emanating from her vagina and the thought she had reluctantly reported at the beginning of the hour about not having a rotting penis.)

6. Actually her *genitals are unprotected and are liable to become diseased*. She feels very upset about the appearance of her genitals because all of her pubic hair was shaved off the morning on which her operation had originally been scheduled. Now her genitals look like those of a child and she feels they are ugly and unprotected. That is probably why she got the recent infection in her vagina. Now she is in danger of picking up more infections. She should not have been shaved because now her tiny penis is exposed, which ordinarily can't be seen when it is hidden by pubic hair. (The analyst remarked on the fact that she was now speaking about her clitoris as though she believed it really was a small penis. He pointed out that her present statement contradicted her earlier assertion that she did not have a penis. The analyst went on to say that her fantasy seemed to be that she has a small penis which is now exposed and in danger of becoming diseased or injured.)

7. *She visualizes a small penis that is eaten away by some disease, like leprosy*. She can recall having read a magazine article a few years ago which made her feel like fainting because it described how leprosy can eat away a person's arms and legs. By "eaten away" she doesn't mean that the penis is eaten by mouth but by some disease.

8. She has an image of a *mouth eaten away by cancer*, so that the person is *left without any lips*. She again recalls that she was once terribly upset, as a little girl, when she overheard her aunt talking to her mother about a woman who was ill (see pp. 45–46). Now she can remember that one of the things her aunt said was the woman's lips were eaten away by cancer. When she heard that remark, she had almost fainted. (The analyst pointed out that throughout the analytic hour she had been recalling numerous incidents in which she had fainted or almost fainted and that she had also described many disturbing thoughts about body mutilation, all of which seemed to reflect her fears of having to be anesthetized and of undergoing the surgical operation on her leg.)

9. There is *something horrifying about the operation* but she doesn't know what it is; all she can think of is a *legless man dancing about on his mutilated stumps*. When she was a little girl she had once seen such

a man with no legs, who climbed in and out of a basket. She had felt horrified. The thought of a man dancing on his bony stumps sends chills up and down her spine. She imagines the stumps as broken bones, excruciatingly painful and highly sensitive, like an erect penis.

10. She has a vivid image of a huge red penis to which she associates violent parental intercourse. Her first visual impression is that of lying in a crib, as a baby, and watching her parents in bed. Then the main visual image is that of an erect penis and the accompanying thought is that father's penis will damage mother. But she also has the impression that the penis looks as though it is painfully swollen and could be easily hurt. She recalls hearing her father groaning, seemingly in pain. She wonders if she had thought that father was tearing mother apart with his penis while, at the same time, mother was painfully destroying father's penis.

The primal scene recollection, fragments of which had come up earlier, was the patient's last preoperative association. At the door, as Mrs. Blake was about to leave, the analyst said he hoped that everything would go well with her in the hospital. Mrs. Blake looked slightly surprised, as though the remark were unexpected, but, as she walked out of the office her expression changed into a smile.

Preoperative Reactions in the Hospital

Upon returning about two and one-half weeks later, Mrs. Blake spent the entire analytic hour talking about her surgical experiences, giving an especially vivid account of her final preoperative reactions. On the night before the operation, she was given the expected enema. In line with her earlier prediction (Session 9), she involuntarily retained the fluid and had no bowel movement whatsoever. She felt slightly chagrined and worried about the self-fulfillment of her prophecy but also had a mixed feeling of pride and embarrassment because of the "amazement" shown by the nurses as a result of the unsuccessful enema.

Upon awakening early the next morning, she immediately realized that the operation was to take place within a few hours. At this time she felt rather indifferent about it. Her bland mood continued until a nurse came in to give her some sedative pills. Shortly afterwards, knowing that she was supposed to rest quietly, Mrs. Blake began to feel increasingly irritable and was unable to relax. While tossing about on her bed for an entire hour, she felt lonely and neglected as well as somewhat jittery. When her husband unexpectedly arrived, her emotions flared up in an outburst of rage. Mrs. Blake felt "furious" at him because, when Mr. Blake had mentioned on the previous night that he would try to come in the morning, she had told him that it was against the hospital rules. When he walked in, she felt that he was intruding at a time when she was supposed to be resting and that he had come only because he enjoyed getting around prohibitions. She was convinced that his main motive was to demonstrate his ability to charm the nurses into allowing him to come to her room. Bluntly, she told Mr. Blake that she was annoyed at his coming, that she was sure he did it only to satisfy himself, not out of consideration of her. Her anger worked up more and more to the point where she blurted out: "Go away, don't bother me!"

This impulsive anger, which was the first of a series of emotional outbursts, soon gave way to agitated feelings of remorse and intense fear. As her husband started to leave the room, Mrs. Blake noticed a hurt expression on his face. His footsteps, as he walked down the hall, sounded to her as though he were sad and disappointed. Suddenly realizing how her husband must be feeling as a result of her rejection, Mrs. Blake burst into tears.

A student nurse, who came into the room during this scene, politely asked Mrs. Blake to stop crying, but the outpouring was completely beyond control: "Panic rose up in me like boiling water." Mrs. Blake felt completely helpless and "scared to death" because her operation was only 15 minutes away. Seeing this uninhibited display of fear, the student nurse evidently became upset and unsuccessfully tried to handle the situation by repeatedly saying: "Mrs. Blake, don't do that, you mustn't cry, everyone will hear you."

The head nurse on the floor finally did hear Mrs. Blake's crying and entered the room. She immediately put her arms around Mrs. Blake and said gently and affectionately: "Sure you're scared, everybody is; go ahead and cry, it will do you good." In her associations to this episode, Mrs. Blake expressed a warmly positive attitude that seemed to derive from her earliest experiences of being mothered:

> She handled me as though I were a baby because she let me put my head against her breast and patted me. . . . She did me so much good, she was so motherly and I just cried hysterically, pouring out fountains of tears. . . . She did much more than my own mother would have done. My mother would be more like that first nurse. She would be disturbed and say, "Come on now, buck up." Anyhow I would never allow my own mother to come that close to me, it would be disgusting. But it was so luxurious and soothing to be held against the nurse's bosom.

Evidently, the strong dependency needs aroused by the threat of the impending operation were satisfied in a very effective way by the head nurse, although, under ordinary circumstances, the patient would not have allowed herself to indulge in any such overt form of regressive behavior. The mothering activity of the nurse enabled Mrs. Blake at least momentarily to overcome her acute fear and to terminate her uncontrollable spasmodic crying. But a little while later she again started weeping when she learned that her operation would have to be postponed until later in the morning. And again she was reassured by the head nurse who said she would stay with her all the way through. Mrs. Blake experienced an especially glowing feeling when, upon asking the nurse how she could spend so much time away from her regular duties, the reply was that "this is more important than anything else."

During this period the surgeon stopped in for a brief visit and asked how she was feeling. Mrs. Blake frankly told him about feeling frightened and he too spoke very reassuringly.

In reporting these incidents, Mrs. Blake said several weeks later:

> I didn't feel the least bit ashamed to let the doctor and the nurses see that I was scared and to ask for their sympathy. But now I feel terribly embarrassed about the babyish way I behaved. I just hope they will forget all about it. Now I'm an efficient business woman again and it's as though all that stuff happened to a different person.

While waiting in her room, after the surgeon's visit, Mrs. Blake felt increasingly drowsy, probably from the sedative. The last preoperative event she could remember was seeing a "loving" look on the head nurse's face as the bed was being wheeled to the operating room.

10.

Causes and consequences of exaggerated fears

According to numerous studies of the way people behave in actual danger situations, exaggerated fears and outbreaks of acute anxiety symptoms are by no means a rare phenomenon.[1]

> On a surgical service the operative procedure often functions as the nucleus about which psychiatric problems are elaborated. The anticipated operation becomes closely invested with the patient's fears, anxieties and wishes, and may precipitate a critical emotional climax. It may also serve as a backdrop upon which sundry unconscious motivations, needs and defenses are portrayed . . .
>
> Many patients envisage the approaching operation as a death threat, usually with no relation to reality. Severe preoperative panic states may be precipitated by the dread of anesthesia as well as possible mutilation or loss of function. (Bernstein and Small, 1951, p. 938.)

Clinical psychoanalysts are accustomed to interpreting the sudden appearance of exaggerated fears as surface indicators—or "derivatives"—of an exacerbated unconscious conflict. As Fenichel (1945) points out, the repressed forces which enter into the conflict may lie dormant for years without occasioning any manifest neurotic symptoms, but they are capable of generating unduly intense emotional spells and related symptoms if mobilized by distressing events. The stress experiences that give rise to neurotic symptoms are assumed to be ones which produce either ". . . an increase in the anxiety that motivates repression or . . . an increase in the repressed instinctual forces." (Fenichel, 1945, p. 123.)

Throughout the entire preoperative period, and especially in the final sessions just described, Mrs. Blake's emotional responses were heavily overlaid with morbid fears. From her free associations on the occasions when she ventilated exaggerated fears, one can discern something of the nature of the repressed conflict stimulated by the external threat.

Latent Content of Surgical Fears

Although capable of arriving at a fairly correct appraisal of the dangerous and benign aspects of the approaching surgical experience, the patient was continually preoccupied with apprehensions stemming from a very early period of her life. Her main preoccupations consisted of unrealistic anticipations of being abandoned by love objects and of being subjected to punitive mutilation. These reactions, although stimulated by the objective dangers of surgery, can be characterized as "neurotic anxiety"; they are symptoms of the very same sort which appear spontaneously, without the provocation of external danger, in persons struggling against the acute *inner* danger of being unable to control unacceptable motives that have been repressed (Freud, 1933, pp. 113 ff.).

The characteristic vagueness and inappropriateness of repressed fears can be readily discerned in the patient's manifest emotional behavior, especially during Session 12. She felt that a horrible fate was in store for her, admitted that the impending surgery almost overwhelmed her with anxiety, but was unable to say what frightened her. Several times she mentioned specific aspects of the anticipated surgical experience as the source of her fears, but it soon became apparent that she was greatly exaggerating the potential dangerousness of relatively benign events. In the sessions during the week preceding her operation, the patient seemed to be searching for an effective way of covering up the repressed content of her fears, trying to find a displaced target onto which she could conveniently project the source of her emotional tension, just as she had done two weeks earlier when she blamed her sleeplessness and agitation on an inconsequential remark made by the analyst (pp. 50–51). In Session 12, she spontaneously produced a series of vivid fantasies of sexual violence and mutilation, asserted that "there's something horrifying about the operation but I don't know what it is," and ended up by complaining that because her pubic hair was removed she had become vulnerable to genital damage.

The patient's morbid fantasies indicate that the anticipated surgery aroused a wide variety of infantile fears of body damage stemming from early phases of her life history. Indeed, the series of associations given to the danger of dissolving (Session 12) could be used to illustrate a psychoanalytic textbook account of the infantile fears associated with each of the successive zonal stages of female psychosexual development: oral fears (destruction of the lips, being eaten away by cancer); anal fears (giving off a repelling stench, suffering from hemorrhoids which require a painful anal operation, possessing rotting organs that must be extracted from inside the body); phallic fears (having an exposed tiny penis, mutilated stumps); feminine genital fears (brutal rape, vagina torn by penis). Her horror fantasies include references to numerous vulnerable parts of her body and to many different ways in which a destructive blow might be inflicted. There is, nevertheless, a single latent theme which repeatedly occurs with only minor variations. In the analytic material from the last three sessions, one can find numerous indications that her unverbalized fears are centered primarily on the *dangers of a sadistic sexual attack with the resulting loss of an important body organ.* The predominance of this latent source of fear becomes more comprehensible, as will be seen shortly, when examined in relation to what was learned in the course of this patient's entire psychoanalysis regarding her psychosexual conflicts. From the psychoanalytic findings on her early life (summarized below, pp. 111–114), it becomes apparent that the current neurotic reactions generated by the anticipated surgery tend to recapitulate the dominant sources of anxiety associated with childhood dangers. The main dangers were those which she had felt to be present during the distressing periods of the first eight years of her life when the nuclear features of her neurotic personality structure were acquired.

The interview data are consistent with the following psychoanalytic hypothesis: An objective threat of body damage will tend to evoke overestimation of the danger and inappropriate fear reactions ("neurotic anxiety") to the degree that it reactivates repressed childhood fears of being mutilated as a punitive retaliation for forbidden hostile and erotic impulses directed toward the parents. The main notion in this hypothesis, although not always formulated in the same way, is frequently alluded to by psychoanalytic theorists. The emphasis on "castration anxiety" in psychoanalytic discussions of surgery (H. Deutsch, 1942; Fessler, 1931; Kaplan, 1956; Musaph, 1950; Nunberg, 1949) embodies the conception that in adult life the threat of being cut by the surgeon's scalpel can readily reawaken buried childhood fears of losing the prized genitals as a punishment for tabooed sexual wishes. Similar concepts are also to be found in psychiatric reports on anxiety symptoms evoked in other circumstances of acute stress, such as the threat of disease, large-scale disasters, and military combat (Coriat, 1946; Kardiner and H. Spiegel, 1947, p. 104; Rado, 1942, p. 366).

Predisposing Factors

The theoretical value of the psychoanalytic conception of exaggerated fear reactions ultimately depends upon whether or not one can specify in observable terms the meaning of the hypothetical constructs which are implied by the phrase, *reactivation of repressed childhood fears.* The main assumption is that the arousal of certain kinds of unverbalized fears stemming from childhood experiences will have certain observable behavioral consequences (exaggerated fears of the current threat). To be useful in a psychological theory of stress, the reactivation concept must be anchored in observable antecedent conditions as well as observable consequences; otherwise, any proposition which employs the concept would remain so vague as to be scientifically worthless because there would be no way of knowing what the crucial evidence might be that could confirm or refute it. To use the hypothesis for predicting whether or not any given human being will actually show the predicted behavioral consequences, it is necessary to specify the circumstances *when* and in *whom* the degree of reactivation will tend to be high or low.

Psychoanalytic literature contains a rich backlog of clinical observations which, although unsystematically recorded, provide data pertinent for extracting supplementary propositions of the kind needed to specify the behavioral consequences of the reactivation construct and to endow the construct with some specific anchorage in antecedent conditions. Fenichel, drawing on the observations of Anna Freud and other psychoanalysts, has formulated the following propositions which are typical of the kind to be found scattered throughout psychoanalytic writings:

> Among a group of persons subjected to the same real danger, those are more likely to react with panic who had no opportunity to master their tension in any other way. Such opportunity may be blocked by external circumstances; it is easier to master anxiety while some task is to be fulfilled or some motions can be made than if one is forced to wait quietly. Or the opportunity may be blocked by internal circumstances, by a state of "readiness for anxiety," due either to antecedent strain or to previous repressions.

This also holds true for children, whose reaction, besides, is also dependent on that of the grownups around them. (Fenichel, 1945, p. 133.)

In such propositions, two major sets of antecedent factors can be discriminated: (*a*) those which describe the external threat situation (i.e., the environmental conditions under which repressed fears are most likely to be stimulated in anyone), and (*b*) those which describe personality predispositions (i.e., characteristics of persons who are likely to react most strongly to any given threat). For the present we shall single out one supplementary proposition pertaining to one type of predispositional factor which may be applicable to many female surgical patients and perhaps to many male patients as well. The case material from Mrs. Blake's psychoanalysis can be used to illustrate the following hypothesis: The probability that an objective threat of body damage will reactivate repressed childhood fears of mutilation is increased if the person retains as a special form of unresolved Oedipal conflict the following two motivational tendencies: (*a*) an unmodified hostile attitude toward the like-sexed parent, as manifested by openly hostile actions and daydreams directed toward the parent or parent-surrogates; and (*b*) a high level of latent guilt and anxiety concerning the execution of acts in line with the sex role, as manifested by overt inhibitions of sexual functions and symptoms of overt anxiety in interpersonal relationships with sex objects.

The meaning of the predisposing characteristics specified by this supplementary hypothesis can best be concretized by examining the particular characteristics of the Oedipal conflicts which seem to underlie the patient's neurotic fear of surgery. Early in the psychoanalysis it became clear that her chronic symptoms and overt disturbances in daily life were closely linked with two basic attitudes: (*a*) incomplete acceptance of the feminine role and (*b*) a strong need to struggle against succumbing to domination by mother or by any mother-surrogate. During the two consecutive years of analysis, the core of the patient's neurosis gradually was uncovered, revealing the repressed impulses, reaction formations, and fantasies that formed the basis for most of her symptoms. Four central factors emerged which helped to explain why she was so exceptionally afraid of being feminine and why she felt that any mother figure was such a threat to her independence.

1. The patient had never fully relinquished a fantasy, developed during early childhood, that she was really masculine rather than feminine. The gist of this fantasy had always been available to consciousness but some of the main elements had been repressed, particularly the details as to how she knew that she was a boy and how it happened that she

had all the actual characteristics and appearance of a girl. As a result of the unrepression produced earlier in the psychoanalytic treatment, certain limited portions of the infantile fantasy would occasionally be openly expressed by the patient during the preoperative sessions. This happened, for instance, when she referred to the "little penis" which was exposed by the shaving of her pubic hair (Session 12) and also when she complained that the operation might rob her of some secret masculine power (Session 10). The main conflict which the fantasy served to alleviate had to do with the ambivalent attitude toward her mother. A major theme in the latent meaning of the fantasy was that as a disguised male she could win her mother's affection more successfully than father or anyone else in the family.

2. The strong wish to be a masculine suitor for mother's affection appears to have functioned as a major defense against the inner danger of striving to satisfy a much more threatening unconscious wish—that of trying to defeat mother in competition for father's love. The defensive effort to concentrate her erotic and affectionate interests exclusively on mother were motivated partly by the felt need to ward off punitive retaliation. The wish for masculinity was also a means for counteracting the dangerous wish to obtain the excited gratification that would come from being attacked sexually by father in the same way that she had seen mother attacked. From infancy until the age of four, the patient had slept in her parents' bedroom and had frequently witnessed parental intercourse. Evidently she was both attracted and repelled by what she saw and heard. Much of the patient's anxiety stemmed from the gross misinterpretation of her parents' excited behavior as acts of mutual destructiveness. This misinterpretation is well illustrated by the vivid, fragmentary memories of the primal scene at the end of Session 12. Similar, though less detailed, memories of parental intercourse had occurred earlier in the analysis at times when the patient was giving associations to a recurrent neurotic symptom, viz., her frigidity during sexual intercourse, which was evoked by observing or imagining the "look" of sexual excitement on her husband's face. This sexual inhibition was clearly linked with an unresolved conflict concerning father. The intolerable "look" on her husband's face reminded her of an excited expression she had seen on her father's face when he was killing chickens during a summer vacation on a farm. She also remembered having had recurrent nightmares as a child in which she awoke terrified by the image of her father's excited expression.

3. During an early period of childhood—probably about the age of three—the patient had been proud of being a girl and had felt that she had won father for herself. The little girl could never be absolutely

certain, however, that father was as indifferent toward mother as she hoped, and at times she consciously harbored the wish that mother would die or go away and never come back (see Session 14, pp. 127 ff.). All this was before the fear of sexual attack became pronounced. But then, at a certain point, the child's erotic interest in father and her hostile attitude toward mother were felt to be extremely dangerous—partly because of witnessing the apparent violence of father's sexual relationship with mother. Through a variety of defensive maneuvers, the child sought to subdue the anxiety and guilt generated by her forbidden longings toward father. These longings had been reinforced earlier by opportunities for close body contact in all sorts of erotically exciting horseplay which, according to the patient's recollection during the analysis, her father had freely permitted. One compromise she subsequently developed was that of adding a frankly masochistic coloring to her wishes, accepting in her fantasies the painful consequences of being brutally attacked by father so that the pleasure would be both hidden and paid for. But her main method of struggling against the forbidden longings eventually became that of object displacement: she abandoned the dangerous competition with mother by regressing to a safer pre-Oedipal orientation, renouncing father and turning back to mother as her main love object (see pp. 128–129 below for additional details bearing on the nature of the patient's conflictful attitude toward her mother and the chronology of distressing childhood events that led up to the wish to be masculine).

4. When she grew older, she went through a number of crisis periods during which the original conflict again flared up. Especially during early adolescence, she was tempted to try to defeat her mother and siblings, to win father's affection exclusively for herself. Invariably the denouement was self-defacing submission to mother, with partially conscious expectations of undergoing punishment so as to regain forgiveness and love. This was the sequence she was repeatedly acting out over and over again throughout her adult life with a succession of older women, each of whom reminded her of mother. An example of this stereotyped sequence is to be found in Session 1 (pp. 44–45), where she described her deliberate efforts to subdue and dominate an older female employee. As usual, her aggressive action against the mother surrogate was followed by a need for expiation. On this particular occasion, however, her conscious guilt feelings were much more intense than usual, presumably as a consequence of anticipating the objective threat of surgery. (See Hypothesis 1A, p. 54.)

Neither the masochistic orientation in her fantasy life nor the defensive displacement were fully successful in alleviating the patient's guilt and anxiety, especially at age four and one-half when a younger sister was born. Subsequently, she developed further compromise formations on which she relied to compensate for acute disappointments as well as to alleviate guilt concerning her dangerous hostile impulses toward mother and libidinal impulses toward father. These compromise formations entered into a very early edition of the masculinity fantasy and were determinants of the crucial repressed details. The main themes in the unconscious childhood fantasy, as reconstructed at the end of three and one-half years of analysis, appeared to be as follows: (*a*) she had secretly stolen a small penis from father (which she sometimes regarded as a loving gift he had been willing to give her); (*b*) the penis gave her the power to attack mother in the same way father did, and, at the same time, carried the guarantee that father could not attack her; (*c*) mother must not become aware of this prized possession, otherwise she would become so envious and enraged that she would take it away or destroy it. This fantasy turned out to be at the root of the patient's recurrent conflict about developing warm, affectionate relationships with maternal figures; her fear that mother, or a mother-surrogate, might take away the cherished possession was often as strong as her fear of losing maternal love and being abandoned.

All of the above psychogenic details are, of course, tentatively inferred from fragmentary memories, associations to dreams, transference reactions, and other such symbol data obtained in psychoanalytic sessions. Since the voluminous interview data in which the indicators of the repressed conflict were manifested are not herewith presented, any reader who is highly skeptical about the validity of reconstructing repressed childhood fantasies from an adult psychoanalysis is certainly entitled to have especially strong doubts about the authenticity of the text of the patient's secret penis fantasy.[2] But even without assuming that all the above inferences are essentially correct, the following facts cannot be overlooked. Throughout the preoperative sessions there are repeated associations indicating that the patient's anxiety reactions are closely linked with a distorted body image and particularly with grossly unrealistic notions about the way in which her body is vulnerable to damage: (*a*) Her initial fear is that the surgeon will require her to undergo an amputation (Session 1); (*b*) she has a preoperative dream about pressing from a pimple on her face a long, bony thing like spaghetti, to which she associates an erect penis and childhood fears of being caught and punished by mother for playing forbidden games in which she used a make-believe penis (Session 5); (*c*) she expresses a current fear-laden fantasy to the effect that the analyst, who at times is equated with the surgeon, threatens to take away some unspecified part of her body (Session 5); (*d*) she manifests violent abhorrence of losing body secretions and of being cleaned out by an enema, which appears to be equated to death or annihilation (Session 9); (*e*) she is afraid that the surgery will somehow result in a loss of her "masculine powers" (Session 10); (*f*) in the final preoperative session she says that her sex organs are diseased and that she has a tiny penis which is exposed and in danger of being damaged (Session 12).

From the above content of her manifest fears of body damage, it seems plausible that her sense of vulnerability during the preoperative period is linked with an underlying fantasy that she has an important body possession, which is located inside her body in the genital region, and which is currently endangered. Thus, some of the main features of the reconstructed childhood fantasy of the illicit penis are indicated by the material from the preoperative sessions.

Similar thematic features were involved in the patient's chronic obsessional symptoms, the repressed content of which was not uncovered until later on, almost a year after the surgical experience. Particularly in her doubts and ruminations about whether to be dominating or submissive toward mother-surrogates, the alternatives turned out to represent, in a disguised form, the same conflict which we have assumed to be involved in the illicit penis fantasy: "Should I give up the precious possession inside my body by letting mother clean me out—like she used to do when she gave me enemas? Or should I fight against her demands and use my masculine powers to attack her—the way father did?"

Thus, the psychoanalytic data provide many different indications that the patient was especially predisposed to overreact with neurotic anxiety to the threat of surgery because she retained in unmodified form a *fantasy of possessing an illicit organ* from which she continued to derive forbidden fantasy gratifications. This fantasy may have left the patient especially vulnerable to threats of physical danger because the symbolic gratification of hostile and envious impulses toward the mother or father generates unconscious anticipations of parental retaliation (S. Freud, 1933 and 1936). According to Hypothesis 5 (p. 91), the threat of physical danger reactivates childhood fears of being abandoned by the parents and thereby creates a strong need for reassurance to counteract separation anxiety. Moreover, in the repressed childhood fantasies of many adult persons, being abandoned by the parents is equivalent to being exposed to a hostile, physically damaging world where they will be subjected to unrelieved suffering. Thus, the patient's inability to reassure herself that she will have the loving care of mother or of mother-surrogates may have prevented her from warding off repressed childhood fears of separation and the accompanying fear of being physically damaged.

Role of Repression in Approach-Avoidance Conflict

In the preceding section, the discussion of predisposing factors centered upon predicting one general consequence of experiencing a reactivation of repressed childhood fears in the presence of an external threat; namely, the tendency to react to the current threat situation with inappropriate or exaggerated fear reactions. Included among such reactions would be tendencies to overestimate the magnitude of the present danger and to display emotional spells of the sort that are regarded by clinicians as symptoms of "neurotic anxiety." In addition, there are other psychological consequences that follow from the stimulation of repressed fears, some of which we shall now examine for the purpose of explicating more fully the implications of the reactivation concept.

One obvious consequence of the arousal of repressed fear is *irrational avoidance behavior*. For example, Nunberg, (1949) describes one of his adult patients who delayed an essential operation by refusing to sign the routine form which is required to permit surgery to be performed. The patient's anxiety was centered on a neurotic fantasy image of the surgeon cutting much more than necessary, reflecting an unconscious fear of being castrated during narcotic sleep. This exaggerated fear was linked with a partially repressed childhood memory of undergoing a circumcision at the age of three. Similar instances of irrational avoidance actions are frequently reported in psychiatric studies of men who are engaged in hazardous occupations. Bond (1952), for example, asserts that repressed fears on the part of noncombat flyers can lead not only to outright refusal to accept a flying assignment but also to overcautiousness, a much more subtle form of avoidance that can impair a flyer's over-all efficiency.

> During the period that the fear remains unconscious, other symptoms make their appearance, the most common being a multitude of physical symptoms, which always undergo exaggeration in flight. One of the least known but very important symptoms—for it is peculiar to flight—is a growing cautiousness in the air, a symptom that can be very dangerous, for it hampers direct action and decision. Often this symptom takes the form of obsessively following one safety precaution to the exclusion of all others. (Bond, 1952, p. 45.)

The heightening of irrational avoidance behavior, which results from the arousal of repressed fears, is well illustrated in the psychoanalytic case material presented in earlier chapters. At times, the patient became strongly motivated to run away from the prospective threat situation, despite her knowledge of the relatively slight risk entailed by the surgical procedure. She knew that much greater harm might result from neglecting the physical impairment of her leg than from having the operation. But her actual behavior was frequently at odds with her intellectual awareness.

The first clear-cut indications that irrational emotional factors were capable of exerting a dominant influence on her overt actions are to be found in Sessions 1 through 5. This was the period when the patient deliberately avoided seeing a physician even though she was suffering from chronic pains and knew that medical attention was needed. Her overt avoidance behavior was closely linked with—and probably was partly caused by—her exaggerated conception of the seriousness of the affliction and of the severity of the corrective measures that would be required. On several occasions after she had overcome her original reluctance to seeking medical aid, the same neurotic distortions reappeared, combined with even more pronounced ones (e.g., the mutilation and death fantasies uncovered at the end of Session 9). And again, these distortions influenced her judgments, although not to the same extent as during the initial period. In Session 10, we learned that even after having fully committed herself to the operation, she was willing to contemplate backing out of it after a nurse at the hospital asked her to help set the date for the surgery. Just as during the period when she had stayed away from her physician, the patient's avoidance tendency was motivated *not by intellectual appraisals* of the alternative risks but by *fantasy notions* that were derivatives of unconscious sources of anxiety.

Vacillating between the alternatives of facing danger or running away from it is not necessarily a consequence of repression. Studies of American combat troops (Stouffer et al., 1949b, Chapters 3 and 4) indicate that many soldiers displayed vacillation tendencies and manifested other symptoms of a conflict between the avoidance motives stemming from fears of being injured or killed and the counteracting approach motives. The latter included conscience demands and social conformity motives directed particularly toward the primary combat unit which was the nucleus of group identification (Grinker and J. Spiegel, 1945a and 1945b; H. Spiegel, 1944). Frequently the combat soldier was acutely conscious of both the approach motives (inclining him to remain in the combat situation) and the avoidance motives (inclining him to escape). The strength of avoidance tendencies in the average soldier was influenced by reality-testing functions involving (*a*) the discrimination of safe versus dangerous battle stimuli; (*b*) the assimilation of information about the nature of the threat; and (*c*) the appraisal of opportunities for minimizing risks. When combat dangers were perceived to be imminent and of great magnitude, the avoidance motives based on fear would tend to become much more powerful. Occasionally, such motives would increase to the point where they greatly exceeded the strength of the counteracting approach motives, as in the rare instances of men who, after being pinned down in foxholes by repeated artillery barrages, felt their plight to be hopeless and either refused to advance or tried to flee from the combat area. More often, signs to the effect that great danger was at hand produced an increase in avoidance motives which eventuated not in actual flight but in more subtle forms of augmented conflict behavior—ruminations about opportunities for escaping by acquiring "a million dollar wound," timidity in executing combat missions, and perhaps even some vacillating attempts to "goof off" on the most hazardous activities in the job assignment (Glass, 1953). Thus, sometimes there were only indirect or covert manifestations of avoidance tendencies if the approach motives remained sufficiently dominant to inhibit actual flight behavior.

The above discussion of conflict among combat troops has referred only to avoidance behavior produced by external environmental signs, i.e., realistic information about impending threats and objective cues of imminent danger. But exactly the same behavioral consequences can occur as a result of the arousal of *repressed* fears. This is indicated by the psychiatric studies referred to earlier (p. 62), which describe the anxiety symptoms of military combat personnel.

The essential point is that repressed fears can increase the tendency to run away from danger just as in the case of fears based on reality-oriented expectations of danger. It seems plausible, therefore, to conceive of the two sources of fear as summating. In other words, our assumption is that the strength of avoidance motivation is determined by the intensity of reality-based fears combined with the intensity of repressed childhood fears reactivated by the external threat.

Illustrative material bearing specifically on this assumption can be noted in the psychoanalytic observations from the last three preoperative sessions. All the external signs, including the authoritative medical information to which the patient was exposed, conveyed essentially the same reassuring story; namely, that the risk entailed by her operation would be very low. She knew it was to be a relatively minor operation involving a routine surgical procedure, that complications rarely occurred, that incision pains would be moderate and controllable, and that fairly rapid recovery was to be expected. If external information about the threat were the only stimuli to which the patient was reacting, her fear would be very slight; she would both think and act entirely in terms of the belief that the important gains from the operation greatly exceeded the slight risks. The approach motives (inclining her to submit to the operation) would be of relatively great strength, reflecting her rational judgment that the operation would alleviate her physical disorder without entailing much danger or loss. In addition, there were powerful social motives which would make for conformity with the physician's recommendations. For any middle-class American, failure to follow the doctor's orders concerning important health matters constitutes a deviation from social norms. Behind the physician is the entire weight of community opinion in contemporary urban society and one cannot disregard the norm without expecting criticism and censure (Parsons, 1951, pp. 437 ff.). To the extent that one internalizes the norm ("Doctors know best"), the thought of not following doctor's orders would stimulate social anxiety and lower self-esteem.

With very powerful motivational forces operating in the direction of approach behavior and with only very weak threats producing the fear that generates avoidance behavior, hardly any manifestations of conflict ought to appear (see Dollard and Miller, 1950, Chapter 22). Under such conditions, the individual supposedly would make a rapid decision to accept the physician's recommendation, display no subsequent vacillation, feel little temptation to postpone the operation, and remain optimistic about the ultimate outcome, although somewhat concerned about the unpleasant experiences that will occur.

The fact that our patient wavered so much and displayed so many symptoms of acute conflict is attributable to repressed fear. The neurotic sources of anxiety in this instance evidently increased the strength of the avoidance tendency to the point where it approached the strength of the approach tendency.[3] In her conscious thoughts, and even in some of her overt actions, the patient showed essentially the same degree of vacillation that would be expected if she had been relatively free from neurotic anxiety but had received authoritative information to the effect that the recommended operation was quite a risky one, that complications might arise which could necessitate an amputation of her leg, or which could even turn out to be fatal. In short, the patient's preoccupations with amputation and death, based on a neurotically determined fantasy, seem to have produced essentially the same conflict behavior as though based on realistic information.

When the patient's conflict situation is viewed from the standpoint of an inner struggle between the incipient desire to run away from the surgery and the stronger need to achieve the anticipated gains from conforming with the physician's recommendation, the necessity for resorting to relatively extreme defenses becomes more understandable. Loosely speaking, one could say that the patient unconsciously relied upon realistic minimization devices to bolster her original decision, so as to maintain the balance of conflicting forces in favor of the approach tendency. In effect, she reduced the magnitude of the avoidance tendency by using repression, suppression, and related denial mechanisms, all of which minimized the anticipated danger; at the same time she sought to augment the magnitude of the approach by developing an exaggerated conception of the compensatory gratifications. The patient's surface attitude of unconcern can be regarded as an attempt not only to avoid awareness of fantasied dangers but also to control inner avoidance motives which could result in objectively harmful consequences. Because of her irrational, repressed fears, she had to exert special efforts to overcome the dangerous tendency to run away from the operation. Thus, her distorted image of the operation as a wholly pleasant opportunity for indulgences may have developed as a secondary consequence of the arousal of repressed fears.

Up to this point the discussion has been focused almost exclusively on the ways in which the behavioral consequences of repressed fears are similar to those of reality-based fears. The main points of similarity are summarized in the following proposition:

Hypothesis 6. *When a person is motivated to approach* (*i.e., tolerate or move toward*) *a threatening situation of potential body damage, the arousal of repressed fears of childhood dangers will have substantially the same effect as the arousal of reality-based fears* (*i.e., fears determined by conscious appraisal of the current dangers*) *with respect to:* (a) *increasing the probability of overt avoidance behavior and* (b) *increasing the degree of vacillation, tension, and other manifestations of acute conflict even when the approach tendencies remain unequivocally dominant over the heightened avoidance tendencies.*

Differences Between Repressed and Nonrepressed Fears

Although repressed and nonrepressed fears may be highly similar with regard to augmenting the strength of avoidance tendencies, as specified in Hypothesis 6, they differ in a number of other important ways. From what is generally known about the effects of repression, we would expect to find fundamental differences in the way in which the two types of fear encroach upon cognitive processes. One such difference, already mentioned several times, has to do with the degree of distortion in the person's perceptions and anticipations of the current danger situation. Misperceptions, distorted judgments, and autistically determined attitudes of overoptimism (as illustrated in our patient's repeated attempts to minimize the threat) are probably much more likely to occur when an avoidance motivation of a given strength contains a large component of repressed fear than when it consists almost exclusively of fear stimulated by clear-cut signs of external danger.

Psychoanalysts regard the occurrence of cognitive distortions as an indicator of the presence of repressed sources of fear in a patient's emotional response to an external threat; repression is characterized as a defense mechanism which ordinarily has damaging effects on the person's reality-testing capabilities (Fenichel, 1945, pp. 130–131 and 148–150). According to psychoanalytic theory and observations, as summarized by Fenichel, an unresolved psychosexual conflict will predispose a person to overreact to objective threats that occur in adult life. The accompanying infantile fantasies are repressed and therefore remain unmodified, despite ample opportunities for corrective learning experiences. Once the repression mechanism sets in during childhood, the person becomes unable to test his unverbalized expectations against reality and is therefore unable to discard childhood misconceptions, such as the notion that the punishment for having a forbidden wish will be the loss of a prized part of his body.

Closely related to errors of perception and judgment are other impairments which, in a moment of great crisis, may result in the inability to dispel fantasied horrors and to maintain control over regressive emotional impulses. We have noted in our patient an especially pronounced tendency to react to the major crises of the preoperative period with uncontrolled emotional outbursts and disorganized efforts to terminate the stress. An outstanding example of regressive emotional behavior occurred just before she was taken to the operating room, when, without provocation, she became enraged at her husband and then wept violently until she was given an infantile form of reassurance (see pp. 105–106).

The most crucial aspect of repressed fear, which differentiates it most sharply from reality-based fear, is its relative imperviousness to corrective information. The psychoanalytic case material suggests the following general proposition:

Hypothesis 7. *When an objective threat of body damage is anticipated, the greater the degree to which repressed fear is aroused the* *lower the probability that sustained emotional relief will ensue as a result of reassuring communications from authoritative persons who are regarded as credible sources of information.*

This hypothesis is consistent with current psychoanalytic conceptions concerning the recalcitrant nature of neurotic fears and the special therapeutic conditions required to alleviate them (Kubie, 1952; Loewenstein, 1954). The hypothesis is also compatible with learning theory formulations of the resistance of repressed fears to extinction under external conditions that normally make for the unlearning of inappropriate emotional habits (Dollard and Miller, 1950, Chapter 11).

From our psychoanalytic case study, it is possible to discern within the same individual a sharp contrast between repressed and nonrepressed fears, as specified by Hypothesis 7. For the purpose of highlighting the differences, a detailed comparison will be made of two specific fears of surgical damage that the patient had expressed in Session 1, before she had been examined by a physician. One was the fear that the operation might involve amputation of her entire leg. The other was the fear that if she were to undergo the surgical repair she would be left with a permanent ugly scar that would ruin the appearance of her leg.

At the time of the medical examination, she learned that both fears were unfounded. After the physician told her about the nature of the operation, she knew that the surgical procedure was to be of a minor character, that there was no question of resorting to amputation, and that the incision would most likely heal in such a way as to leave no obvious scar. The latter reassurance appeared to have set her fear of possible disfigurement completely at rest. She accepted what the physician told her and never again expressed any serious doubts about it. Even when she noticed that the scar was highly visible shortly after the operation, she became only mildly concerned and retained her confidence in the physician's reassuring prediction. In general, the patient's reaction consistently indicated that her initial fear of being disfigured by the incision scar was eliminated by the authoritative information.

Not so, as we have seen, in the case of her fear of amputation. Intellectually she believed the reassuring medical information and, for a while, felt relieved, but after a few days, the fear reappeared in full strength. Even after the operation was over, she remained haunted with doubts as to whether her leg would be spared. Later on we shall see that this fear reached a very high intensity when she experienced postoperative pains, even though her physician had told her that such pains were to be expected in the normal course of recovery; on more than one occasion during the postoperative period she was unable to dismiss the intense fear that her blood vessels were so badly impaired that this time she actually would have to undergo the amputation (see Session 16, p. 156).

The difference between the fear of amputation and the fear of a disfiguring scar appears to be essentially a matter of high versus lower degree of neurotic involvement. The patient's fear of disfigurement consistently meets the criteria that analysts use when they refer to an attitude as being "within the conflict-free sphere of the ego" (Hartmann, 1951). The patient showed no evasion, distortion, or circumlocution in discussing the possibility of being disfigured. Neither before nor after seeing the physician did she show any disinclination to give free associations on this topic. For many women the danger of being marred by an incision scar represents a profound narcissistic injury and can stimulate powerful unconscious conflicts (Hill and Silver, 1950); but there is no evidence of any such reaction in our patient. Before the operation, her neurotic fantasies had never focused on the theme of disfigurement, and during the period of the operation her fears in this particular sphere appeared to be a direct reflection of her conscious expectations derived from the information that was available to her. We assume that the relative absence of repression in this instance is an important factor in explaining why the fear of disfigurement could be cleared up so rapidly and completely by the reassuring medical information she received from her physician.

The fear of amputation, on the other hand, cannot be expected to respond in the same way if the main source of the fear is not to be found in the external reality situation. We have already seen in the psychoanalytic evidence from Sessions 1 through 12 that behind the fear of amputation were partially repressed expectations of body mutilation as a retaliation for forbidden impulses that had remained unmodified since early childhood. Long before the period of the operation, the patient had referred to morbid fantasies about losing a leg and had shown considerable reluctance to talk about these fantasies. From the sparse associations she gave, the analyst had surmised that the manifest content of the fantasy was associatively linked with a profoundly distressing inner conflict involving repressed sexual desires toward her father. For instance, one of her childhood memories concerning erotic horseplay with father included the specific detail that, on more than one occasion, she had contrived to rub her leg against father's penis, pretending that it was an unnoticed accident. This memory was reported during the first month of analysis and was amplified during the subsequent year, particularly in associations which showed that the secret bodily contact with father was a major source of her fear of being detected and of being savagely punished by mother. Thus, long before the current prospect of undergoing surgery touched off the fear of having her leg cut off, there were definite indications of a predisposing neurotic attitude concerning the danger of undergoing punitive mutilation in this region of her body.

A final comment is necessary to clear up a possible source of misunderstanding concerning the distinction between repressed and nonrepressed fears. Whenever a person is confronted with external dangers, unconscious sources of fear are likely to enter into the emotional picture even though his reactions may be determined largely by external information about the threat. Probably it is best to assume that both repressed and nonrepressed components of fear will be aroused to varying degrees whenever anyone encounters a severe external threat of body damage. In our discussion of Hypothesis 5, we have assumed that at least one kind of repressed fear (of parental abandonment) is apt to be very widespread, if not universal, among people in our culture whenever there is a serious threat of injury or death. Repressed fears of punishment for forbidden use of sexual organs and related body fears, such as those referred to when we speak of an "unresolved Oedipal conflict," are also likely to enter into everyone's latent attitude toward body damage, to some extent. Thus it would be oversimplifying matters to assume that some people react with repressed fears while others do not. Rather it is a question of the *degree* to which the repressed fear component is a determinant of the person's emotional responses.

The various hypotheses presented in this chapter should be understood as referring to instances where the repressed fear component is aroused to such a high degree as to become the dominant factor in the person's emotional behavior. At times it may be exceedingly difficult to ascertain the relative strength of the repressed fear component in a given individual exposed to an external threat. Nevertheless, in some instances—as in the psychoanalytic sessions with Mrs. Blake—the observer can readily discern that information about a mild external threat situation evoked a disproportionately great emotional turmoil and that the disparity between the mild external stimuli and the intense emotional response was attributable to the arousal of repressed fear. Similar cases in which such disparities occur (some of which will be described in Chapters 20 and 23) can provide fairly clear-cut data for testing the hypotheses put forth in the present chapter.

Notes

1. For bibliographic references concerning the acute anxiety symptoms observed among persons exposed to various types of stress situations—surgery, chronic illness, childbirth, large-scale disasters, and military combat—see note 1 of Chapter 5, p. 62.

2. Secret fantasies of the type that emerged from Mrs. Blake's free associations seem to be encountered frequently in the psychoanalytic treatment of female patients (Fenichel, 1945, pp. 99 ff.; S. Freud, 1933, pp. 170 ff.). The tenaciousness with which such secrets are guarded may be indicative of their importance as a substitute for forbidden Oedipal wishes (Gross, 1951).

3. Technically the conflict should be conceptualized as "double-approach avoidance." (Dollard and Miller, 1950, Chapter 22.) For simplicity the term "approach" is used for all pro-operation motives and "avoidance" for all antioperation motives that are activated at a given time point. The relative strength of approach and avoidance motives is assumed to vary with changes in perceived incentives which increase the positive or negative value of the given decision. It is assumed that these incentive values or "valences" are, in turn, influenced by external communications and events and also by internal psychological occurrences such as memories, thought sequences, and unverbalizable fantasies.

11.

Emotional relief during early convalescence

This chapter will deal with the patient's emotional reactions during the first week following her operation. The observational material was obtained from the retrospective accounts and associations given about two weeks later, when she returned for treatment (Sessions 13 through 16). According to her own account of the recovery period in the hospital, Mrs. Blake was able to achieve some of the psychological gratifications to which she had been looking forward with so much longing before the operation. By and large, the initial phase of her postoperative recovery was characterized by a self-indulgent attitude, euphoric feelings, and preoccupation with erotic fantasies concerning the surgeon. However, the elated mood proved to be of relatively short duration. As will be seen in Chapter 14, after the elation subsided (by about the eighth or ninth postoperative day), it was replaced by depression and irritability. In the present chapter attention will be focused on those descriptive statements and the accompanying free associations which help to illuminate the underlying dynamics of the patient's transient episode of reactive elation.

RETROSPECTIONS FROM SESSIONS 13–16: THE ELATION SYNDROME

Immediately upon awakening from the anesthetic, Mrs. Blake was somewhat disturbed to realize that her surgical wounds were more extensive than she had anticipated. Nevertheless, within a few hours she was in a mildly euphoric state, despite the usual discomforts from the surgery. When nurses and visitors began to arrive, she was spontaneously warm and friendly toward them. She felt completely relaxed, as though having "awakened from a nice deep sleep." Her conception of herself—"for the first time in years"—was as a completely feminine woman who could be extraordinarily appealing to men. She took pains to make a good appearance and deliberately chose to wear an expensive, fluffy bedjacket which she knew would be attractive. When a male co-worker from her office came during visiting hours, she was "thrilled because he said, 'You look positively ravishing.' " At this time she felt friendly and sexually attracted toward him, whereas, previously, she had thought of this man as a despicable, dangerous competitor who was constantly belittling her work and trying to get her fired.

In her elated mood, she was convinced not only that she had again become attractive to men but also that she was admired and loved by the nurses and other women with whom she was in contact: "I felt like a completely different person—young, attractive, well liked by everyone."

One of Mrs. Blake's key associations to the temporary period of euphoria—produced in Session 14, about a week after the elation subsided—provides an important clue as to the psychogenic origin of her elated reactions:

> The feelings were completely familiar except that I couldn't identify them. But then in yesterday's session I suddenly realized that I felt as though I were Joyce and now I know that it was just like the way I felt when I was three years old.

Joyce was a much admired woman in Mrs. Blake's current circle of acquaintances. Many times earlier in the analysis, Joyce had been depicted as the epitome of successful femininity—universally admired, seemingly passive, but with complete self-confidence in her power to attract and influence any man who came within her orbit. Several months earlier in the treatment, Mrs. Blake had referred to Joyce as being at the opposite pole from herself: "I don't have that special something that she has—that spark that makes a woman really attractive to any man; and I lack something that is essential for being a good mother."

Mrs. Blake had also asserted in an earlier session that there had been only one time in her life when she had felt "self-confident and completely feminine, just like Joyce." That was when she was three years old, the year preceding the birth of her younger sister. Throughout her analysis she had repeatedly described it as the "golden age" of her childhood, a period when she felt happy, well loved, and highly self-confident because of having won the affection of her father. According to her vivid fantasy conception of family relationships at that time, she had completely defeated her mother as well as her older sisters in the competition for father's affection, while simultaneously being protected from their hostility by virtue of a "secret marriage" to father. In free associations concerning this idyllic arrangement, she asserted that one of the main sources of gratification from the fantasied marriage was that it supposedly put at her disposal all of father's "prized possessions" and his "enormous masculine powers."

When she was about four years old, the budding feminine conception of herself was rudely shattered by two major events—the birth of her younger sister and the near-drowning of her mother. Evidently she had succeeded in not being aware of her mother's pregnancy, or, perhaps, she was able to deny it. In any case, the sister's birth shocked her into realizing that mother was still the main woman in father's life. The child not only felt betrayed and forsaken by father, but suddenly had a distressing sense of being left helpless to protect herself against mother's rage.

The drowning episode occurred at a beach, a few months after the baby sister was born. The four-year-old girl heard mother call for help but calmly continued to play in the sand without looking in the direction of all the commotion, quietly saying to herself, "*mother will not be saved.*" This combined wish and command was thwarted by father, who promptly went to mother's rescue. When the little girl looked up and saw father carrying mother out of the water, it seemed to her that "he was a strange and different man." According to her repeated recollections about the events of her early life, this episode marked a decisive change in the girl's personality. From this point on she no longer thought of herself as feminine. Gradually she became more and more compulsive with respect to adhering to her mother's demands, and unconsciously imitated the hostile and aggressive components of her mother's personality.

With this developmental context in mind, the analyst surmised from what Mrs. Blake said about her postoperative period of elation, that she had been able temporarily to abandon her guilt-laden identification with the threatening mother imago. The temporary regression to age three seemed to be a matter of returning to the period before the occurrence of the death-wish episode and before becoming too guilt-stricken to allow herself to compete openly for father's affection. In describing her guilt-free feelings during the recovery period, Mrs. Blake added the information that when her elation ended, her conception of her sex role simultaneously changed: "Now I'm not carefree any more and I'm not like Joyce any more; I'm my usual self again—a supposedly efficient business woman, a sexless neuter, neither man nor woman."

An outstanding feature of Mrs. Blake's elation, which highlights the fact that she could temporarily conceive of herself in a feminine role without feeling guilty, was the tremendous upsurge of erotic interest. Her mental life throughout the first week of convalescence seems to have been filled predominantly with vivid daydreams about love-making and intercourse. These fantasies and the accompanying sexual feelings were directed mainly toward the one person who plays the most active role in the dramatic events of a surgical operation—the surgeon himself. In Session 13, Mrs. Blake reported that she had been:

> . . . swamped by sexy feelings toward him. It was nice because I had thought those feelings were gone forever. All during the time I was in the hospital I was constantly thinking about him. After I came home, for several days I still had those daydreams and voluptuous feelings.

Mrs. Blake had met the surgeon many years earlier and had occasionally been examined by him for minor disorders. During all the time she had known him, she had never felt particularly attracted to him nor had there been anything of a flirtatious nature in their relationship. In Mrs. Blake's analytic sessions prior to the operation, she had occasionally referred to the surgeon but not in the way she spoke about any of the various men who at one time or another stimulated her erotic fantasies. The first time the surgeon was ever mentioned as an object of sexual interest was after the operation.

The fantasied love affair seems to have been stimulated, probably quite unintentionally, by the way the surgeon behaved on his first post-operative visit. Mrs. Blake reported that her sexual interest in him began when they were talking together a few hours after she awoke from the anesthetic. The surgeon had come to her room for a routine check on her condition and, after a brief physical examination, he had begun to ask a few questions about her usual daily life activities. It seemed to her that the surgeon was very much interested in hearing about her husband's various physical defects, particularly after she mentioned that her marriage was not very satisfactory at present:

He kept asking me more and more questions about my marriage setup and he really seemed personally interested in me. Suddenly I realized that this was a real flirtation we were having. I felt very pleased about it. After he left the room I remembered having heard years ago that this doctor wasn't getting along with his wife. And then I started to wonder where our flirtation was going to lead.

Whether or not there actually was something flirtatious in the surgeon's behavior, the fact is that Mrs. Blake displayed a considerable readiness to develop a strong erotic attachment in response to minimal encouragement. A few minutes of questioning about the state of her marital relationship was sufficient to complete the transformation of her former conscious attitude of sexual indifference toward the surgeon into an intensely excited infatuation.

Part of this readiness, as has already been suggested, probably stemmed from the temporary reduction in guilt feelings, and the accompanying freedom to indulge in hedonistic satisfactions that characterized the early part of Mrs. Blake's convalescence. But it obviously was not simply a matter of normal sexual motives being released and asserting themselves. Despite the fact that she was continually preoccupied with voluptuous thoughts about a love affair with the surgeon, Mrs. Blake reported having experienced little sexual excitation and no wish to masturbate. This was in marked contrast to the way she had reacted during the preceding year on those rare occasions when she had had similar erotic daydreams about the analyst and other men.

FREE ASSOCIATIONS FROM SESSIONS 13–16: LATENT ATTITUDE TOWARD THE SURGEON

Mrs. Blake's free associations during the analytic hours in which she spoke about the infatuation episode clearly revealed that her interest in the surgeon was more closely tied up with needs for affection and protective reassurance than with sexual needs. An attitude of intense dependency is revealed by the following series of associations in which Mrs. Blake expressed her wish for a substitute protector:

Before the operation I didn't want to leave you. I felt I needed to come here for analysis to escape from the jungle outside and this was the only place I really felt safe. I even wanted to postpone the operation because I hated to give up coming here. Then in the hospital Miss M. (the head nurse) took your place and she helped me get through that awful time just before the operation. After the operation was over I concentrated all my feelings on the doctor—and I hardly thought of you at all. You weren't available then when I needed you, but he was. Besides I felt ready for a love affair and I knew that you wouldn't have an affair with me.

These associations, and others to be described shortly, suggest that Mrs. Blake's attitude toward the surgeon must be understood in relation to the transference reactions that had arisen in the course of psychoanalytic treatment. In her postoperative erotic fantasies, the manifest content expressed only the positive components of the patient's general attitude toward the important men in her life. But, as has been repeatedly pointed out, the transference reactions toward the analyst always were strikingly ambivalent during all phases of her analysis, and especially during the period just before she underwent the operation. Underneath the positive exterior attitude was an interior attitude of covert fear and hostility that was ready to come to the surface whenever the therapist said anything which she construed as a threat of punishment. For example, several months earlier when the analyst made a passing reference to an impending vacation period, Mrs. Blake's reactions were: "You just want to get rid of me . . . you'll never come back . . . you'll be killed." At times when she displayed these reactions, her associations invariably led to expressions of guilt and anxiety concerning her parents (see Session 8, pp. 49 ff., for a typical sequence of such associations). The same dominant theme was repeated in endless variations: She is always destined to undergo severe punishment and to lose whatever satisfactions she might momentarily manage to get out of life because of her past bad behavior toward mother and father.

Given the fact that ambivalence was so clearly manifested in the transference reactions toward the analyst, it was not surprising to discover similar negative components in her affective responses to the surgeon. Certain of Mrs. Blake's associations clearly showed that the surgeon also became endowed with the attributes of a punitive parent figure. Rather than expressing exclusively pleasant erotic feelings, her associations to the daydreams about the surgeon led to profoundly disturbing fantasies which revealed a deeper layer of infantile anxieties. From this material we can see the remarkable way in which the postoperative infatuation was overdetermined.

Upon resuming analytic treatment (Session 13), Mrs. Blake's description of the infatuation was given in the context of associations which clearly expressed anxiety about vague dangers. Her first association was that she currently felt afraid of going to the surgeon's office for a follow-up examination. In the next session (14) she revealed some extremely uncomplimentary notions about the surgeon which had dominated her thoughts during the first few postoperative hours. Shortly after awakening from the anesthetic, she had looked at her bandages and realized that the operation affected a much greater area than she had expected. Not only was there an incision at the site she had known about but there was also a separate large incision in an adjacent area as well. This unexpected occurrence was very disturbing. It reminded her of the novel *King's Row*, in which, according to her description, "a sadistic doctor cut off a man's leg without anesthetic; his face conveyed a love of the thrill of torturing a person just for the fun of it." After relating to the analyst some of the gory details from *King's Row*, Mrs. Blake's associations explicitly equated the sadistic physician in the novel with her own surgeon: "He most likely did much more cutting than necessary, just for the fun of it; probably he would like to amputate my entire leg if he could get away with it."

Thus, the infatuation appears to have served partly as a means of camouflaging her deep suspiciousness and fear of the surgeon. From what the patient reported, one gets the impression that, at the moment when the surgeon had come into her room, she had begun to distrust him as a powerful, dangerous authority figure. But during the brief conversation with him she evidently found a way of warding off the fear of his punitive intentions so that, by the time he left the room, her attitude of aversion had been transformed into the opposite. Her infatuation with the surgeon, therefore, seems to have functioned partly as a defensive means of escaping from her growing fear of his sadism.

In a subsequent analytic hour (Session 16), the source of the sadistic conception of the surgeon became apparent. She began by referring to one of her favorite dichotomies: "the two types of men, those who *take the lead*, and those who *follow my lead*, like a child." As usual, her husband was placed in the latter category and was characterized as being "shy most of the time and sensitive, like father." The surgeon, on the other hand, was represented as being the sort of man who ruthlessly dominates people.

> He is much more sexually attractive because of his masculine qualities. He is insensitive and cruel and wrapped up in himself and tough, just like my mother. She was always much more masculine than my father and I never liked those qualities in her. But in the doctor I loved those qualities.

These and numerous other associations suggested that the intense fear of the surgeon, and the sadistic attributes with which he had been endowed, had their origin in an unconscious attitude toward her mother. The particular way in which Mrs. Blake managed to cope with the fear of the new, dominant, knife-wielding adult seems to have duplicated an important bit of her developmental history from the very same crucial period of her childhood already implicated in the analysis of her postoperative elation. As discussed earlier, a series of profound disappointments in her father had occurred at the age of four, following which she had displayed a dramatic shift in attitude toward her mother. Feeling no longer protected by her father, she developed an exaggerated conception of the damage she had caused to her parents' marriage; correspondingly, she expected to be subjected to merciless retaliation at the hands of the seemingly all-powerful mother. Her defense against the accompanying guilt and anxiety was to appease the angry mother by becoming a loving, highly conforming child who would no longer compete for her father's affection. At the same time she strove to overcome the threatening emotional attachment to her father by redirecting her erotic as well as affectionate impulses toward her mother.

Essentially the same sequence of psychological events had already been repeated more than once in her transference reactions toward the analyst. From time to time she would regard the analyst as a powerful, punitive figure who, like the mother imago at age three or four, could be appeased only by complete submission. At such times she would display a reconciliatory trend. For the moment the analyst would become an object of effusive affection and erotic longing, whereupon her fear and hostility would temporarily subside. The fantasied love affair with the surgeon appears to have been another recapitulation of the same infantile emotional cycle.

12.

Attitudes toward danger-control authorities

The term "danger-control authority" is introduced to refer to anyone who is perceived as having the power to help or hinder one's chances of escaping exposure to the full impact of external danger. A person's attitude toward a danger-control authority obviously can have a marked influence on the way he behaves under stress conditions, as is repeatedly emphasized in discussions regarding the role of leadership in averting panic and disorganized behavior (Cantril, 1943; MacCurdy, 1953; Stouffer et al., 1949a and 1949b).

When entire communities are threatened by a tornado, a flood, or a wartime bombing attack, the disaster-control personnel who are most likely to become the dominant authorities in the eyes of the affected population are those state and local officials who announce or attach their names to public warnings and directives. In military combat, infantrymen usually regard the officer in charge of their platoon—rather than a higher echelon colonel or commanding general—as the dominant danger-control authority, probably because he is the one who communicates the orders that are perceived as determining their fate under the hazardous conditions of frontline fighting. His power, backed up by the full weight of the military hierarchy, is usually felt by the men as giving them no choice but to remain in combat and to carry out dangerous missions under enemy fire; his skilled judgments and his interpersonal attitudes are generally regarded by those under his command as crucial factors determining their ultimate chances of survival (Grinker and J. Spiegel, 1945a and 1945b; MacCurdy, 1953; W. Menninger, 1948).

For surgical patients, the surgeon will generally be perceived as fulfilling a parallel role. Like the leader in military combat, the surgeon possesses the twofold powers of danger control in the eyes of his patients: First, as the physician who makes the final decision about the necessity for the operation, he is likely to be regarded as an authority who is impelling one to undergo exposure to the surgical assault; moreover, as the man who actually does the cutting, he is apt to be irrationally apperceived as a source of danger, an ominous being who will inflict pain and injury. Second, in so far as the patient consciously judges that the surgery is essential for his well-being or survival, he tends to regard the surgeon as a potential benefactor who can help him to avert danger. If he has confidence in the surgeon's professional qualifications, he is inclined to regard the surgeon as a source of reassurance, a protective agent who can skillfully counteract any dangers that may arise in the operating room or any complications that may develop afterwards. However, both the positive and the negative evaluations of the authority figure are apt to be overlaid by irrational beliefs and misconceptions stemming from the powerful anxieties stimulated by the threat of body damage.

In the case of Mrs. Blake, none of the negative feelings about the surgeon's danger-control powers became apparent until after the surgery had been completed. Before the operation, the manifest content of her vivid fantasies of being mutilated never specifically implicated the surgeon as a source of danger, although her free associations contained numerous clues to a latent negative attitude (see Session 12, pp. 100 ff.). One of her first conscious thoughts after awakening from the anesthetic, however, was that the surgeon might be a sadist. In the preceding chapter we have seen that her postoperative fantasies and free associations in Sessions 13 through 16 clearly revealed a strongly negative attitude as well as a positive one. She projected onto the surgeon essentially the same punitive intentions as she had attributed to her mother after the series of disturbing events which, at age four, seemed to have frightened her into overt submission. Her latent negative attitude toward the surgeon evidently had been repressed during the preoperative period, when anxiety was maximal, but came to the surface while the surgeon was still a dominant danger-control authority with regard to the stressful period of postoperative recovery.

Just as with her mother, the patient's intense fear of the surgeon was temporarily held in check by the fantasy that he was sexually interested in her and would become her lover. Thus, the psychoanalytic observations indicate that she was using once again the mechanism of *defensive libidinization of a potential aggressor*—a means she had originally adopted during the Oedipal phase in order to deal with comparable fears of a punitive mother. The unconscious choice of this infantile mechanism was undoubtedly fostered by other psychological factors which involved the lowering of her level of guilt during the postoperative period. Probably one reason why she permitted herself to indulge in pleasurable erotic fantasies was that she experienced a momentary sense of relief at having paid off old superego debts through submitting to the surgery. (See the discussion below of Hypothesis 9, pp. 143–145). The choice of the surgeon as a new love object during the convalescent period was also fostered by the heightened need to cling to this authoritative figure as a source of realistic reassurances at a time when there were some objective grounds for fearing prolonged physical suffering and permanent bodily impairment. But, although psychological factors of this type may have entered into the erotic attachment to the surgeon, the analytic material cited in the preceding chapter shows that any account of the motivations underlying the fantasied love affair would be grossly incomplete if it overlooked this patient's defensive need to combat her *irrational fears of the surgeon's hostile and punitive intentions.*

Perhaps a similar constellation of motives, including the need to counteract a fear-producing conception of the authorities' intentions, underlies the readiness with which people who are exposed to a danger situation will develop strong feelings of dependency and affection toward danger-control personnel (Blanton and Kirk, 1947; Glover, 1942; MacCurdy, 1953; Ruesch and Bowman, 1948; Wittkower, 1952). Even when the childhood history does not so uniquely dispose a person to adopt exactly the kind of defenses habitually employed by Mrs. Blake, it seems quite possible that many individuals might, nevertheless, have undergone similar, albeit less dramatic, formative experiences that would incline them to develop a counterphobic attitude toward authority-figures and to behave in a similar way (see Fenichel, 1939, pp. 269–270).

Clinical psychoanalysts are likely to be quite familiar with defensive tendencies of the type noted in Mrs. Blake's relationship to her surgeon, because the same phenomena can be readily observed in the transference reactions of most psychoneurotic patients undergoing psychoanalytic treatment (Braatoy, 1954; Fenichel, 1941; S. Freud, 1905b and 1930). At times when a patient is suffering from intense feelings of guilt—whether stimulated by external events or by internal pressures to ward off forbidden impulses—the punitive power of the analyst is apt to become grossly exaggerated. The latent content of the patient's fantasies then takes the form of expecting to be punished by the analyst in retribution for superego violations. In effect, the analyst becomes a threatening authority figure to whom the patient's own superego demands have been projected. When this occurs, many patients begin to display signs of a defensive need for a love relationship. What predominates on the surface, however, may be the heightened erotic or affectionate interest directed toward the person of the analyst. Only later on, by means of free associations, will it become apparent that the attachment is defensive in character and stems from self-punitive tendencies which are being projected.

Thus the unconscious components in Mrs. Blake's reactions to her surgeon, rather than being highly idiosyncratic residues of her unique life experiences, might prove to be a somewhat extreme occurrence of a more or less typical mechanism that many people use to cope with superego conflicts stimulated by external threats of punishment.

The preceding discussion of the psychoanalytic observations bearing on the patient's latent attitude toward her surgeon offers some basis for expanding the dependency concept in Hypothesis 5. From the additional observations, the following set of interrelated propositions is suggested:

Hypothesis 8A. *In adult life, when danger to body integrity is perceived to be imminent, the emotional attitudes which develop toward danger-control authorities are largely determined by transference reactions which give rise to reality-distorting apperceptions and judgments.*

Hypothesis 8B. *The main components of the transferred attitudes derive from early life experiences in which one (or both) of the parents had been perceived as being responsible for the onset and termination of suffering or deprivation and typically include the following:* (a) *overestimation of the authority's personal power to increase or decrease the amount of exposure to danger;* (b) *excessive uncertainty and preoccupation as to whether the authority's intentions are benevolent or malevolent;* (c) *heightened dependency on the authority (i.e., increased need for direct or symbolic contact with the authority combined with greater sensitivity to the authority's communications of approval and disapproval).*

All three of the latent attitude components specified in Hypothesis 8B were manifested in the patient's relationship with her surgeon. Although in Session 9 the patient had ventilated her extreme fears of the impersonal dangers of surgery (e.g., the possibility of developing a fatal embolism), her comments in subsequent preoperative sessions indicated that she had developed a highly personalized view of the chances of a successful outcome. Whenever she alluded to this topic she spoke as though everything depended on only one factor, namely, the surgeon's willingness to help her. After the operation was over, she revealed (in Sessions 13–16) that she had been struggling to ward off a basic distrust of the surgeon's intentions. In conscious postoperative thoughts and daydreams about the surgeon, she first projected the attributes of a dangerous sadist and then those of a flirtatious paramour.

The patient's emotional dependency is most clearly revealed by the preoccupying fantasies which brought her into continual symbolic contact with the surgeon. The incidental conversation which gave rise to her exaggerated conception of his personal interest in her provides an extreme example of the way in which a predisposed patient will seize upon any indication in the surgeon's behavior which could be construed as a sign that the relationship had more to it than the impersonal contact involved in obtaining his professional services.

In general, the diverse components in Mrs. Blake's complex attitude toward her surgeon illustrate an emotional regression of the type implied by Hypotheses 8A and 8B. The guilt feelings, fears, and hopes which characterize early childhood attitudes toward the parents will be temporarily reawakened in severe stress episodes of adult life and will tend to be focused on the danger-control authorities.

13.

Constructs for a theory of reactive elation

What accounted for the general state of euphoria, the reduced guilt, the self-indulgent behavior, and other components of the patient's temporary elation during the first week of convalescence? In what ways was the elation induced by the conditions of stress to which the patient had been exposed? In some respects the patient's mood and actions were similar to the pathologic elations observed in episodes of mania and hypomania among psychotics and neurotics (Fenichel, 1945, pp. 409–414). In other respects, however, her postoperative elation resembled the nonpathologic elated reactions displayed by disaster survivors when emotional relief sets in as they realize that the danger is past and they have emerged unscathed (M. Wolfenstein, 1957, pp. 181–198). In the present theoretical analysis, a major assumption is that the psychodynamics of the temporary syndrome of poststress elation are not necessarily the same as those of pathologic mania and hypomania.

When one examines the extensive psychiatric literature in which cases of elated affect and behavior are described, it soon becomes obvious that there are considerable individual differences in the degree to which the elation is attributable to external environmental happenings.

Just as with depressions, there is a considerable range from one extreme, where the so-called precipitating event obviously is of little etiological importance (e.g., recurring psychotic mania touched off by trivial occurrences), to the other extreme, where the occurrence of some unusual event appears to be an outstanding causal factor. Of special interest in the present discussion are those cases of elation in which one or another feature of a *stress episode* can be identified as a clear-cut *precipitating event* and assigned a significant causal role, at least as a contributory etiological factor. Thus, the instances of primary concern are those in which a person's elated emotional state, in all probability, would not have materialized if an unusual stressful event had not occurred, even though he or she may be more or less predisposed to be highly influenced by any event of the given type. All such instances can properly be called "reactive" elation, in the same sense as "reactive" depression.

It is assumed that episodes of reactive elation, like reactive depression, may vary considerably in their diagnostic significance, some episodes being symptomatic of a chronic emotional disorder and others being benign and transient in character.

In Fenichel's (1945) and B. Lewin's (1950) surveys of the psychiatric literature on reactive elations, one finds numerous indications of at least two major subtypes which need to be distinguished because they have somewhat different causes and consequences, even though they may have a few genetic and dynamic features in common.

1. *Pseudo elation as a defense against painful inner stimuli.* Sometimes a reactive elation is essentially a part of the individual's defensive efforts to ward off intense guilt, low self-esteem, or other affective disturbances evoked by the precipitatory event. After the death of a parent, for example, an adult may react with a temporary elation which constitutes a "denial of affect" (B. Lewin, 1950) and which involves postponing the painful work of mourning (Lindemann, 1944). In patients with acute disseminated lupus erythematosus, a marked tendency to minimize symptoms as well as an artificial cheerfulness has been noted during periods of restricted activity when reactions of depression would have been expected (McClary et al., 1955). Similar reactions of pseudo elation have been observed in patients suffering from cancer, tuberculosis, and other diseases (Schilder, 1938; Sutherland and Orbach, 1953;Wittkower, 1952). *Inappropriateness of the affect* to the external provocation is one of the indicators (though not a ubiquitous characteristic) of a defensive type of elation. Another diagnostic indicator is *forced hyperactivity*, i.e., the individual displays an insatiable need to

engage uninterruptedly in one seemingly gay activity after another, with marked uneasiness and tension at moments when he attempts to relax. A third indicator, more dependable than the other two, is the occurrence of *momentary breakthroughs of weeping, agitation, or depressive mood*, betraying the artificiality of the surface euphoria and the unsuccessful character of the attempted denial.

2. *Emotional relief following the termination of stress.* Reactive elations often appear to be genuine euphoric reactions—evoked by the perception that an anticipated danger or deprivation has not materialized or has been successfully averted. In such instances, the indicators of defensive pseudo elation are absent. The person displays a consistently benign mood of exhilarated relief, uncomplicated by any compulsive need for distraction or hyperactive gaiety. Self-esteem is relatively high, feelings toward people in the immediate environment are exceptionally warm and friendly, periods of calm relaxation succeed periods of high energetic motility. The onset of the relief reaction is, of course, most easily discerned when it takes the form of an explosively joyous release of pent-up tension. If the source of inner or outer stress abates gradually, however, the onset of emotional relief may be correspondingly gradual, but, eventually, the full syndrome of elated relief may become as apparent as when the onset is more abrupt and tumultuous.

Earlier, we had an example of defensive pseudo elation in Mrs. Blake's exaggerated response to the postponement of her operation (pp. 98–100). When she learned that she would have to leave the hospital without undergoing the surgery and would have to wait a few more days until the operating room would be available, she may have felt some genuine relief that the operation was deferred. But she became extraordinarily gay and compulsively hyperactive; her surface elation was punctuated by spells of disturbing affect evoked by minor occurrences that "spoiled everything" by reminding her that the danger was not really over.

In contrast to the preoperative pseudoeuphoria, the elation after the operation appears to have been essentially a reaction of genuine emotional relief (although some defensive functions, such as counteracting the latent fantasy of being further assaulted by the surgeon, may have also entered into its formation).[1] From the patient's lengthy retrospective descriptions in Sessions 13 through 16, it seems that the elation was primarily an inner celebration of having emerged practically unscathed from the operating room. In contrast to the pseudoeuphoric reaction to the preoperative postponement, her postoperative emotional state seems to have been consistently cheerful and free from tension, at least during the entire first week of convalescence. Evidently there were no momentary outbreaks of depression or anxiety. While in the hospital, her affable attitude toward the people around her led to the development of several new friendships which continued long after her convalescence was over. Her feelings toward her children, her husband, and even her business associates (e.g., the male co-worker who came to the hospital during visiting hours) seemed to involve more emotional warmth than at any other time in recent years.

Before the operation, she had developed a compensatory fantasy, as we have seen, concerning the way she would be indulged in the hospital: She would be the center of attraction, everyone would treat her affectionately and would cater to her whims. During the period of elation, she permitted herself to make deliberate efforts to bring about this blissful state of affairs and she felt that she was actually succeeding. All during this period she felt extraordinarily self-confident about her ability to elicit the affection and admiration of others. This was in marked contrast to her usual self-critical attitudes ("I am an ugly and nasty person") and her chronic obsessional ruminations ("Why do all those people continue to be friendly, what can they see in me?")

The change in the patient's mood and social attitudes after the operation was over resembles in many salient respects the behavorial changes observed in numerous large-scale community disasters and in many types of personal stress situations. An expansive, euphoric mood combined with friendly interpersonal relationships and a satisfying sense of group cohesion is a common syndrome following the termination of any objective danger situation (Committee on Disaster Studies, 1955; Glover, 1942; Kirk, 1949; J. Spiegel, 1953). Speaking about the reactions of surgical patients, H. Deutsch (1942) reports: "Many patients say that every time they recover from such a state of unconsciousness, particularly from general anesthesia, they have the exhilarating feeling of having returned to life." Temporary reactions of emotional relief occur, of course, not only after escape from external danger but also after the completion of difficult work assignments, important school examinations, public performances and other such stress experiences in which the person feels threatened by the loss of social esteem or by other nonphysical dangers. (Fenichel, 1939a and 1939b.)

Some clues to the determinants of poststress elation can be discerned in the psychoanalytic case study data. Two main hypotheses are suggested, the first bearing on the role of *conscious* anticipations and the second on *unconscious* anticipations. The two hypotheses, together with several interrelated assumptions, are put forth as a tentative theory for explaining the reactive elations of subtype 2 above.

Hypothesis 9. *At the termination of an episode of stress impact, the affective status of the person (on a continuum of euphoric versus dysphoric mood) will depend upon whether the amount of perceived suffering and loss (victimization) is more or less than he had consciously expected before the onset of the stress episode: If the amount of victimization is more than had been expected, the mood will tend to be dysphoric; if less than had been expected, the mood will tend to be euphoric (provided that no further impact of severe danger or deprivation is anticipated in the near future).*

During the preoperative period, as we have seen, the patient's fears of what the operation would do to her were greatly exaggerated: She was afraid that her leg might have to be amputated, that she might not come out of the anesthetic, and that she might die from a blood clot. Shortly after awakening from the anesthetic, she examined the bandages over her incision, noted that the surgical wound was much more extensive than she had been told it would be, and felt extremely worried about the amount of body damage that had been inflicted upon her. In line with her dire preoperative fantasies, her thoughts were centered on the possibility that she had been brutally mutilated by the surgeon and that she might be in further danger of being victimized by his sadistic assaults. At this time, she was uncertain about how much victimization she had undergone and her mood was far from euphoric.

During the next few hours, however, the patient had the opportunity to obtain reality-oriented information as to what her physical condition really was. Gradually she came to realize that she was physically intact and, from the nurses and the surgeon, she learned that her large incision did not imply any serious complications. It was at this time—probably toward the end of the surgeon's reassuring visit—that her mood began to change. Although the marked change in attitude toward the surgeon was partly defensive in character, all the other major components of the patient's elation syndrome, as already noted, had the characteristics of genuine emotional relief. During the succeeding hours and days, as she experienced a rapid physical recovery with only slight pains and discomforts, her positive evaluation of the postoperative situation continued to be reinforced.

Much of her elation seems to have been an inner celebration of having survived the threat of possible mutilation, pain, and death at the hands of the surgeon. Presumably she experienced much more emotional relief—and psychologically had more cause to celebrate—than had her preoperative anticipations and fantasies been more in line with what reality actually held in store for her.

In this connection, it is instructive to compare Mrs. Blake's reactions with those observed in the 30 surgical patients included in the case study series to be described in Chapters 18 through 25. Mrs. Blake's conscious expectations of the magnitude of the threat would place her at the extreme negative end of the range; in intensive preoperative interviews of the 30 patients, only three or four expressed comparable fears about the dire fate that might await them in the operating room. But with respect to the actual amount of victimization experienced, Mrs. Blake was at the opposite extreme. During the first week of her convalescence she had relatively little pain, discomfort, or impairment of physical functions as compared with the majority of patients in the case study sample, most of whom had undergone major abdominal or chest surgery. Mrs. Blake's euphoric mood, in turn, appears to have been somewhat more extreme than that observed in any of the thirty cases. These rough comparisons suggest the following proposition, which is a more general statement of Hypothesis 9:

The greater the positive (or negative) discrepancy between the magnitude of the anticipated threat and the amount of victimization that is subsequently perceived to have occurred, the greater the degree of poststress euphoria (or dysphoria).

The discrepancy factor specified by Hypothesis 9 can be conveniently represented by the following symbols: $V_e - V_o$, where V_e refers to amount of victimization expected prior to exposure to the danger situation and V_o refers to the amount of victimization perceived as having been obtained as a result of exposure to danger stimuli. (The term "victimization" is meant to include all forms of deprivation, loss, and suffering.)[2]

According to the above extension of Hypothesis 9, the greater the positive value of the discrepancy, the greater the intensity of the euphoria. (Discussion of negative values of the discrepancy as a determinant of dysphoria will be postponed until Chapter 15, which is devoted to the psychodynamics of reactive depression.)

Although the discrepancy factor may prove to be an important component, it can at best be regarded only as a part of the general formula for the emotional relief syndrome. An additional factor which seems to be a necessary condition for poststress elation is the awareness of reality signs that serious danger or unbearable deprivation will not occur in the immediate future. Only when Mrs. Blake felt convinced that recovery from her operation would be without serious complications did her elation begin. In the next chapter we shall see that a week later, when she began to interpret the slowness of her recovery as an indication that she might need another operation, her elation ceased. Thus, a second factor which must be included in the formula for poststress elation is the degree of potential danger or deprivation expected in the near future (D_e). Even if $V_e - V_o$ is a large positive value, one would not expect elation to occur if D_e is a substantially high value. The discrepancy specified in Hypothesis 9 is intended to be a determining factor only when D_e approaches zero; this notion is expressed by the phrase ". . . provided that no further impact of severe danger or deprivation is anticipated in the near future." [3]

So far we have considered mainly the conscious (or preconscious) anticipations which influence a person's poststress mood and behavior. The following hypothesis, which also bears on the way in which the termination of a stress episode can bring about a marked emotional change, introduces a much more subtle determinant involving unconscious (unverbalized) anticipations suggested by the psychoanalytic observations.

Hypothesis 10. *If the degree of perceived victimization is less than had been expected and if no immediate recurrence of severe danger or deprivation is anticipated, the termination of danger impact will tend to be unconsciously assimilated to the reconciliation experiences of childhood which followed the termination of overt parental punishment; the individual's emotional state will be dominated by reduced guilt from a sense of having paid the penalty for past misbehavior and will involve a relaxation of inner superego demands with a corresponding increase in self-indulgent behavior.*

A dominant feature of the patient's postoperative elation was an unusually marked reduction in guilt, particularly with respect to chronic unconscious conflicts that centered upon her mother. During the days immediately following the operation, the inner commandments and prohibitions—which ordinarily played such a crucial role in her daily compulsive rituals, in her acutely ambivalent relationships with other women, and in her sado-masochistic fantasies—were relaxed to the point where she was relatively free of many chronic neurotic symptoms (see pp. 127–129). For the moment she could indulge in an emotional regression to a childhood paradise which antedated the establishment of pathogenic superego controls. Thus she could permit herself to feel self-pride and to identify with a woman (Joyce) who symbolized successful femininity.

During the preoperative period, when her level of guilt was exceptionally high, the patient's free associations frequently equated the operation to parental punishment (see pp. 47–49). Of particular importance are the associations in Session 9 concerning the enema that she knew would be given on the night before the operation. She spoke explicitly about the enema as a punishment, and likened it to a spanking that would "wash away all my sins." These punishment associations occurred immediately after the expression of a transference attitude which had led to the fantasy of being spanked by the analyst: ". . . and the baby screams, and then is cuddled, and there is a reconciliation." Following her operation, the patient seemed to be reliving this fantasy. Once the punishment was over, she welcomed being "cuddled"; and when describing her unusually affectionate attitude toward the surgeon and nurses, her associations led to reminiscences of childhood reconciliations. The internal change seemed to involve a marked alteration in superego functioning: After she had submitted herself to the punishment of surgery, her elation may have been partly a reactivation of earlier celebrations which had occurred on those rare occasions when she had "appeased" the angry mother imago, leaving her momentarily free from any need for further self-punishment.

Hypothesis 10 is offered as a potential explanation for the reduction in guilt frequently noted in people after they have undergone severe hardships or physical suffering (H. Deutsch, 1942; English and Pearson, 1945, pp. 101 ff.; S. Freud, 1919b, p. 397 ff.; Flugel, 1945, pp. 301 ff.). This hypothesis must be considered in relation to Hypothesis 1, which specifies the conditions under which the opposite sort of reaction will occur. According to Hypothesis 1A, the expectation of danger in the near future (D_e) will produce heightened self-scrutiny and more rigid adherence to superego standards, especially with respect to aggressive behavior. Hypothesis 1A implies that during the poststress period, when D_e again approaches zero, the tendency toward excessive inner control over forbidden impulses will be dissipated and the person's superego vigilance will tend to return to its prestress level. But Hypothesis 10 asserts that something more than that will happen during the poststress period: The level of superego vigilance will drop well below the individual's normal level (provided that $V_e - V_o > 0$). In other words, the termination of stress will result in a pendulum swing toward the opposite extreme, resulting in less self-criticism, less conscientiousness, and more self-indulgence in modes of gratification that are normally felt to be imprudent or immoral.

Part of the explanation for the relationship specified in Hypothesis 1A was provided by Hypothesis 1B, which is predicated on the assumption that threats of external danger are unconsciously interpreted as a repetition of childhood punishments. The reader will note that it is essentially the same assumption that enters into Hypothesis 10, to account for superego relaxation following the termination of danger.

Notes

1. The two subtypes of elation, although arising from different psychological causes, need not be considered as mutually exclusive. It is quite possible for a reactive elation to be "overdetermined" in the sense that the etiology involves defensive processes combined with genuine emotional relief. For example, following their release from combat duty, some soldiers appeared to develop a genuine euphoria in response to the termination of their arduous danger assignment but, at the same time, showed hyperactivity and forced gaiety which appeared to be a defense against low self-esteem and guilt about abandoning their comrades (Grinker and J. Spiegel, 1945a, pp. 278 ff.). In the case of Mrs. Blake, the presumption that her postoperative elation was genuine is based on numerous indications, such as the fact that she was temporarily free from her chronic obsessional symptoms and was able to acquire some new and lasting friendships. That her elation may also have served a defensive function is suggested by the fact that her euphoric fantasies about the surgeon were found to be defensive in character and, moreover, when the period of elation ended, it was followed by an obvious depression. It seems quite possible that the patient's elation may have been partly motivated by defensive needs even though the most salient characteristics suggest that it was primarily a reaction of genuine emotional relief. In general, it should be anticipated that in many instances of reactive elation, a mixture of the two subtypes may occur. In such instances, it is still useful to take account of the distinction between the two, because the etiology may be predominantly that of one subtype rather than the other.

2. The discrepancy factor, $V_e - V_o$, as a determinant of euphoria and dysphoria, is similar to the concept of "relative deprivation" which has been used by social psychologists and sociologists to account for high and low morale among military personnel and industrial workers (Merton and Kitt, 1950; Stouffer et al., 1949a, pp. 124–130, 250–254, 172–182). If $V_e - V_o$ were regarded as psychologically equivalent to the relative deprivation factor, Hypothesis 9 could be generalized to apply to the milder varieties of stress stimuli which give rise to favorable and unfavorable morale attitudes. The relationship between the discrepancy factor and the concept of relative deprivation requires further theoretical analysis.

3. If, after having undergone a surgical operation, a person anticipates that a bearable amount of pain and only minor deprivations will persist for several days, the D_e factor is not likely to reduce the elation tendency produced by a positive value of the $V_e - V_o$ factor. But if the D_e factor is relatively high, e.g., if unrelieved pain is anticipated, the elation tendency may be completely counteracted. (See the earlier discussion of Hypothesis 1, pp. 53–58, and also the discussion of Hypothesis 13, pp. 173–176 below.) The assumption that D_e can counteract the

elation-evoking tendencies of the discrepancy factor, even when $V_e - V_o$ is substantially greater than zero, may account for the fact that few people became intensely elated or engaged in hedonistic celebrations following large-scale air attacks during World War II, despite the fact that large numbers of remote-miss cases experienced less victimization than they had anticipated.

"People who are facing the prospect of illness, unemployment, or any extreme form of deprivation will often attempt to ward off the danger by making sure that they do not deserve to be punished. Evidently, this was one of the dominant types of reaction among the bombed population of Britain. Stringent self-control and efforts to live up to purified moral standards seem to have submerged incipient hedonistic strivings. Perhaps the latter tendencies are likely to break through only under special conditions, such as those found in European displaced persons' camps after the defeat of Germany, where an uprooted population without reliable or respected leadership was facing an uncertain social and economic future after having already undergone intense suffering and hardship. At any rate, the increased asceticism noted in England, together with the observations of high behavioral conformity in Germany and Japan . . . implies that hedonistic abandonment of social restraints rarely occurred among people faced with the threat of an attack. Certainly there are no indications that common moral standards were swept away in any mass outbreaks of greed, lust, or violence. On the contrary, what little evidence we have consistently points to fairly rigid conformity to social norms and increased efforts to adhere to conventional morality." (Janis, 1951, pp. 169–170.)

This quotation suggests that there is another factor which may foster self-indulgences and normally forbidden gratifications: *temporary separation* from one's primary groups and from other persons who reinforce adherence to the norms of conventional morality. In this respect, the surgical ward of a hospital may resemble a displaced persons' camp. Surgical patients are temporarily uprooted and put in a new social milieu where old norms and conventions, especially with regard to body exposure and manipulation, are no longer valid.

Among the additional factors which probably play an important role in determining the degree of poststress elation, are those which affect the person's *sense of mastery* over the sources of danger. Psychoanalytic accounts emphasize that elated states are characterized by a regressive sense of "omnipotence," which refers to childlike expectations of magically being able to dominate or control the environment (Fenichel, 1945; B. Lewin, 1950). There are also more rational considerations of one's ability to cope with anticipated danger which, like the irrational feelings of omnipotence, may influence one's cognitive and affective responses to a stress situation. For instance, a person might expect grave danger in the immediate future without becoming emotionally disturbed if he were given convincing, authoritative information that he can easily master the danger.

Expectations of mastery may have a considerable effect upon the way a person will react to a large positive discrepancy between anticipated victimization and obtained victimization ($V_e > V_o$). If a person has been expecting a great deal of suffering and hardship which would tax all his resources, he might feel somewhat "let down" if the challenging situation proved to be one in which practically no danger or deprivation materialized. When $V_e > V_o$, elation might occur only if V_o were not such a low value that it turned out to be no challenge at all. Thus there may be some optimal value of V_o ($V_e > V_o > 0$) which enables the person to feel not only that he has suffered less than he had expected but also that he has mastered a truly difficult situation. The optimal values of V_o, and the occurrence of positive or negative self-evaluation of one's degree of mastery, are undoubtedly a function of personality predispositions as well as situational factors.

14.

Affective disturbances during prolonged convalescence

From the patient's associations and dreams, numerous indications were obtained concerning the determinants of the affective disturbances which superseded her temporary elation. The psychoanalytic observations help to answer a fundamental question which may have important implications both for some practical problems of mitigating adverse effects of human disasters and for the theoretical problems of explaining a major pathological consequence of severe stress episodes: *Under what conditions does exposure to danger and deprivation tend to induce reactive depression?*

SESSION 13: AVOIDANCE OF AFFECTION

By the time Mrs. Blake resumed analysis, two and one-half weeks after the operation had been performed, her manifest attitudes and feelings had changed markedly from what they had been (according to her own account) during the first week after the operation. The expansive, friendly mood which had characterized her contacts with people when in the hospital had been replaced by an attitude of emotional indifference and even a mild degree of annoyance. In the first postoperative session (13) she was acutely aware of the change:

> During those days I felt so warm and friendly and close to all the nurses and the other patients. When I began walking around, I would visit the other patients. They were always glad to see me and I was glad to be able to talk with them. I made loads of friends there. But now I don't feel that way toward people anymore. Why can't I be just as friendly with the people where I work? They're the same kind of people as the people in the hospital. But I just don't give a damn about anyone; I just want people to stay out of my way. I've become like a policeman. My only interest in people is to see that they do what they are supposed to, to control them enough so they won't bother me, and so they will stay out of my way.

The tendency toward emotional constriction applied equally to her daily interpersonal relationships and to her inner thoughts about significant persons in her life. We have already noted that the strong erotic attachment to the surgeon was short-lived. When she visited his office for a postoperative checkup, she felt afraid that he might not have a strictly professional interest in her and again became suspicious that he might take pleasure in hurting his female patients. The head nurse, whose warm maternal handling had evoked such a positive response, was still regarded affectionately but was now someone to be avoided because Mrs. Blake felt she would be embarrassed to see her again. Within her immediate family, there were frequent quarrels with her children as well as with her husband, for which Mrs. Blake admitted feeling that her own behavior was largely to blame. For instance, she reported that on the previous day one of her children had justifiably accused her of being a neglectful mother because she ignored an invitation to attend Parents' Night at school. Under the pressure of the child's protest, Mrs. Blake went to the school after supper, but, while there, became "fidgety," suffered from incision pains, and ended up feeling somewhat resentful toward the child for having "forced" her to go.

The clearest indications of Mrs. Blake's attempts to turn away from love objects were revealed in her attitude toward the analyst in Session 13. The first emotion she expressed was one of anger toward the analyst for not having been in his office at the moment when she had first tried to phone on the preceding day to report that she was well enough to resume treatment. When the analyst asked if there had been any provocation on his part to account for her anger, she reluctantly gave the following explanation: What she really felt resentful about was coming back to the analytic sessions, where she received neither sympathy nor affection from the analyst but was required to subject herself to the humiliation of having to reveal all her thoughts. She then went on to express similar feelings of resentment toward her mother, blaming her for being cold and indifferent. The specific charge was that three weeks earlier, just before the operation, her mother had failed to acknowledge receiving an unusually affectionate letter she had sent her and instead, responded only by sending back a short, cold letter dealing with family business matters. This particular complaint was actually without foundation inasmuch as Mrs. Blake was forgetting the subsequent discovery that her mother had mailed the business letter *before* receiving the affectionate letter from her. As a matter of fact, her mother had promptly sent back an equally affectionate reply which arrived two days after the business letter. When the analyst reminded her of what had actually happened, Mrs. Blake said: "I guess I didn't want to think of that. The truth is I don't love my mother any more. I want to boil at her, just like I did at you a little while ago."

In the same analytic session there were a number of indications that Mrs. Blake's readiness to become resentful toward both her mother and the analyst was motivated, at least in part, by an unconscious effort to avoid giving in to her intense longings for a close dependent relationship. One of her complaints was that the analyst never told her how to please him and did not directly ask her to give him anything. Her associations to this complaint led first to the recurrent wish that the analyst would demand sexual intercourse, and then was followed by thoughts and fantasies which revealed a strong latent fear that out of love for the therapist she might yield to the temptation to give up all her neurotic symptoms. In further associations she elucidated on the dangers of becoming too dependent: She might succumb to a state of abject helplessness in which she would be vulnerable to extreme disappointments and would "go completely to pieces."

SESSIONS 14 AND 15: ASSOCIATIONS TO A POSTOPERATIVE DREAM

Further evidence of the motivations underlying Mrs. Blake's emotional constriction and resentment came from a postoperative dream reported in Session 14. This dream clearly revealed her latent fears of becoming a victim of her own powerful dependency longings. At the beginning of the analytic hour she repeated her complaints against mother and analyst. The dream was recalled immediately after the analyst had remarked that "you seem to be especially afraid right now of allowing yourself to feel any affection either toward your mother or toward me." The patient stated that the dream had occurred ten days earlier (on the eighth day after the operation) but she still remembered it vividly:

> My sister Gertrude was inside a snowball, rolling down a hill toward a lake. I watched her from on top of the hill. At first I was going to let her go, but then I rushed to let her out before she reached the lake and drowned.

Her first association after relating the dream was the recollection of a childhood episode in which her father had saved her from drowning in icy water. The lake in the dream reminded her of the one in which her own near-drowning had occurred. She had been walking on the ice at a short distance from the other members of her family when suddenly she stumbled into a hole. Her father had quickly pulled her out. Dripping and chilled, she was brought home in her father's tight embrace. This incident occurred when she was about five years old, at a time when she was still estranged from her father. Evidently it reawakened once again her deep attachment to him, but had left her feeling disappointed because he had not become as sympathetic and affectionate as she had hoped.

Her next association pointed to the day's residue that had entered into the formation of the dream: Her sister Gertrude had actually arrived from out of town on the preceding day and had spent several hours visiting her. As had happened so many times in the past, Mrs. Blake felt that Gertrude was scrutinizing her behavior in a critical manner. Secretly she had wished her sister to go away and leave her alone. Nevertheless, she had behaved in an unusually friendly manner and even told Gertrude something about her fantasies concerning the surgeon's personal interest in her.

In Mrs. Blake's next association, the erotic fantasies were linked to the snowball in the dream. She referred once again to her preoperative expectations concerning the indulgent treatment she had hoped to receive in the hospital:

> I felt it would be like dropping into a deep *featherbed or snow.* That was the mood I was actually in when I felt myself to be so feminine, when everyone was so nice and people responded so affectionately to me.

Then, in referring specifically to her daydreams about the surgeon, she used the phrase, "These voluptuous ideas began to snowball." When her attention was called to the fact that in her dream the person inside the snowball was in danger of drowning, she said, "Yes, but I changed my mind and saved her before it was too late."

At this point Mrs. Blake described how surprised she had been at her own behavior in the surgeon's office when she had come for the routine postoperative checkup. The appointment was for five in the afternoon. Upon her arrival, the surgeon had greeted her affably and made a joking reference to the fact that they were entirely alone in the building. Instead of feeling pleased, Mrs. Blake reacted with anxiety. She again felt consciously afraid that the surgeon might be a dangerous sadist and her only impulse was to end the flirtation as rapidly as possible. She reported having automatically behaved in such a cool, prim fashion that the physician promptly responded to her chilliness by dropping his friendly attitude. From then on his manner was thoroughly businesslike, abrupt, and impersonal.

Mrs. Blake again discussed these reactions in the next analytic session (15). This time she asserted that her anxiety was stimulated by the realization that her erotic daydreams might come true. She had a vague sense that all sexual behavior was forever forbidden to her because of her past misdemeanors. She could not even allow herself to daydream about sex any more because of the danger that she might be tempted to engage in love-making. Sexual intercourse with her husband was now out of the question. The mere thought of seeing him become aroused, with "an excited look on his face," filled her with dread.

Here the patient was referring to a specific detail that entered into her recurrent frigidity, which was the "sex problem" she had wanted to overcome just before the operation. Loss of sexual desire usually occurred during love-making if she saw "signs of sexual desire" in her husband's facial expression. When she did not actually see his face during intercourse, she sometimes had obsessional fantasies in which she would imagine the look on his face, with the same result. To keep this symptom secret from her husband, she often pretended to have a full orgasm when, in fact, she had an aborted one or remained totally frigid.

She now felt convinced that she would remain permanently frigid, adding that the fear of her husband's facial expression was due to her guilty feelings about having committed "criminal acts" of unfaithfulness in the past. She was "all through" as far as her sex life was concerned: with her husband she was frigid, and with any other man an affair would entail too much suffering. Psychoanalysis, she announced, could no longer help her and by continuing the treatment she was "paying a fiendish price" for her former sexual escapades.

After giving many associations which linked various elements in her snowball dream to guilt-laden sexual desires and frigidity, Mrs. Blake spontaneously recognized that the person inside the snowball might represent herself. The fact that in the dream the person was supposed to be her sister led to the recollection that at the age of five she had told this same sister about her secret game of imagining all sorts of exciting things while lying in bed before falling asleep; the older child's response to this revelation had simply been, "That's a lot of foolishness." This recollection, in turn, led Mrs. Blake to assert that her sister's comment would be an appropriate way to characterize the recent fantasied love affair with the surgeon, which she had also started to reveal to her disapproving sister. It was at this point that she reported having turned to the surgeon as a substitute for the analyst:

> Before the operation, I didn't want to leave you. I couldn't bear the thought of not coming here. Then, when I was in the hospital I switched all my feelings onto him and hardly thought of you at all. I knew it was hopeless to try to have a love affair with you and that's the main reason I went all out for him.

Although several different layers of latent content could be discerned in the associations to the dream, the analyst confined his comments to pointing out that a central theme had to do with wishing to escape from a strong desire to sink into the dangerous featherbed of a deeply affectionate relationship with him. At the same time, he reminded her how often in the treatment her direct expressions of ambivalent feelings (e.g., "I hate to come here every weekday to see you but I can't stand the weekend because I won't see you") had led to associations which showed that intense longings—originally directed toward her mother in very early childhood and toward her father during later childhood—were being directed toward the analyst. The main assumption behind this interpretation was that, to a large extent, the dream work involved reassuring herself that the moralistic, critical part of her personality, which she symbolically represented by her sister, would not be submerged by her erotic and affectionate transference reactions. There was also a markedly pathognomonic feature in this dream, however, the implications of which might have been overlooked by the analyst had it not been for the unusually intense emotional display which occurred in a subsequent session when Mrs. Blake gave further associations to the same dream.

SESSIONS 16–20: THE EMERGENCE OF ACUTE DEPRESSION

The pathognomonic feature of the postoperative dream was the allusion, only thinly disguised in the manifest content, to the danger of self-destruction. From the material in Sessions 16 through 20, it became increasingly apparent that, along with the patient's intense fear of being overwhelmed by powerful longings for a dependent relationship, there was a marked tendency toward depression. The first clues had already been noted in the first session after she returned, especially in the attitude she expressed toward psychoanalysis. All during this period she continued to refer to the analysis as a form of "torture," a "punishment" for her moral transgressions. In Session 16 she again assured the analyst that her neurotic condition was hopeless and that she would never derive any real benefit from the treatment. In the same session she expressed an extremely pessimistic view of her postoperative physical condition. The operation, she felt, was such a complete failure that she would end up becoming a cripple. All it had succeeded in doing was to increase her pain and to add new discomforts. Her blood vessels were so badly damaged that sooner or later her leg would have to be amputated.

In Session 17 the theme of hopelessness was reiterated and, finally, when the analyst said that something must be causing her to feel depressed, she admitted "weeping a lot" since having left the hospital. Once this fact was mentioned, Mrs. Blake was no longer capable of controlling her emotions. She burst into agitated weeping.

The associations which accompanied her weeping highlighted the sense of guilt underlying her depression. She described herself as feeling "like the snowqueen in the fairy tale, who would melt into nothingness if she ever became warm." Further associations to the snowqueen led her to recall the dream symbol of being inside a snowball, which, in turn, brought to mind her present problems of being withdrawn, unfriendly, and sexually frigid. At this point the analyst intervened with an interpretation which again pointed out the defensive aspect of her emotional constriction, emphasizing her strong wish to ward off the anger and guilt that would ensue if she were to allow her frozen emotional impulses to thaw out. She responded with the assertion that she felt like the woman in the Bible story who violated God's explicit commandment by looking back upon the destruction of Sodom and Gomorrah. Like the biblical character, her destiny was to be transformed into a pillar of salt: "The salt would be all that would be left of me after I had melted down." This image led to a variety of ruminations about guilt-laden recollections from very early childhood which she had already started to recall earlier in her analysis. Included were memories of witnessing parental intercourse from her crib, these memories having been partially recovered just before the operation. Partly remembering and partly re-experiencing the disturbing event, she produced a wealth of associations, showing once again that she had misinterpreted her parents' sexual behavior to be an act of mutual destruction which endangered her (the forbidden view of Sodom and Gomorrah). Her specific fear of "dissolving into a spot of salt or nothingness," according to these associations, was linked to a profound sense of being abandoned, which is the way she recalled having felt at the time when she witnessed the "horrible" act. (See the account of Session 12, pp. 101–104, in which the same fear was expressed, somewhat more obtusely, when she was recovering the same memory.) In the same session and in the next three sessions, Mrs. Blake made explicit references to suicidal inclinations, asserting that she really had nothing to live for and that she felt tempted at night to take an overdose of sleeping pills.

The next two weeks of analytic sessions were devoted mainly to dealing with her depression, her fear of emotional thawing, and various related unconscious tendencies that had been condensed into the snowball dream. During this period there were obvious signs that the acute affective disturbance was beginning to subside. The end of the postoperative depression—and of the exacerbated symptom of sexual frigidity—was heralded by her having a pleasant dream of lying in bed, luxuriously covered by a folded electric blanket, feeling quite comfortable while "melting under many layers of heat."

Gradually, thereafter, the patient's symptoms of acute depression cleared up. By session 22, she no longer felt so guilty and unloved; she was able to re-establish friendly relationships with people about her, and her concern about sexual guilt diminished to the point where she could again experience occasional orgasms in intercourse with her husband.

It is important to note, however, that even after the postoperative depression lifted, some of her major neurotic symptoms showed no remarkable change from what they had been at the beginning of the preoperative period. Six weeks after the operation, when she experienced sporadic pains in the region of the surgical incision, she displayed exactly the same kind of exaggerated fears as during the period which preceded the operation:

> My leg hurts and I'm afraid to find out what's the matter. It kills me when it hurts but if I go to the surgeon, I'm afraid he'll say it has to be amputated. . . . Or maybe he will laugh at me and say that he had already explained that I would have some pains like this. But I really think that there is something horribly wrong because I've never had a pain like that before. I think that gangrene is developing and I'm going to lose my leg. I know that a sensible person would go to the doctor but I'm afraid he'll laugh at me.

She had not forgotten the reassuring information the surgeon had given her many weeks earlier concerning the fact that postoperative pains might recur from time to time even though the leg was healing normally. She acknowledged that if she had her leg examined, she would undoubtedly be given some medication to alleviate the pain and that she would not be scolded or humiliated. The surgeon no longer was assumed to be a powerful, sadistic assailant. But something within the patient herself, which she had not yet relinquished, continued to make her afraid of becoming a helpless, masochistic victim.

15.

Constructs for a theory of reactive depression

In Chapter 13 the psychoanalytic data bearing on the early period of convalescence were explored for the purpose of gaining more insight into the role of unconscious factors in the etiology of reactive elation. The corresponding task remains to be carried out for reactive depression: What are the crucial psychological processes that account for the occurrence of depressive symptoms when a person is exposed to external circumstances of prolonged deprivation?

The Biphasic Character of Stress Impact

Surgery, like many other crises and catastrophes, involves two main phases of stress impact. First comes the phase of *acute danger impact.* When a person undergoes major surgery, this phase occurs in the operating room, where, in a short period of time, he faces the possibility of being severely damaged or annihilated by a twofold physical assault—exposure to a strong dose of a general anesthetic and to the cutting of body tissue by surgical instruments. For the average surgical patient, the potential psychological impact of this initial phase is, of course, markedly dampened because, while on the operating table, he is in a state of partial or complete unconsciousness. Postoperative elation is assumed to be a psychological reaction that sets in when the patient discovers that he has successfully passed through the ordeal of the acute danger phase. But then, a second major phase of stress impact gradually develops as a result of accumulating pains, discomforts, and frustrations during convalescence. While undergoing the latter type of stress impact, which will be referred to as the phase of *prolonged deprivation*, the danger to life and limb may be more or less in abeyance. The essential feature of the second phase is unrelieved exposure to a continual succession of physical irritations, body dysfunctions, and restrictions of motility. In addition, there is a profound, albeit temporary, loss of many major sources of gratification that are ordinarily felt to be necessary to "make life worth living." (See pp. 214–216.)

The two phases of stress impact occur in almost all large-scale community disasters. When the initial danger of a tornado, flood, bombing explosion, or some other destructive event is over, it is usually followed by a secondary impact phase of prolonged deprivation. During the second phase, large numbers of survivors are likely to experience an accumulation of noxious stimuli and frustrations resembling those encountered by the convalescing surgical patient. Similarly, a pattern of emotional response has been observed in a sizeable number of disaster survivors which bears a striking resemblance to the reactions observed postoperatively in the psychoanalytic patient and in a number of surgical ward patients included in the case study series (to be described in Chapters 18 through 21). The emotional pattern is biphasic in character: First, there is an elated reaction of emotional relief and then a gradual development of reactive depression. The latter affective disorder, as observed in disaster victims, includes the following component symptoms: feelings of hopelessness, low self-esteem, loss of pleasure in usual social activities, resentment, constriction, and irritability in daily interpersonal relationships.[1]

One factor which is assumed to play a causal role in euphoria or dysphoria was specified in Hypothesis 9, namely, the discrepancy between the degree of victimization expected (V_e) and that perceived to have been obtained (V_o). Hypothesis 9 could be applied to the emotional sequence of euphoria followed by dysphoria if one assumes that there is first a positive discrepancy ($V_e > V_o$) at the termination of the acute danger phase, followed by a negative discrepancy ($V_e < V_o$) during the second stress phase of prolonged deprivation. This psychological sequence can be clearly discerned in Mrs. Blake's postoperative reactions. During the first few days after the operation, she was relieved that the damage sustained was much less than her dire fantasies had led her to expect. But then, in her elated state, she seemed to have assumed that there would be nothing more to it, that she would soon be fully recovered and out of the hospital. A week later, although already back at home, her convalescence was far from over. She was still suffering from sporadic incision pains and was not yet in a condition to resume many of her normal daily activities. Thus, there was a negative discrepancy between expected and obtained impairment during the postoperative period when her depression developed, in contrast to the positive discrepancy which characterized the period of elation.

The discrepancy factor, however, is at best a necessary condition, but not a sufficient condition, for the onset of reactive elation and reactive depression. When someone develops a dysphoric mood as a consequence of a negative discrepancy between expected and obtained victimization, it does not necessarily mean that the person is displaying the syndrome of reactive depression. The dysphoric mood is only one component of the syndrome; unless other components, such as self-punitive tendencies, are also clearly manifested, the person would not be diagnosed as markedly depressed (Fenichel, 1945; E. Jacobson, 1946 and 1953). In the aftermath of a community disaster, there are sometimes thousands of victims who suffer unexpected personal losses and undergo unanticipated deprivations. A high percentage may react with depressive feelings, but only a relatively small percentage develops a clear-cut depression or any other form of acute affective disorder (Lindemann, 1944; Titmuss, 1950). The conditions under which acute reactive depression develop in response to stress experiences are certainly not fully specified by Hypothesis 9, which applies only to the occurrence of a dysphoric mood. In order to arrive at a more complete explanation of the etiology of stress-induced depression, it is necessary to seek additional causes that can account for the entire set of component symptoms and, above all, for the severity of the disturbance in interpersonal relations.

Aggrievement Reactions

Although many important psychoanalytic observations and insights can be found in the writings of Freud, Abraham, H. Deutsch, E. Jacobson, and other clinical investigators, the psychoanalytic theory of reactive depression remains somewhat vague and incomplete, especially with regard to relatively transient varieties of depression that follow in the wake of stressful events. Most of the theoretical propositions that have been put forth deal with pathological personality predispositions. Such propositions help to explain why some persons react with a severe depression under stressful circumstances, whereas other persons, exposed to essentially the same circumstances, do not. Much less attention has been paid to the problems of delineating the situational variables which determine the affective disturbances induced by stress stimulation. The situational variables are the ones with which the present chapter is primarily concerned. What are the environmental conditions which increase or decrease the probability that a normal individual (holding personality predispositions constant) will develop a temporary depressive reaction? What types of stress experiences are most likely to induce transient depressions in persons who are strongly or weakly predisposed? Why do certain stressful circumstances give rise to a relatively high incidence of transient depressive reactions among clinically normal persons, whereas other, seemingly similar circumstances do not? What are the critical stimuli in stress situations that determine whether a depressive reaction is more likely to occur in the average person than some other type of affective disturbance, such as phobic anxiety or externalized hostility?

Although speculative answers to these questions abound in the existing psychoanalytic, psychiatric, and psychological literature, little empirical evidence can be ferreted out. In theoretical discussions of the dynamics of mourning and melancholia, based on psychoanalytic and psychiatric studies of depressed persons, there is one major type of event to which paramount importance is attached as a precipitating cause of acute depressive reactions: *the loss of a cathected object* (Bibring, 1953; Fenichel, 1945; Freud, 1917; E. Jacobson, 1953; B. Lewin, 1950). This includes not only the loss of loved persons through death or separation but also the loss of any cherished part of one's own body, the destruction of one's home or separation from any other possession which is symbolically apperceived as being part of the self.

In the discussion which follows, an attempt will be made to carry the theory of reactive depression one step further by delineating additional causal factors which determine whether a given stress episode resulting in object loss will produce a greater or lesser degree of depression. Certain of the factors to be considered may help to explain why it is that even when a stress episode occurs without inflicting any great loss, people will sometimes display as severe a reactive depression as though they had been seriously bereaved. The theoretical formulations, although derived from the psychoanalytic observations described in the preceding chapter, are essentially reconstructions based on inferences from free associations; they attempt to account for outstanding features of the patient's postoperative depression in terms of the reactivation of rage and grief which originally had been evoked by profound disappointments in childhood.

The tentative hypotheses to be put forth obviously do not provide a complete theory covering all causes of stress-induced depressions. Of the many different stress variables that might conceivably play a causal role, only a few will be singled out for discussion because of their apparent importance in accounting for the case material at hand. First, a set of hypotheses will be presented which state the general psychological conditions under which a stress episode involving a given degree of victimization will produce a strong rather than a weak affective disturbance. Then, two sets of supplementary hypotheses will be formulated, specifying situational variables which determine whether the affective disturbance elicited by a stress episode will take the form of externalized aggression or self-aggression. All of the hypotheses employ theoretical constructs referring to changes in the person's inner psychological state produced by certain classes of environmental circumstances. An adequate test of their validity will require long-range "panel" studies of fixed groups of people, so as to determine whether or not the occurrence of certain external stimuli regularly increases the probability of depressive reactions (or of alternative affective disturbances) when personality predispositions are held constant.

Hypothesis 11A. *If an episode of stress impact produces actual physical suffering and if the degree of perceived victimization is greater than had been expected beforehand, the episode will tend to be unconsciously assimilated to early victimization experiences which had evoked in the child feelings of intense disappointment concerning the behavior of one or both parents. The disappointments that are rearoused stem from painful episodes which had been interpreted by the child as excessive punishment caused by an angry or rejecting parent and which did not terminate in the usual degree of reconciliation.*

Hypothesis 11B. *The reactivated disappointment will be manifested as an "aggrievement" reaction (a combination of rage and grief) and will be externally directed toward danger-control authorities (resentment and retaliation against parent-surrogates) and/or inwardly directed toward the self (lowered self-esteem, self-punitive asceticism, feelings of hopelessness).*

During the first few sessions after psychoanalytic treatment was resumed, the patient was highly pessimistic about her future, manifested a marked tendency toward asceticism, felt guilty about past moral transgressions, and displayed related symptoms of a depressive nature. Still suffering from sporadic incision pains and chafing under the limitations imposed on her daily activities, she had begun to doubt that the disagreeable convalescence would soon be over or that she would ever be fully restored to good health. The surgery was judged by Mrs. Blake to be a total failure, allegedly having made her worse rather than better, and the same adverse outcome was expected from the psychoanalytic treatment. Her symptoms of hopelessness and self-aggression soon became so severe as to constitute an acute depressive disorder.

While still in the incipient phase, however, the depressive symptoms were interwoven with aggrievement reactions of quite a different character. Toward the surgeon, who only a week earlier was the main object of her passionate sexual and affectionate longings, she began openly to express an attitude of distrustful aversion. In her daydreams he was now a vile sadist who would misuse his professional prerogatives to attack her. Moreover, feelings of resentful aggrievement were directed against both the patient's mother and the analyst. On a very flimsy basis, she accused first one and then the other of being neglectful. Finally, she became aware of an irrational urge to "boil" at both. The content of her grievances (the mother's alleged failure to answer her affectionate letter, the analyst's absence from his office when she telephoned, both of them lacking sympathy) directly conveyed the theme that the parent and parent-surrogate failed to appreciate her suffering and withheld the affection she needed.

The main inference is that the basis for her aggrievement reactions had to do with a reactivation of early parental disappointments. This was first suggested by associations in which she referred to the dangers of becoming too dependent on the analyst. She complained that the analyst refused to tell her what to do to please him and then expressed the vague fear that if she were to give up her neurotic habits out of love for him, she would end up being utterly disappointed and overwhelmed by a sense of abandonment. Her attitude seemed to be that of an emotionally burnt child whose bitter disappointment in mother (and perhaps also father) inclined her to keep away from any warm object relationship. ("I just don't give a damn about anyone; I just want people to stay out of my way.")

Clues to the psychogenic origins of the combined grief and rage reactions are contained in the patient's free associations to her postoperative dream. Her first recollection, elicited by the dream image of a lake in which the person inside the rolling snowball might drown, was of a place where long ago she herself had nearly drowned. What stood out most vividly in her memory of the near-drowning was the reconciliation with her father which the rescue had started to bring about. But she explicitly pointed out that it ended up in a sharp disappointment for her because nothing ever came of it. Earlier in the analysis, the same near-drowning episode had been recalled; in her associations, the disappointment in her father was linked with her guilt-laden disappointment and hostility at the time of her mother's near-drowning, which had occurred earlier, after the birth of a sister (see pp. 128–129). The text of the dream actually contains a direct reference to another sister and there are various dream elements which lend themselves to interpretation as symbolic references to birth: e.g., emerging from inside an enclosed circular space (being "let out" of "the snowball") and approaching the water ("rolling toward a lake"). Thus, the symbols in the postoperative dream, considered in relation to the patient's immediate associations and the previously noted associations linked with the screen memory of being rescued by her father, point to a specific phase in her early life history. That is, the latent content of the dream probably refers to longings and disappointments generated *at the time when her next youngest sibling was born.*

Additional associations to the snowball dream indicated that an outstanding latent theme was the danger of becoming too warmly affectionate toward parent-surrogates (surgeon and analyst). Finally, recollections of overwhelming shock and disappointment in her parents emerged very clearly in a subsequent session when, after an outburst of depressive weeping, she elaborated on her guilt feelings and on the self-destructive implications of the snowball dream. While ventilating her fear of "dissolving," her main associations were to the biblical story of Sodom and Gomorrah, which led to painful memories of a primal depression. She recalled—and seemingly relived—the feelings of annihilation and abandonment which evidently occurred very early in life as a result of the unassimilable shock of seeing her parents engaged in violent sexual intercourse.

Thus, there is a common theme of parental disappointment which seems to run through all the main associations to the postoperative dream. The dream material suggests that there may have been a defensive motivation underlying her resentful attitudes toward parent-surrogates and her constricted withdrawal from love objects; *viz.*, an urgent need to remain frigidly aloof from all potentially warm relationships so as to counteract the danger of being, once again, overwhelmingly disappointed.

In the above discussion, only a cursory summary has been presented of the manifold ways in which the patient's postoperative depressive and aggressive reactions were linked with profound disappointments in her mother and father during the early years of her life. From the patient's fantasies and free associations, the analyst surmised that much of the intensity and content of her disappointment reactions during the prolonged convalescence came from the symbolic meanings evoked by the current deprivations. Although the actual degree of physical suffering was relatively slight, the emotional impact seemed to be enormously amplified by the reawakening of old memories and the reopening of old emotional wounds. This *amplification* phenomenon, noted time and again as the patient seemingly "relived" on the analytic couch one or another of the painful episodes of her childhood, provided the main basis for putting forth the concept of reactivated childhood disappointments in Hypothesis 11A.

The statement of the conditions for reactive depression in Hypothesis 11A sounds rather symmetrical with that of the conditions for reactive elation in Hypothesis 10. But the former hypothesis should not be regarded as the converse of the latter. Each of the two hypotheses can be tested independently; it may turn out that one is confirmed while the other is not. The nonreciprocal relationship of the two hypotheses stems partly from the fact that their dependent variables—elation and depression—are not exhaustive opposites. To describe a person as "nonelated" does not mean that he is necessarily depressed; nor does the term "nondepressed" necessarily imply "elated." In common psychiatric and psychological usage, both elation and depression are deviations from a middle category of clinically "normal" affective status (neither elated nor depressed) which might characterize the way most people feel most of the time.

Another reason why the two hypotheses should not be regarded as semantically equivalent is that the two mediating variables, which refer to the reactivation of childhood emotional experiences, also are not exhaustive opposites. Here the assumption is that at least three different categories of victimization experiences in childhood can be differentiated according to the way in which they affect the *cohesiveness*[2] of the child's relationship to one or both parents:

Type I. Extreme Augmentation of Cohesiveness. A punishment or deprivation deviates from the norm (see Type II) in that its termination evokes an exceptionally high degree of affection and amiability (e.g., an episode in which reconciliation takes place following a period of estrangement, as a result of a dramatic demonstration of the parent's love and protectiveness).

Type II. The Normal Degree of Cohesiveness. The average punishment or deprivation episode during childhood, eliciting neither an exceptionally high or low degree of cohesiveness.

Type III. Extreme Diminution of Cohesiveness. Unusually severe or unexpected victimization experiences giving rise to estrangement or withdrawal from one or both parents (e.g., a painful accident which the child misinterprets as a deliberate punishment or as an act of abandonment by the parents).

All three types of events presumably occur during everyone's childhood and any one of the three could be reinstated by a given stress episode in adult life. Hypothesis 10 states some of the conditions and consequences of reinstating Type I; Hypothesis 11 does the same for Type III. By implication, it follows from the two hypotheses that if reinstatement of Type II were to occur, the consequence would be a relatively neutral affective status, i.e., markedly less elation than Type I, and markedly less aggrievement than Type III.

Hypotheses 10 and 11 refer to only *one class of environmental factors* which may determine whether a stress episode will be assimilated to childhood experiences of Type I or Type III; the propositions are not intended as comprehensive statements which summarize *all* the major causal factors. Predispositional factors undoubtedly play an important role and may sometimes interact with the environmental factors in such a way as to obscure the effects of the latter.

Externalized Rage and Resentment

There are certain indications in the psychoanalytic data which suggest that situational factors as well as predispositional factors influence the probability that rage rather than grief will become the dominant response to an episode of prolonged deprivation. In the case of Mrs. Blake, the childhood memories of aggrievement experiences that were aroused at times when externalized rage was her dominant response seemed to differ from the memories aroused at times when grief was predominant. The patient's transference reactions, dreams, and associated recollections suggest that it may be useful to postulate at least two subtypes of childhood aggrievement situations (Type III), each of which may produce low parent-child cohesiveness, but with quite different emotional consequences for the child.

Type IIIA. Active Alienation. Usually severe or unexpected victimization experiences which elicit indignation or animosity in the child, thus resulting in a temporary lowering of motivation for cohesiveness with the parents; the parents are felt to be unfair and blameworthy but the child remains sufficiently confident about their basic affectionate attitude to allow himself the risk of aggressively protesting or retaliating for their "bad" behavior.

Type IIIB. Passive Estrangement. Unusually severe or unexpected victimization experiences as a result of which the child perceives the parents as having abandoned him, and he develops feelings of hopelessness ("primal grief") concerning the prospects of returning to the former state of parent-child cohesiveness (e.g., the child undergoes a traumatic physical separation and thinks that he has irrevocably lost the parents' love and protectiveness through his own bad behavior.)

Whether a punishment episode is of Type IIIA or IIIB, the child's disappointment in the parents is apt to involve some degree of anger against them and some loss of self-esteem. Nevertheless, the main assumption is that in so far as the disappointment experience approximates the conditions specified in Type IIIA, externalized aggression will tend to be a more dominant reaction than grief; whereas, a Type IIIB experience will tend to induce a predominance of depressive reactions (grief and self-aggression).[3] Type IIIB may be regarded as including any parental punishment for misbehavior which elicits grief or guilt, even though it may have little or no effect on the child's later personality development. Most instances of Type IIIB, however, are likely to be experiences of childhood despondency over object losses which are capable of having profound effects on personality development (see E. Jacobson, 1946; M. Klein, 1952; B. Lewin, 1950).

A sequence of Type IIIA and IIIB reactivations appear to have occurred during the sessions when Mrs. Blake was displaying postoperative disappointment reactions. In Sessions 13 through 15, her predominant reactions were those of externalized aggression. Her associations in those sessions centered about childhood ambivalent feelings toward her parents. This tendency is epitomized by the vivid recollections of the way her father treated her at the time of a childhood accident. She recalled her positive feelings of being protected and indulged by him and, at the same time, the negative feelings of disappointment because of his failure to show more affection and to bring an end to her estrangement from him. The latter complaint, in turn, was a consequence of an antecedent disappointment, the birth of a sibling, to which she had reacted with only mild grief but with considerable rage, protest, and retaliatory withdrawal from both parents. Thus, childhood memories of Type IIIA were predominant in the analytic material during the sessions when Mrs. Blake was giving associations to her postoperative feelings of resentment and irritability.

In Sessions 16 through 20, about a week later, her grieflike depressive symptoms were predominant, and a similar correlation was noted between these symptoms and the rearousal of memories of Type IIIB experiences. The outstanding memory recollected during this period, fragments of which had come up in several earlier sessions, was of a traumatizing scene, witnessed from her crib, of violent parental intercourse. As already noted, at times when this memory occurred she displayed intense abreactions of the kind that can be called emotional "reliving" of the experience. Her mood on these occasions was that of horror and hopeless despair. Her symbolic allusions to the destruction of Sodom and Gomorrah, together with numerous related associations, indicate that much of the traumatizing effect of the experience had to do with a painful alteration of her conception of the parents and of their relationship to her: They were suddenly transformed from safe love objects into dangerous beasts who might destroy her. Having lost her "good" objects, she felt abandoned, like "a spot of nothingness." [4]

Hypotheses 12 and 13, which will be discussed in the remainder of this chapter, state some of the main inferences drawn from the psychoanalytic observations concerning the way in which the patient's current aggressive and depressive reactions were linked with antecedent stress experiences of childhood, as reconstructed from her free associations.

Hypothesis 12A. *Given a stress episode of unexpectedly high victimization* ($V_e < V_o$)*, the probability that disappointment reactions will take the form of externalized rage toward danger-control authorities (or toward other parent-surrogates) will be increased by the presence of any external cues which tend to reactivate childhood experiences of resentment against the parents for unwarranted punishment.*

Hypothesis 12B. *The effective cues which tend to reactivate childhood resentment experiences include any action on the part of a danger-control authority which is perceived as deficient behavior and which resembles the apparent deficiencies of one's parents at times when seemingly unfair, excessive, or undeserved punishment was inflicted.*

This hypothesis attempts to carry the explanation of disappointment reactions further than Hypothesis 11 by setting forth certain of the psychological conditions under which outward directed resentment, rather than inward directed depression, will tend to become the predominant disappointment reaction. The hypothesis should not be construed as implying that the *only* basis for stress-induced resentment is the reactivation of a certain type of childhood punishment episode. The reactivation construct is introduced mainly to help explain the *irrational* resentment and *unprovoked* rage that has been noted in the clinical material and that has been repeatedly observed in large-scale disasters, even among survivors who are fully aware that the target of their aggression is not really at fault (Glover, 1942; Sorokin, 1942; Tyhurst, 1951; Veltfort and Lee, 1943; Vernon, 1941).

One need not resort to any such explanatory concept to account for the obvious increase in aggressive protest that is provoked when danger-control authorities perform actions that are patently negligent or self-aggrandizing at a time when people are counting on them to function as effective leaders in a crisis (see the account by Stouffer et al., 1949a, pp. 369 ff., on resentment toward officers among enlisted men in the U. S. Army). Hypothesis 12 is intended to supplement, not to replace, the existing propositions about the dynamics of aggression in relation to environmental frustrations and provocations. (See Dollard et al., 1939; Himmelweit and Pear, 1950.) Because the well-established propositions concerning the determinants of aggression do not offer a full explanation of rage and recrimination in response to minimal provocation, an important theoretical gap remains to be filled. As a tentative theoretical construction to help fill this gap, Hypothesis 12A introduces the notion that when a given frustration or provocation to aggression occurs, the intensity of resentment reactions will vary depending upon the presence or absence of certain types of situational events. According to Hypothesis 12B, the events which energize current emotional reactions of anger are those deficient actions on the part of danger-control authorities which reinstate childhood episodes of undeserved punishment on the part of the parents.

In stress episodes of adult life, the following are assumed to be typical of the perceptible deficiencies which are likely to operate as effective reactivating cues (for most persons in modern society): (*a*) The danger-control authority fails to give advance warning about the magnitude of the punishment (i.e., about the danger or deprivation that actually materializes) or fails to give any prior information as to how one can avert it; (*b*) the danger-control authority misinterprets or refuses to acknowledge one's special efforts to be "good," (i.e., to conform with authoritative demands and wishes); (*c*) the danger-control authority shows little interest in observing or obtaining information about the magnitude of one's subjective suffering; (*d*) the danger-control authority, although generally continuing to act in accordance with his protective role, refuses to listen to one's protests or unsympathetically rejects one's personal pleas for aid or reassurance.

The reinstatement of episodes of undeserved punishment (Type IIIA) is assumed to arouse not only the affective components of the original experiences but also the habitual aggressive responses which the child developed as a means of coping with the parent's unacceptable behavior. When unfairly or overseverely punished, a child is apt to struggle against the maltreatment—and against incipient guilt feelings about having committed an offense which evoked strong parental disapproval—by angrily protesting, aloud or silently, e.g., "I don't deserve this, you didn't warn me that I was doing anything wrong; you don't love me anymore so I don't love you; you are the bad one, not I."

Mrs. Blake's postoperative sessions provide numerous examples of excessive aggressiveness in response to nonprovocative actions on the part of parent-surrogates, and her reactions seem to involve a reactivation of childhood resentments and protests. Her conception of the surgeon as a dangerous sadist first occurred when she discovered that the area of her surgical wound was larger than he had told her it would be (see pp. 131–132). The same exaggerated misconception of the surgeon recurred about ten days later, at which time the only basis for her suspicions was the fact that she was currently suffering much more pain and discomfort than she had expected. We have already seen that similar feelings of resentment toward the analyst clearly pointed to reactivated childhood disappointments at the hands of her parents (see pp. 151–156). From the beginning of her analysis, she had repeatedly complained about the analyst's adherence to the standard rules of psychoanalytic treatment; but in the postoperative sessions the complaints were blown up into accusations that the analyst had no intention of helping her, was taking no cognizance of her suffering, was ignoring her efforts to be a "good girl," and wanted only to get rid of her as soon as possible. These negative transference reactions were closely linked with an irrational need to "boil" at her mother and with various indications of a more generalized sense of resentment toward all authority figures. The formulation of Hypothesis 12 derives mainly from the numerous indications in the psychoanalytic data concerning the way that the patient's current exaggerated complaints were traceable to childhood resentments against her parents.

One of the major implications of Hypothesis 12 pertains to individual differences in sensitivity to ostensible errors and misbehavior committed by danger-control authorities. Any given deficient act may have little or no effect on some people but may engender intense resentment in others, as a consequence of exposure to different patterns of parental punishment. To understand why an authority's action elicits exceptionally strong protests or resentment in a given individual, one would need to know exactly which actions on the part of his parents were the ones that, during his childhood, had made him feel he was being unjustly punished. Insofar as parents are idiosyncratic in their punishment practices, marked individual differences would occur in their children's subsequent responsiveness to the behavior of group leaders and other parent-surrogates. But within any given culture, there are likely to be social norms which define the forms of parental discipline and the occasions when punishment of a child is "fair" or "warranted." When parents deviate from the norms by administering "unfair" or "unwarranted" punishment, they are likely to behave in certain characteristic ways that are quite different from those when they are administering "warranted" punishment. It is therefore to be expected that there will be some degree of homogeneity in parental punishment practices. For instance, it is mainly at times when parents become very angry that they are most apt to overpunish their children for minor offenses, or to blame them for offenses they did not commit. Parental anger, whether in America, Europe, or even Asia, is likely to be accompanied by some characteristic forms of excited behavior, including unusually precipitous action without regard for what the child is trying to communicate in his efforts to prevent unearned retribution. Thus, there may be some degree of commonality the world over in certain modes of parental action at times when excessive or unwarranted punishment is being inflicted.

Much of the above discussion of Hypothesis 12 should be regarded as a first approximation toward the specification of general classes of parental behavior that may give rise to common cues to unwarranted punishment within our culture. Obviously, these tentative formulations will require modification and elaboration as more information becomes available concerning subcultural, ethnic, and social class differences.[5]

Grief and Self-aggression

The limitations which have just been discussed apply equally to Hypothesis 13, which provides a tentative formulation of the types of external events likely to reactivate childhood experiences of passive estrangement.

Hypothesis 13A. *Given a stress episode of unexpectedly high victimization* ($V_e < V_o$)*, the probability that the disappointment reaction will take the form of acute depression will be increased by any external cues which tend to reactivate childhood episodes of hopeless grief in which the child felt that it "deserved" to be punished and thought it was being physically abandoned (isolated) or psychologically abandoned (irrevocably rejected) by its parents.*

Hypothesis 13B. *The set of effective cues which tend to reactivate childhood experiences of hopeless grief includes any signs of abandonment by parent-surrogates, i.e., sustained physical isolation from affectionate persons or occurrences which are perceived as the product of their sustained rejection.*

Hypothesis 13C. *The probability of exposure to signs of abandonment, as specified in Hypothesis 13B, is a function of the temporal duration of the stress episode:* (i) *The longer the duration of a deprivational episode involving physical confinement or low mobility, the greater the degree of actual and perceived separation from most or all persons in one's prestress milieu, including those who function as affectionate parent-surrogates;* (ii) *the longer the duration of suffering and deprivation, the higher the frequency of apparent failures on the part of danger-control authorities to mitigate discomfort or to produce the expected rewards for conforming with their demands; hence, the greater the likelihood that they will be perceived as unappeasable parental figures who have withdrawn their power to alleviate suffering.*

Just as with Hypothesis 12, this hypothesis is to be understood as designating unconscious factors (in the etiology of reactive depression) which have an effect over and beyond the direct psychological impact of any current circumstances (e.g., object loss, disabling disease) that may be responsible for provoking or precipitating the emotional disturbance. Guilt, low self-esteem, and pessimism may be elicited by a variety of provocative occurrences during exposure to prolonged stress. Among the major sources of hopelessness and guilt that may arise during the convalescent period following surgery are the following: (*a*) Ambiguous signs suggesting that one's illness might be incurable; (*b*) development of new organic complications which increase one's incapacitation; (*c*) authoritative information that one's present condition is attributable to past misbehavior or failure to adhere to medical orders; (*d*) an accumulation of minor tribulations which are regarded by others as trivial or ridiculous, rather than as serious deprivations requiring heroic fortitude. There are also various types of guilt-provoking occurrences which bear no relationship to one's current suffering but which, on the basis of religious, ideological or superstitious beliefs, may be felt as a source of retribution from the deity, from fate, or from supernatural powers (See Glover, 1942; M. Schmideberg, 1942; M. Wolfenstein, 1957). One would expect to find exceptionally intense reactions of guilt and self-recrimination if the patient, only a short time before falling ill, had indulged in an action which violated his own moral code.

Similar psychological consequences may ensue when a surgical patient, in a temporary state of elation over having survived the operation, engages in unconventional, self-indulgent behavior. During the later stages of convalescence, as deprivations accumulate, he may begin to interpret his suffering as a punishment for his recent moral lapses. Thus, when people undergo exposure to the successive phases of stress, *the greater the relaxation of superego controls while celebrating the termination of the first (acute danger) phase, the greater may be the chances of reacting with guilt and self-recriminations during the second (prolonged deprivation) phase.* Perhaps it is for this reason that some surgical patients who display salient postoperative elations become depressed within a short time after the elation subsides. The same hypothesis might also help to account for a positive correlation between initial elation and subsequent depression following exposure to large-scale physical disasters or other catastrophic occurrences (M. Wolfenstein, 1957).

The events and circumstances referred to in the above discussion include various "realistic" and "unrealistic" sources of self-blame which may contribute to depressive reactions partly because they sometimes reinstate early episodes during which the child felt that it deserved to be punished, as specified in Hypothesis 13A. However, if the signs of abandonment specified by Hypothesis 13B are also present, childhood grief experiences are much more likely to be reactivated. One of the main implications of Hypothesis 13B is that any event in adult life which stimulates pessimism or guilt feelings will tend to produce a much more profound effect if it occurs in a social environment where one is socially isolated or where there are signs of rejection by parent-surrogates. This implication is consistent with observational reports that social isolation augments the intensity of reactive depressions (Greenson, 1949; Robinson et al., 1956; Segal, 1954; Strecker et al., 1938; Sutherland and Orbach, 1953), and also with various recommendations concerning the importance of social stimulation and of a friendly, personalized approach in the psychological handling of hospitalized patients (Kennedy, 1950; Lawton, 1956; Ochsner, 1950; Reiss et al., 1953).

From the above discussion of Hypothesis 13, it appears that in any deprivational situation there are two main types of external events which, when combined, augment the probability of a reactivation of childhood episodes of passive estrangement (Type IIIB): (*a*) signs conveying that the person's suffering is a consequence of his own shortcomings or past misbehavior, and (*b*) signs of abandonment by an authority figure, a protective friend, or anyone else who functions as a parent-surrogate. Hypothesis 13 is most directly applicable to those disproportionately intense reactions of depressions which occur even though the person realizes intellectually that his current suffering and frustration will terminate sooner or later with no residual loss or victimization. A sick person may know that his chances of regaining his health are exceedingly high, but an irrational sense of hopelessness may, nevertheless, become the pervasive mood as a consequence of the unconscious assimilation to which Hypothesis 13A refers. For example, a patient with a broken leg may believe his orthopedist's prediction that the bones will fully mend within five or six months, but, nevertheless, may become inordinately depressed when week after week he repeatedly experiences periods of social isolation, unrelieved discomfort, and related deprivations which are apperceived as the equivalents of childhood experiences of prolonged punishment.

In the case of Mrs. Blake, the temporal duration of the stresses of convalescence seems to be a major factor related to her shift from optimism to pessimism and the corresponding development of an attitude of hopelessness. In order to elucidate this point, it may be helpful to summarize the sequence of the patient's main postoperative reactions.

1. Her first postoperative week was characterized by high self-confidence, optimism, and elation, despite the fact that she was subjected to sporadic pains and continual discomforts.

2. By about the tenth postoperative day, her attitude and mood became dominated by a general sense of disappointment, which appeared to be centered on the fact that the pains and discomforts were continuing and her recovery was obviously still far from complete. Over the next two weeks her attitude was predominantly extrapunitive: she suspected the surgeon of being a sadist, she behaved in an irritable, belligerent fashion toward her husband and children, and she showed an increased tendency to withdraw from social contacts in general. It was during this period (in the middle of the third postoperative week) that

she resumed psychoanalytic treatment. Her sessions were filled with complaints and recriminations, and her associations led to memories of childhood resentments against her parents.

3. During the fourth postoperative week, she became increasingly pessimistic about the chances that the pain and disability would ever let up. She referred to her operation as a total failure and expressed a thoroughly gloomy outlook concerning her entire future, including the prospects of gaining any help from the psychoanalytic treatment. During this final phase of convalescence, overt depressive symptoms gradually became dominant and her associations led to the revival of childhood memories of being abandoned by her parents (e.g., recollections of the childhood disappointments connected with the birth of a sibling and of an infantile depression precipitated by witnessing the primal scene).

The above sequence of emotional reactions not only suggested the way in which the psychological preconditions for resentment may differ from those for depression, as formulated in Hypotheses 12A and 13A, but also suggested the importance of the temporal duration factor, as specified in Hypothesis 13C.

Notes

1. Symptoms of reactive depression have been reported following exposure to a wide variety of stress situations, including: (*a*) peacetime disasters (Cobb and Lindemann, 1943; Committee on Disaster Studies 1955; Wallace, 1954; M. Wolfenstein, 1957); (*b*) wartime bombings of the civilian population (Glover, 1942; Janis, 1951; Thouless, 1941); (*c*) military combat (Grinker and J. Spiegel, 1945a, 1945b; Hastings et al., 1944; Kardiner and H. Spiegel, 1947; Lidz, 1953; A. Wilson, 1941; Wright, 1946); (*d*) imprisonment or concentration camp confinement (Arntzen, 1948; Bettelheim, 1943; Bondy, 1943; Greenson, 1949; Nirembeski, 1946; Segal, 1954; Strassman et al., 1956); (*e*) unemployment and loss of social status (Ginsburg, 1942; Jahoda-Lazarsfeld and Zeisel, 1932); (*f*) chronic illness (Shands, 1944; Strecker et al., 1938; Wittkower, 1949, 1952); (*g*) postoperative convalescence (Bernstein and Small, 1951; Lindemann, 1941; Sutherland and Orbach, 1953; Sutherland et al., 1952).

Commenting on the ubiquitousness of reactive depression in times of deprivation, Bibring (1953, pp. 35–36) asserts that it is ". . . essentially 'a human way of reacting to frustration and misery' whenever the ego finds itself in a state of (real or imaginary) helplessness against 'overwhelming odds.' "

2. The term "cohesiveness" is borrowed from the social psychological literature on group dynamics.

"One of the key concepts, which has been the subject of much experimental investigation is that of *cohesiveness.* Intuitively, cohesiveness refers to the forces which bind the parts of a group together and which, thus, resist disruptive influences. Hence, the study of conditions affecting group cohesiveness and of the effects upon group functioning of variations in group cohesiveness is at the heart of the study of group life.

". . . The force acting upon an individual to remain in the group may derive from the attractiveness or positive valence of the group, the negative valence of not being in the group, and/or barriers or restraints against leaving the group. . . ." (M. Deutsch, 1954, pp. 214–215.)

3. An important set of questions concerning psychogenetic determinants is posed by the distinction between the two types of reactions to disappointment: What factors—in the personality of the child, in the interaction between the child and its parents, and in the external frustration situation—will determine whether a given disappointment during the early years of life will turn out to be an instance of active alienation (Type IIIA) or of passive estrangement (Type IIIB)? Such questions are beyond the scope of the present inquiry; the answers will have to be obtained from systematic studies of child development as well as from psychoanalytic research on the emotional impact of childhood events. For present purposes, the assumption is made that every child experiences at least a few instances of both types of reaction (Types IIIA and IIIB) in response to childhood illnesses, injuries, punishments, and other such victimization episodes.

To understand the dynamics of reactive depressions in surgical patients and in disaster victims, it may be useful to attempt to answer the following question: Under what conditions will Type IIIA as against Type IIIB be *reactivated* by a given victimization episode *in adult life?* This is the central question on which the theoretical analysis in the last part of Chapter 15 is focused.

4. It is noteworthy that precisely the same type of reaction to witnessing the primal scene is singled out as one of the sources of primal depression in Abraham's (1924, pp. 464–470) classical account of affective disorders. Elsewhere in the psychoanalytic literature on reactive depressions, one finds concepts that are somewhat similar to those introduced into the present discussion of the reactivation of childhood disappointments. For example, M. Schmideberg (1942) asserts that among many people who were exposed to the air blitz against England, "being bombed was felt as a repetition of parental punishment and often produced a . . . reaction of docility." B. Lewin (1950, pp. 35–36) asserts that: "The first reaction to object loss is an indignant rebellion, and when the rebellion fails, there comes an attempt to move the object by contrition, remorse, self-punishment and expiation." Similar theoretical formulations are presented in psychoanalytic accounts of depression by Flugel (1945), E. Jacobson (1946 and 1953), M. Klein (1952), and Schilder (1942).

5. Hypothesis 12A carries the implication that any group differences in parental punishment practices are likely to produce their counterpart in differential sensitivities to the apparent deficiencies of danger-control authorities. Suppose, for example, that among certain sectors of the American middle class, parents typically offer detailed verbal explanations when they administer punishment, except on those occasions when they are so aroused as to lose emotional control. In a crisis situation of adult life, how would the offspring brought up under such a

regime react to the bald announcement by community authorities that in order to cope with a community crisis a curfew or some other restrictive measure was to be imposed upon them? For such persons, the absence of a detailed explanation as to why the undesirable restrictions are essential is apt to function as a cue which reinstates experiences of arbitrary, unwarranted parental punishment. But the presence or absence of such explanations probably would make little or no difference to persons brought up in an ethnic group or social class which does not share the tradition of giving elaborate verbal explanations to children when punishment is inflicted.

16.

A paradoxical effect of stress: unrepression

One of the best-known facts about psychological stress is that a severely traumatizing experience can give rise to various functional disorders, including retrograde amnesias and related memory disturbances. Many psychiatric studies of traumatic neurosis, especially among military combat personnel, have emphasized the severity and persistence of memory loss (Culpin, 1940; Grinker and J. Spiegel, 1945a and 1945b; Kardiner and H. Spiegel, 1947). Sometimes the survivor of a harrowing combat mission represses not only the memory of the danger episode but also associatively linked memories from earlier periods of his life. The amnesias produced by exposure to traumatic danger stimuli will occasionally clear up spontaneously, but often the memory gaps will persist indefinitely unless hypnosis, hypnotic drugs, or other special therapeutic techniques are employed to overcome the repression. When people undergo relatively minor emotional shocks, involving much less severe stress than military combat, memory distortions are of frequent occurrence. Even when exposed to only mild sources of danger which do not give rise to traumatic neuroses, many people fail to recall the painful events or alter their recollections of the stress episode in such a way as to skip over the most anxiety-producing details (Freedman et al., 1952; Kardiner, 1941; Maskin, 1941).

In view of the well-known adverse effects of stress experiences on memory functioning, it seems paradoxical to assert that stress experiences can also have the opposite effect of "unrepression," enabling the individual to regain memories that had previously remained unconscious. And yet it is precisely this paradoxical outcome which becomes salient when one searches through the psychoanalytic case record to determine what effect, if any, the surgical experience had on Mrs. Blake's psychoanalytic progress.

The phenomenon of unrepression would be quite understandable as a reaction to environmental stress if it occurred when there was a relaxation of superego censorship, i.e., during the poststress phase of elation, after the person had undergone suffering and was experiencing a temporary relief of neurotic symptoms (see English and Pearson, 1945, pp. 101 ff.; Flugel, 1945, pp. 156–159). But the main instances of unrepression were observed during two periods when superego pressures were by no means relaxed: (*a*) before the operation, at a time when the anticipation of danger led to an apparent increase in guilt and more rigid adherence to superego standards (see pp. 100–104); (*b*) during the depressive phase of convalescence, at a time when the patient displayed symptoms of intense aggrievement, including a variety of self-derogatory attitudes and suicidal fantasies which implied a heightening of superego tension (see pp. 155–157). Thus it seems somewhat puzzling to encounter an extraordinarily large amount of recovery of repressed material at precisely the time when all indications show that the person is reacting to external threats with a heightening of both superego anxiety and objective anxiety.

The present inquiry began with two main questions: (1) Did the stress episode facilitate or interfere with the essential steps in the analytic work of uncovering repressed material? (2) Did the stress episode have any sustained positive or negative effects on the patient's neurotic disabilities (i.e., on the form of her overt symptoms, on the intensity of her subjective neurotic suffering, on her capacity to control and to sublimate conflictful infantile impulses)? In order to give objective answers to these questions, it is necessary to compare the quality and rate of the patient's analytic progress in the twenty sessions during the period of the surgical episode with comparable time samples during the remainder of her three and one-half years of psychoanalysis.

Although fairly comprehensive notes had been kept throughout the patient's entire analysis, the records were not always sufficiently detailed to warrant any attempt at systematic, precisely quantified comparisons. Nevertheless, there is one outstanding comparative finding from the case study observations which the author regards as a conclusion that can be reported with fairly high certainty in answer to the first of the above two questions: *During the period when the stresses of surgery were in the focus of attention, the patient recovered, to an extraordinary degree, details of childhood memories which up until that time had been repressed.* During the two-month period of the surgery episode, the quantity of recovered memory material was not only greater than during any comparable time period of the patient's three and one-half years of psychoanalysis but was greater than during all the rest of the sessions put together.

When conducting a character analysis with a patient who has pronounced obsessional and compulsive traits, one can hardly expect to encounter very many clear-cut instances of recovery of repressed childhood memories. Indeed, many analysts report that even though they try to help all their patients to reconstruct the details of formative experiences, few of them achieve any remarkable recovery of lost childhood memories. Evidently, among the predominantly obsessive-compulsive personalities of our time, it is quite rare to dissipate childhood amnesias on the analytic couch, unlike the early days of psychoanalysis when most patients were being treated for acute hysterical symptoms (Kris, 1956, pp. 78 ff.). In the case of Mrs. Blake, unconscious wishes, apprehensions, and emotional impulses were constantly being unrepressed throughout her entire treatment by means of the standard techniques of analyzing her resistances, nocturnal dreams, daydreams, and transference reactions; nevertheless, it very rarely happened that she became able to recall any fragments of childhood experiences which had not been available to consciousness before analysis.

In the twenty sessions bearing on the surgical operation (described in Chapters 4, 6, 9, 11, and 14), there was a total of eleven different childhood recollections containing details never before recounted to the analyst. Not all of them, of course, can be classified as definite instances of unrepression because there is insufficient evidence to ascertain whether they were previously inaccessible to consciousness, and, hence, one cannot be sure they were originally repressed. The following are the eleven instances in question, all of which refer to objective or subjective occurrences in the patient's life prior to age seven:

1. Subjective feelings and fantasies evoked by the sight of the cripple boy observed from a train window.

2. Attitudes and fears connected with playing the penis-stick game.
3. Observation of father relieving himself at night when sleeping in her parents' bedroom.
4. Episode of homesickness when sent off to camp for first time.
5. Observation of a basket amputee hobbling on his leg stumps.
6. Details of the episode of near-drowning in icy water and of the subsequent near-reconciliation with her father.
7. Content of a reprimand from her sister Gertrude on an occasion when she confided secret daydreams.
8. Specific content of the illicit penis fantasy developed during the crisis periods of age three or four, when she became extremely fearful of her mother's retributions.
9. The triangle scene at the beach, when mother and father were ignoring her because of their preoccupation with the flirtatious New York lady.
10. Her aunt's "spooky" comments about cancer of the lips, on the occasion when she saw her aunt's genitalia.
11. Visual perceptions and emotional turmoil evoked when witnessing parental intercourse from her crib.

Only a few of the above examples, it will be noted, pertain to obviously traumatic events; the others refer to mildly disturbing experiences (probably "screen memories"), most of which were subsequently found to be associatively linked with crucial anxiety-provoking events in the patient's early life history. Among the first seven items on the above list, there may have been several which had been hitherto repressed, but there is insufficient evidence to make a definite judgment. In the case of the last four items, however, the evidence of unrepression is quite clear-cut. When recalling these particular memories, the patient showed one or more of the characteristic signs of the lifting of a retrograde amnesia: emotional excitement, visual impressions of almost hallucinatory clarity, and sudden organization of piecemeal and disjointed memory fragments into a coherent pattern which fitted in with previously known facts and events. In the case of each of the latter four memory items, the patient herself reported that she never before had been aware of the material. Moreover, each of the four events had been partially brought up in earlier sessions, at which time the analyst had observed that the account was confused and incomplete and that the patient was unable to fill in the gaps. The reader is already familiar with the example in Session 1 of the patient's failure to recollect what disturbing things she had overheard at the time when she observed her aunt's genitalia; subsequently, in Session 12, when she managed to remember what her aunt had said, it became clear that the patient was filling in the missing details, obvious derivatives of which had appeared in her free associations and fantasies only a short time earlier when it was inaccessible to consciousness.

At first the patient was inclined to doubt the genuineness of her sudden recollection of the early childhood fantasy of possessing a secretly stolen penis, and she remained skeptical about having observed parental intercourse. But many weeks later in her analysis, after she repeatedly produced the same memory fragments and gave additional elaborations, both the patient and the analyst felt quite sure that these memory details could not be spurious. (See the reconstruction concerning certain of these memories, made at the end of the analysis, pp. 111–115.)

Especially in the light of the known facts about the patient's neurotic conflicts, the psychoanalytic observations bearing on the four memories in question lead to the conclusion that these were genuine instances of unrepression. Earlier it was pointed out that, in contrast to the twenty sessions of the surgery period, the remainder of the patient's analysis was relatively devoid of such examples. In the remaining 580 sessions, the patient made considerable therapeutic progress but there were only two instances of the recovery of childhood memories which were comparable to the four just discussed.

After obtaining and examining the above psychoanalytic evidence, the author became fairly well convinced that the surgery period was one of marked acceleration in the patient's progress with respect to becoming aware of repressed childhood experiences. Nevertheless, the author was inclined at first to consider the entire phenomenon as having little general significance for understanding the psychology of stress. One consideration was that toward the end of her second year of treatment the patient might have reached an especially productive stage of her analysis in which the loosening of repressions would have been manifested in any case, the occurrence of the surgery at that time having been sheer coincidence. Another consideration was that, even if the surgical stress experience could be assigned a causal role in augmenting the patient's capacity to overcome childhood amnesias, the phenomenon might nevertheless be attributable to unique characteristics of her personality which predisposed her to be stimulated by the threats of surgery in an unusual way. Thus, the lifting of repressions in this particular case might be a unique phenomenon—one that would hardly ever occur in anyone else under comparable conditions of stress.

What altered this view was the fact that an equally dramatic occurrence of the very same phenomenon was encountered in another psychoneurotic patient, a 35-year-old man, whose motivations, interests, and personality characteristics differed markedly from the first patient. Under psychoanalytic treatment of several years' duration, this man had repeatedly ruminated about an exceptionally disturbing experience involving an illness that had occurred when he was about five years old. The illness had begun while he was in Europe with his mother and his brothers. They were on their way back to America from the Continent, where they had lived for several years because of the father's employment in the United States diplomatic service. The father had already returned to Washington. The rest of the family, upon arriving at Liverpool, were required to remain in the emigration center for several days because of the boy's contagious disease. After he had been examined by several physicians, his mother was informed that she would have to postpone the trip even longer to enable the boy to undergo a minor surgical procedure. A few days after the operation was performed, the boy was well enough to travel, and they boarded the ship. After several days of confinement in the family stateroom, the boy had recovered sufficiently to enjoy the sea voyage.

The recollection of the hours spent in the emigration office at the steamship dock and of his mother's agitation over the postponement of the trip had been verbalized several times during his analysis and was invariably accompanied by vague feelings of anxiety and depression. Despite numerous attempts to discover the source of disturbance, the patient completed his analysis without ever understanding why the memory was such a painful one.

Several years later a specific answer came, not from the application of psychoanalytic techniques but from a severe stress experience similar to the one at age five. A sudden flood of memories, including the missing parts of the Liverpool story, occurred at a time when the patient was suffering from a serious organic illness, following the completion of a long series of treatments for which he had been hospitalized. It happened on the day he was brought home from the hospital, at a time when he was feeling exceptionally weak, depressed about the prospects of a long and painful convalescence, and slightly resentful toward the doctors who had failed to cure him.

The patient had begun to confide his inner feelings about being sick and bedridden to a friend who had come to visit him. The friend was a professional colleague with whom personal matters had never before been discussed. While ventilating feelings of pessimism and self-pity, the patient suddenly found himself choked up with intense emotion as he began to recall in vivid detail the scene in the Liverpool emigration office of some thirty years earlier. For the first time he realized that, while he had been lying sick on a cot, he had interpreted his mother's worried conversation with the doctors to mean that he was going to be left behind at Liverpool because all the rest of the family would go on the boat back home to America. He now recollected that he had felt overwhelmed with grief, fear, and self-pity because he had thought that as a result of his illness he would be left to suffer alone among strangers and would never see his family again. This forgotten part of the episode came back so vividly that the patient felt he was "reliving" it.

The specific content of the unrepressed memory, it will be noted, provides an excellent illustration of the concept of "reactivated childhood fears of abandonment," as elucidated in earlier discussions of Hypotheses 5 and 13 (pp. 91 ff. and 173 ff.). What is of special interest here, however, is the stimulus situation in which the unrepression took place. As in the case of Mrs. Blake, exposure to severe stress seems to have had the effect of loosening the repression of disturbing childhood material, facilitating the vivid recall of memory details which had resisted being uncovered by earlier analytic efforts.

Upon encountering the evidence from the second case, the author proceeded to re-examine his protocols of pre- and postoperative interviews obtained from surgical ward patients[1] and from professional acquaintances who had volunteered to be interviewed at a time when they were about to undergo a surgical procedure. Several suggestive examples were noted in which the interviewee expressed surprise about having unexpectedly recollected a stressful childhood event. For example, a prominent psychoanalyst, when interviewed on the day after undergoing oral surgery, informed the author that the preoperative interview (conducted a few hours before the operation took place) had produced a remarkably therapeutic effect. He explained that, as a result of being questioned about his feelings and expectations concerning the impending tooth extraction, he had become aware of the fact that he was "all poised and emotionally aroused as though it would be terribly painful," even though he realized from prior experiences with the same dental surgeon that it would not be a painful procedure. (During the preoperative interview he had described a "feeling of appointment with destiny" and had freely admitted that what he feared most was the emotional tension at the moment of the extraction: "I'll be holding myself in check, to prevent myself from screaming or striking out, or refusing, or displaying furious behavior at the moment when I shall be helpless—helpless partly through my own will to go through with it.") After the interview was over, he suddenly had a vivid recollection of an early dental episode in which, as a small child, he was firmly held down by his father while the dentist, inflicting much pain, pulled a tooth.

In the postoperative interview, the interviewee stated that the recollection was followed by a feeling of emotional relief. He reported, however, that this particular experience had been recollected and verbalized many years before when he was undergoing a personal didactic analysis, and at that time he had gained some insight into its connection with irrational components in his attitude toward his father. But never before had he thought of this childhood event in connection with his chronic dental anxiety. The preoperative interview, in his opinion, had stimulated a remarkably successful piece of self-analysis, enabling him to see a connection between a memory and an affect which had hitherto remained isolated.

To find such a phenomenon in a few cases is still far from warranting any conclusion about the psychological effects of stress experiences in general. Nevertheless, after considering the clear-cut indications in the psychoanalytic case material together with the additional examples of seemingly related occurrences in other cases, the author felt encouraged to entertain the notion that unrepression is facilitated by exposure to external stress stimuli. This led to a search of the literature on stress behavior to see if there were any indications as to the possible generality of the case study findings. The observational reports, although fragmentary and incomplete, contain numerous additional examples of persons who, while exposed to conditions of severe stress, recollected vivid memories of earlier stress experiences. There are even some vague but suggestive indications that the tendency to regain repressed memories might possibly form an experiential basis for the popular belief that, at the moment of facing death, a person's entire past life will suddenly flash before his eyes. What is directly indicated by the observational reports, however, is that exposure to stress will sometimes have a markedly stimulating effect on: (*a*) the recall of disturbing events of one's past, and (*b*) the production of self-revealing introspections.[2]

The reports found in the literature appear to be compatible with the psychoanalytic observations of unrepression described above, but do not provide sufficient information to indicate whether the recollections of past experiences can be regarded as memories that had been repressed. A few examples will suffice to show the nature of the observational reports concerning the memories elicited under conditions of exposure to extreme danger and deprivation.

Bernstein and Small (1951) describe a 35-year-old man who was referred to a psychiatric clinic because of his intense fear of submitting to an urgently recommended pulmonary operation. During the psychiatric interview, he reported an extremely vivid recollection of an accident at age four when his father took him to a hospital to be treated for a laceration over the right eye; he recalled having fled from the hospital in terror after having caught sight of the needles. He also had vivid recollections of two other accidents he had seen when he was about three years old, one involving his sister's eye being injured by a kitchen knife and the other involving his mother's eye being struck by the edge of the swing on which he was riding.

Schilder (1938) also speaks about psychiatric interviews in which patients revive memories of past accidents or traumas at times when they are threatened by actual danger. He cites the case of a man who, just before undergoing an appendectomy, "relived" a wartime episode of being gassed during an enemy attack. Similar recollections can be found in the account of the "last thoughts" of a drowning man, recorded by Thurmond (1943) at a time when the victim was still in a state of delirium and was apparently reliving the entire experience. According to the verbatim record of the spontaneous "re-enactment" of the drowning episode, the young man had been swept out to sea when caught by an undertow while jumping the breakers at a Pacific Ocean beach. Some of his thoughts took the form of making a specific plan to tread water beyond the breakers until the tide turned; but, after several hours of fatiguing effort, he was feeling somewhat pessimistic about surviving. At this time he began to recall a series of disturbing past experiences, including one incident of being horrified by the sight of the mutilated corpse of a drowned man, and another incident of being injured, and "almost killed," in a serious automobile accident.

It is difficult, of course, to assess the reliability of the case material and anecdotal reports found in the literature, and, as mentioned earlier, one cannot be certain that they involve valid instances of unrepression. In order to make a definite determination as to whether or not a person shows an actual increase in ability to recall formerly repressed memories, it is necessary to make observations before as well as during the stress episode, and to conduct the investigations under circumstances where a person will readily verbalize memories of intimate personal details of his life history. Probably the investigators best-suited to meet these conditions are psychoanalysts who employ standard Freudian procedures and psychotherapists who use intensive interview procedures derived from psychoanalytic techniques. Unfortunately, however, such investigators have rarely reported any data concerning the psychological effects of external stress situations which arise while their patients are under treatment. The implications of the psychoanalytic observations described in the present chapter could be tested fairly readily if a number of psychoanalysts and psychoanalytically oriented therapists became sufficiently interested in the problem to keep careful records of their patients' verbal behavior as observed during interview sessions before, during, and after exposure to conditions of stress (see Chapter 2, pp. 18–20). Accordingly, the following hypothesis is put forth as a comprehensive generalization, with the expectation that this provocative formulation will have the merit of stimulating psychoanalytic investigators to record and report the pertinent data needed to confirm, refute, or modify it:

Hypothesis 14. *Exposure to any stress episode involving the threat of body damage will facilitate the revival of disturbing childhood memories, which, up to that time, had been wholly or partially repressed. Thus, a person's early memories of danger episodes are more likely to be unrepressed under conditions where fear is strongly aroused by signs of approaching danger or deprivation than under ordinary, relatively stress-free conditions.*

If subsequent research indicates that the unrepression effect occurs fairly frequently, even though not necessarily as ubiquitously as the above hypothesis asserts, a number of important theoretical problems may be illuminated concerning the relationship between fear and memory functioning:

1. To what extent is the paradoxical decrease in defensiveness a consequence of general "weakening of the ego" which facilitates the "return of the repressed"? Perhaps the fear, anxiety, and guilt stimulated by external stress impair the capacity to maintain one's usual defenses, reducing the efficiency of internal censorship to the point where traumatic memories and associated screen memories can break through into consciousness. One testable implication of this explanation is that unrepression should be found to occur more frequently with increased length of exposure to severe stress in situations like military combat where, as Grinker and Spiegel put it, the ego defenses are gradually "weakened by constant pounding under stress" to the point where "the ego loses its power to maintain its functional efficiency" (1945a, pp. 82–83).

2. Does the arousal of fear act like a catalyst, allowing one to regain partially or weakly repressed memories which can become accessible only when one encounters pertinent memory cues? A current stress experience may trigger off the recall of certain types of memories because it provides salient external (threat) cues and internal (emotional) cues which "remind" the person of similar experiences in the past. The

memories that are affected may be those on the borderline, so to speak, between preconscious and unconscious. Ordinarily, a person may fail to recall such experiences because, in the absence of threat stimuli, the effective memory cues are never present.

3. Does the unrepression phenomenon serve a defensive *expiation* function, involving an unconscious attempt to gain forgiveness from the "powers that be" so as to mitigate the anticipated punishment? Most examples of unrepression encountered so far involve an element of "confession" in that the hitherto buried memories were communicated to an analyst or friend at the very moment when they were recovered. Even the drowning man, as he was recollecting his earlier auto accident, addressed his statements to God, much in the manner of a childish religious confession (Thurmond, 1943). And perhaps, too, it is no accident that the main examples of unrepression refer to events which could furnish a potential justification for feeling hostile toward one or both parents. Consider, for example, Mrs. Blake's misconception of her parents' sexual passion as a brutally destructive action which threatened her. By remaining uncorrected, such a misconception of her parents' behavior, at a later stage of her development, may well have served as an excuse for her own childish destructive impulses toward them. In the second example, the man evidently had retained from childhood a repressed (hence uncorrected) misconception that his mother was capable of abandoning him in Liverpool. Such a misconception, entering dimly into consciousness through disguised derivatives, could have helped to make him feel justified in occasionally harboring childish retaliatory sentiments toward her. Similarly, the man who remembered being held down in the dental chair by his father may have felt some vague sense of justification for becoming "furious" on occasions which reminded him of the earlier assault, provided that his affective tendencies remained isolated from the content of the memory.

In each of the instances just cited, a series of recurrent disturbances in the child's relationship to its parents may have been condensed into a single "prototypic" memory. The release from repression of any such memory (or of the affect connected with the memory) may be tantamount to renouncing secret grudges from the past, especially those that had been maintained unmodified by being kept secret from consciousness. If so, the self-revelations may turn out to be a special case of the same unconscious process referred to in Hypothesis 1B, the product of a need to confess as a means of seeking expiation.

4. Does the unrepression phenomenon serve a defensive *reassurance* function involving an attempt to reduce fear, anxiety, or guilt by discounting the potential impact of the impending danger or deprivation?

The recollection of past traumas may serve not only as a warning but also as a consolation (Schilder, 1938). Under conditions of stress, a person may become strongly motivated to remind himself of past dangers which, after all, had been somehow surmounted, since he had managed to survive more or less intact. Thus, despite all the emotional disturbance that may be momentarily reawakened from recalling a painful memory, the person may nevertheless gain considerable reassurance (e.g., "That horrible experience seemed even worse than this one, but still I lived through it and came out of it alive.") The emotional tension created by remembering shocking and distressing events of the past might therefore be tolerated—as a lesser evil, so to speak—because of a more powerful need to gain reassurance about what is going to happen in the immediate future. For example, in the case of the sick man who suddenly recalled the painful childhood memory of being (seemingly) abandoned by his mother at Liverpool, the unrepression might have come about not from any weakening of his capacity or motivation to maintain the repression but, rather, from a more powerful competing motivation to reassure himself by means of an analogy to a past event: Once before he had suffered and felt afraid; but it turned out that his dire expectations were based on misunderstandings and his exaggerated fears never materialized. In the case of Mrs. Blake, the same urgent need for reassuring analogies might help to explain the unrepression of details of the traumatic experience of witnessing parental intercourse. Here again is an instance of an overwhelming emotional experience that was based partly on a gross misunderstanding of what the parents were actually doing; when it was all over, the apparent danger to her parents and to herself disappeared without producing the destructive effects the child had expected. This type of reassurance may also be involved in the other examples of unrepression of distressing memories which contained the element of having developed unwarranted fears because of misinterpreting the source or magnitude of the danger. Thus, it seems plausible to consider, as an alternative explanation of the paradox of unrepression, that under conditions of impending danger or deprivation a person may seek to gain reassurance by recalling memories of analogous threats of annihilation from which he had managed to escape in the past. According to Fenichel (1945, p. 145), there are times when a person will develop a "hunger for screen experiences." So, too, the circumstances of external stress might create a hunger for memories of past experiences of stress, especially for those in which the person's fears turned out to be unwarranted or in which he achieved some degree of mastery.[3]

In summary, the above discussion has singled out four different causal factors which remain to be investigated as plausible theoretical leads to account for the unrepression phenomenon described in Hypothesis 14: (1) The weakening of ego defenses resulting from exposure to conditions of stress; (2) the reinstatement of external (threat) cues and internal (emotional) cues which may help to overcome the obstacles which ordinarily interfere with the recall of similar stress episodes from the past; (3) the motivation to mitigate anticipated punishment by confessing, and thereby renouncing, secret grudges or resentments against a parental figure, which had been harbored in unmodified form since childhood; (4) the motivation to gain reassurance about impending danger or deprivation by recalling past experiences of horror or suffering which turned out to be not as bad as they had seemed at the time.

We turn now to the possible *consequences* of unrepression. When a patient who is undergoing psychoanalysis regains childhood memories that formerly had been repressed, there is sometimes an accompanying clinical improvement, manifested by the disappearance of one or another of the patient's neurotic symptoms [see Freud's early account of psychoanalysis (1904, p. 269) in which curative effects were attributed to the recovery of unconscious memories]. Did any such therapeutic effect occur in relation to the unrepression phenomenon observed under conditions of stress? This brings us back to the second main question stated at the beginning of this chapter: "Did the stress episode have any sustained positive or negative effects on the patient's neurotic disabilities . . . ?"

During certain phases of the surgery episode, notably the first week following the operation, the patient experienced a brief remission of various chronic neurotic symptoms. Subsequently, however, she showed the reverse effect, including a depression that was more acute than any she had experienced during the preceding two years of psychoanalytic treatment. But, when the episode was over, the patient reverted to essentially the same neurotic status as before the operation. Perhaps there was some slight abatement of neurotic disturbances achieved by the analytic sessions during the two-month period of the surgery episode, but it was not noticeably greater than for any other two-month period during her psychoanalytic treatment.

The absence of any marked improvement immediately following the surgical episode in this case suggests that the unrepression phenomenon is not necessarily a sign of therapeutic progress. At the time, the patient was evidently unable to make much effective use of the additional self-insight that came from the unrepression of childhood memories and fantasies. Moreover, she showed no apparent gain from the other opportunities for corrective emotional learning, during that same period. For instance, as part of her postoperative elation, she went through a phase of "benign regression," returning to a feminine conception of herself which she had abandoned since the age of three (see pp. 000–000). Her new-found feminine attitude led her to behave in a relatively warm, nonaggressive manner, and she was gratified to see how responsive people were to her femininity. And yet, despite the fact that her new mode of behavior was socially rewarded, she failed to show any definite change in attitudes or actions until after more than a year of additional treatment.

Thus, the patient's neurotic symptoms remained impervious to the postoperative opportunities for new emotional learning, just as during the preoperative period her neurotic fears failed to be influenced by the surgeon's reassuring statements. Before the operation, she had displayed an irrational fear of having her leg medically examined, based on the neurotic fantasy that she would be required to undergo an amputation. The discovery that her fear was unfounded had no apparent effect in the long run (see discussion of Hypothesis 7, pp. 121–124). Six weeks after the operation, as we have seen, she displayed exactly the same avoidance behavior based on the same neurotic fantasy. All of this simply points once again to the well-known fact that psychoneurotic habits rarely are influenced by a single cogent interpretation or self-insight, even when accompanied by clear-cut demonstrations via impressive life experiences. Probably for the same reasons, it takes a good deal more than the recovery of a few repressed memories to improve a chronically psychoneurotic personality. As Freud has pointed out in his later writings, the therapeutic gain from psychoanalysis comes about only after a patient has recovered the affect connected with the repressed memories and has "worked through" all the related feelings and impulses.

> For we find that even after the ego has decided to relinquish its resistances, it still has difficulty in undoing the repressions; and we have called the period of strenuous effort which follows . . . the phase of "working through." (S. Freud, 1936.)

Over a period of many months following the surgical episode, Mrs. Blake continued to work on the memories which had been recovered during the stressful period, gradually becoming more and more aware of the profound anxieties and longings with which they were associated. Thus, although the instances of unrepression led to no immediate therapeutic gain, they might have contributed, in the long run, to the marked clinical improvement which the patient eventually showed.

Notes

1. In later chapters, when the case studies of the surgical ward patients will be presented, additional instances will be encountered in which the person spontaneously recalls a childhood memory and reports that he had not previously remembered the event. (See, for example, the associations given to a postoperative dream by Case H–4, pp. 332–333.)

2. The following statement by Rickenbacker (1943), concerning the way he and his companions reacted while undergoing the ordeal of being stranded on a life raft in the Pacific Ocean at a time when there was little prospect of rescue, illustrates the strong self-revelation tendency that may be aroused by situations of extreme danger and deprivation:

"My companion clearly began to think of what lay beyond death and to think of it in terms of their own lives.

"They began to tell of what they had experienced in life: their hopes, fears, ambitions, their achievements, their mistakes. I suppose it takes the imminence of death to release one completely from inhibitions. The talk was entirely honest and, I am sure, entirely frank. What was said will always be locked up in our minds. As far as I am concerned, no hint of those long, man-to-man conversations will ever be revealed. I am sure of one thing, that it did us a great deal of good."

3. According to psychoanalytic theory, repression is essentially a defense against forbidden impulses or drives; this form of defense in the adult personally has as its model certain types of defensive avoidance reactions developed during the early years of life as a means of coping with what appeared to the child as overwhelming threats of mutilation or annihilation by the parents or by other outside sources of danger (S. Freud, 1933 and 1936). Commenting on the "unrepression" phenomenon, K. Wolf (1957) has remarked that it can be explained in a way that is consistent with this theory if it is assumed that when an outside danger reaches a high magnitude during adult life, the person may apperceive the external threat of annihilation as a greater threat to his integrity than certain of the inner dangers which, under normal circumstances, constitute a dominant source of anxiety. A conflict may be postulated (within "the ego") between: (*a*) the sources of anxiety (or "countercathexes") which motivate the repression of certain memories and (*b*) the temporary need to gain reassurance through the recollection of past escapes from threatened annihilation. If the latter motivation is momentarily more powerful than the former, unrepression will occur. This implies a temporary reduction in ego defense against certain specific memories, notably those which convey the reassuring notion that "I survived that time so I will survive again this time."

Taking account of Hypothesis 1, the most effective reassurances might be memories of those childhood incidents in which the external threat of annihilation was thought to be a punishment for forbidden impulses ("I thought I deserved annihilation that time but the punishment was not so bad after all"). In order to gain this type of reassurance, it is necessary for the person to relax temporarily his involuntary censorship with respect to certain repressed impulses so that he will be able to remember some occasions when external punishment did not have the anticipated consequences. However, there need not be a complete relaxation of all censorship with respect to the repressed experiences; the internal dangers which the child feared on those occasions would not necessarily be unrepressed. As a matter of fact, in all instances of unrepression found in the psychoanalytic case study during the period of external stress, the patient was able to remember some of the external features of the danger situation but did not become aware of the inner dangers which presumably had been a major source of anxiety. Thus, the unrepression of childhood memories induced by exposure to threats of physical danger seem to be quite incomplete. The *partial* unrepression may be limited to that portion of the repressed material which the person currently needs for the purpose of gaining reassurance.

Another factor that may contribute to the person's ability to tolerate certain memory details which had formerly been repressed was mentioned in connection with the "expiation" hypothesis (p. 189). In so far as the instances of unrepression involve a renunciation of childhood grudges against the parents, the internal censorship might be somewhat less stringently enforced. In general, the content of the fragmentary memories that are unrepressed can be plausibly interpreted as a compromise formation, reflecting the influence of both the chronic repressing forces and the temporary wish for reassurance created by the external threat of annihilation.

17.

Summary of part I: Major psychodynamic hypotheses

In the preceding Chapters of Part I, a large number of propositions were formulated concerning the dynamics of stress behavior. These propositions generally deal with the causes and consequences of various types of emotional reactions and adjustment mechanisms that are frequently activated when people are exposed to severe environmental threats, dangers, or deprivations.

Certain of the propositions, designated by being numbered and italicized, were singled out because they appear to be theoretically plausible hypotheses which are at least partially supported by the evidence presented. Such hypotheses were arrived at by a complex set of procedures involving the use of psychoanalytic data for the purpose of drawing inferences about psychological processes which mediate "typical" reactions to threat and danger. In Chapters 2 and 3, a detailed exposition and rationale of the research approach was given, indicating how and why the available psychological and psychiatric studies concerning the behavioral effects of exposure to physical danger were taken into account. "Typical" stress reactions, as against idiosyncratic ones, were identified on the basis of comparative data from a number of different sources: studies of surgical patients, hospitalized patients with chronic illnesses or incapacitating injuries, military personnel exposed to the hazards of combat, civilians exposed to wartime bombing raids or to peacetime disasters, such as industrial explosions, floods, and tornadoes. Against the general background of such information, a detailed study was made of the depth-interview data obtained from a female psychoanalytic patient before and after she was hospitalized for a surgical operation. The primary goal of the psychoanalytic case study was to discover mediating processes which would help to explain the occurrence of stress reactions of the type observed in at least a sizeable minority, if not the majority, of cases exposed to comparable stress situations. The observations of the patient's affective changes, dreams, fantasies, and free associations were subjected to a "microscopic" examination, so to speak, in order to understand better some of the characteristic "macroscopic" reactions to extreme environmental conditions.

In the present chapter, the main inferences derived from the psychoanalytic study are recapitulated. The numbered hypotheses from Chapters 5, 7, 8, 10, 12, 13, 15, and 16 are reproduced so that they can be read consecutively as a general summary of the main theoretical content of Part I. This summary may prove to be especially useful for reference purposes when the reader encounters the frequent allusions to the numbered hypotheses in the chapters of Part II.

Each of the numbered hypotheses is followed by one or more supplementary propositions. The latter are highly tentative hypotheses for which there is, as yet, even less substantiating evidence than for the numbered hypotheses. They are restated here in order to summarize the main assumptions, corollaries, and implications which were presented in the earlier chapters devoted to theoretical discussions of the psychodynamics of stress behavior.

There is a common theme which runs through all the numbered hypotheses and most of the supplementary propositions as well. The common theme pertains to the regressive effects of severe stress experiences and can be formulated as a general theoretical postulate: *In adult life, exposure to any signs of potential mutilation or annihilation will tend to reactivate the seemingly outgrown patterns of emotional response which had originally been elicited and reinforced during the stress episodes of early childhood.*

Whenever a situation of physical danger arises, marked individual differences in affective reactions, unconscious attitudes, and overt regressive behavior are to be expected because of constitutional factors (e.g., innate sensitivity to pain) and unique formative experiences (e.g., actual infantile traumas, unusual circumstances that prevent the child from gaining mastery over recurrent threats, and idiosyncracies in the parent's ways of handling the child's fears, disappointments, and physical suffering). It is assumed, however, that predispositional factors are not the only determinants of stress behavior. That is to say, specific situational factors and general changes in the environment are assumed to play a significant role in increasing or decreasing the probability that one or another type of stress reaction will occur. Most of the hypotheses refer to the effects of situational variables or specify the unconscious psychological changes that are likely to occur, despite differences in predisposition, among a substantial proportion of people exposed to severe physical dangers.

Hypothesis 1A. *Exposure to a threat of body damage (as in the case of an impending surgical operation) tends to sensitize the individual to unacceptable hostile and destructive tendencies in his own aggressive behavior, so that even relatively minor aggressive actions, which are normally tolerated without affective involvement, are consciously or unconsciously felt to be violations of inner superego standards.*

Hypothesis 1B. *Any objective threat of body damage, even though consciously appraised as an event that cannot be influenced by one's own behavior, will tend to be unconsciously assimilated to childhood threats of parental punishment for bad behavior: The individual will strive to mitigate his fate in the same way that, as a child, he succeeded in mitigating the parent's punishment—primarily by controlling his aggression and by making sure that he gives no cause for provoking the maximum penalty.*

Supplementary Propositions

The unconscious assimilation of external threats of physical danger in adult life to childhood threats of parental punishment probably also is a major determinant of two other types of reactions which have been frequently observed in circumstances where large numbers of people are threatened with an impending physical disaster: (*a*) increased adherence to conventional moral standards pertaining to sexual behavior and governing other sorts of pleasurable or self-indulgent activities; and (*b*) the development of new verbal taboos which are consciously felt to be an insurance against "tempting" fate or Providence. Insofar as endangered people are afraid of being unable to control their own destructive aggressive impulses, the anticipatory fear evoked by the external danger situation is augmented by fear of an internal danger. The latter can be regarded as an essentially irrational or neurotic type of fear, especially since people facing physical dangers rarely have much difficulty in inhibiting violent, antisocial, or hostile impulses. In most danger situations, overt aggressive behavior is typically limited to either: (*a*) energetic protective action or (*b*) socially harmless verbal complaints.

Hypothesis 2. *When a person faces an objective threat of body damage, he will spontaneously attempt to alleviate guilt and anxiety by thinking of compensatory gains, the content of which derives from fantasies which functioned as effective reassurances in childhood threat situations.*

Supplementary Propositions

Compensatory fantasies help to bolster the person's decision to face impending danger rather than to turn away from it. Such fantasies may be especially effective in reducing fear because they enable the person to have a conception of himself as an *active participant* rather than as a *passive victim.* By concentrating on anticipated rewards, the impending exposure to danger can come to be regarded as a matter of one's own choosing instead of a wholly undesirable event toward which one is being pushed by external social pressures or by physical restraints.

Hypothesis 3A. *The closer an anticipated threat of body damage is perceived to be (in space or time), the greater will be the individual's motivation to ward off anticipatory fears by minimizing the potential danger or by intellectually denying that he will be seriously affected by it.*

Hypothesis 3B. *When a person attempts to minimize the danger after becoming aware of a potential threat, fear reactions are not extinguished but, rather, are temporarily held in check only so long as no clear-cut signs of danger are brought to his focus of attention.*

Supplementary Propositions

Denial tendencies are manifested by overoptimistic expectations which: (*a*) minimize the probability that the potential danger will actually materialize; (*b*) minimize the magnitude of the potential danger; (*c*) maximize one's own ability to cope with danger; (*d*) maximize one's chances of receiving adequate help from others to mitigate the danger; (*e*) maximize the gains or gratifications to be derived from the potential danger situation. All such attempts at intellectual denial will have the effect of successfully inhibiting overt fear symptoms provided that the denial conceptions are not refuted by external reality signs or called into question by impressive communications from other people. At best, attempts at intellectual denial can succeed only in reducing the total frequency of overt emotional outbursts. Even when a denial conception enables a person to be calm and unconcerned for a long period of time, the predisposition to react with intense fear in response to inescapable signs of impending danger will remain intact as a powerful emotional habit; the full-blown fear reaction can be repeatedly evoked whenever there are external cues which momentarily prevent the person from being convinced that he is unaffected by the danger.

Hypothesis 4. Under conditions where a person is strongly motivated to deny an impending danger, he will tend to rationalize his self-perceptions of residual emotional tension by mislabeling his affective state and attributing it to other, less fear-arousing circumstances.

Supplementary Propositions

Judgments and expectations which tend to deny potential dangers in the future are the joint product of suppression, repression, rationalization, and related adjustment mechanisms which operate together to create and maintain pseudo-optimistic attitudes. In addition to intentionally avoiding information about an impending outer danger and deliberately suppressing thoughts and fantasies about it, a person will display parapraxes, displacements, and other *unintentional* curtailments of his own thought processes which involve some of the same defense mechanisms that are used when one is struggling to ward off neurotic anxiety generated by the inner danger of releasing unacceptable sexual or hostile impulses. Among the unconscious modes of defense which may be used to ward off anticipatory fear of external dangers are the following two interrelated mechanisms: (*a*) *reaction formations* against one's passive submissive tendencies, expressed in fantasies that one will become aggressive, dominant, or stubbornly negativistic and (*b*) *identification with the aggressor*, which involves denying one's own passivity and helplessness by fantasying that one can inflict the feared damage upon others. Rationalizations which displace the apparent source of affect enable a person to escape thinking about the causes of his emotional tension at those crucial times when other adjustment mechanisms momentarily fail to be effective. If denial tendencies are strongly aroused and if the person is momentarily unable to inhibit obvious manifestations of anticipatory fear, he will try to escape thinking about the anticipated danger which is arousing this affect by concentrating his thoughts upon a different source of danger which, from prior learning experiences, he unconsciously or preconsciously anticipates will evoke much less emotional tension.

Hypothesis 5. When faced with potential body damage, a person is likely to experience a reactivation of childhood fears of parental abandonment, as a result of which he will have an unusually high need to be reassured that he is affectionately regarded by love objects and by other persons upon whom he is emotionally dependent.

Supplementary Propositions

Regressive fears of parental abandonment constitute a major source of motivation underlying a variety of changes in social behavior which characteristically occur during periods when dangers or deprivations are anticipated—heightening of primary group cohesiveness, increased valuation placed on relationships with authority figures, and a general upsurge of interest in symbols and tokens of one's affiliative connections with formal groups and with the social community at large. The wish for reassurance about not being abandoned by love objects is likely to be a dominant latent theme in the dreams and free associations of a surgical patient.

Hypothesis 6. When a person is motivated to approach (i.e., tolerate or move toward) a threatening situation of potential body damage, the arousal of repressed fears of childhood dangers will have substantially the same effect as the arousal of reality-based fears (i.e., fears determined by conscious appraisal of the current dangers) with respect to: (a) *increasing the probability of overt avoidance behavior and* (b) *increasing the degree of vacillation, tension, and other manifestations of acute conflict even when the approach tendencies remain unequivocally dominant over the heightened avoidance tendencies.*

Supplementary Propositions

Repressed childhood fears reactivated by an external threat of body damage will summate with reality-oriented expectations of danger, so that the strength of avoidance motivation is determined by the combined intensity of the two sources of fear. Both repressed and nonrepressed components of fear will be aroused to varying degrees whenever a person is in the presence of an external threat of body damage.

When a person intellectually believes that only very low risks are entailed in facing the danger but, nevertheless, feels strongly impelled to run away, or becomes hesitant about what to do, the conflict is attributable to a powerful component of repressed fear. In such instances, an extraordinarily strong attempt at intellectual denial and various other efforts (e.g., fantasies of compensatory rewards) may be made in order to overcome a socially unacceptable impulse to take flight. The probability that an objective threat of body damage will reactivate repressed childhood fears of mutilation is increased if the person retains, as a special form of unresolved Oedipal conflict, the following two motivational tendencies: (*a*) an unmodified hostile attitude toward the like-sexed parent, as manifested by openly hostile actions and hostile daydreams directed toward the parent or parent-surrogates, and (*b*) a high level of latent guilt and anxiety concerning the execution of acts in line with his or her sex role, as manifested by overt inhibitions of sexual functions and symptoms of overt anxiety in interpersonal relationships with sex objects. In general, an objective threat of body damage will tend to evoke overestimation of the danger and inappropriate fear reactions ("neurotic anxiety") to the degree that it reactivates repressed childhood fears of being mutilated as a punitive retaliation for forbidden hostile and erotic impulses directed toward the parents.

Hypothesis 7. *When an objective threat of body damage is anticipated, the greater the degree to which repressed fear is aroused the lower the probability that sustained emotional relief will ensue as a result of reassuring communications from authoritative persons who are regarded as credible sources of information.*

Supplementary Propositions

Misunderstandings of authoritative communications, apperceptive distortions of reality signs of danger, errors of judgment, and autistically determined attitudes of overoptimism or overpessimism are much more likely to occur when an avoidance motivation of a given strength is based on a comparatively large component of repressed fear than when it is based largely on fear stimulated by reality-based estimates of the magnitude and probability of the external danger. Cognitive errors are most likely to occur in those neurotic personalities whose conflictful Oedipal strivings are symbolically gratified by a latent fantasy of possessing a secret body organ or appendage, illicitly obtained against the wishes of one or both parents. Such persons, when confronted with an objective threat of body damage, are predisposed to develop exaggerated fears that are relatively impervious to corrective information.

Hypothesis 8A. *In adult life, when danger to body integrity is perceived to be imminent, the emotional attitudes which develop toward danger-control authorities are largely determined by transference reactions which give rise to reality-distorting apperceptions and judgments.*

Hypothesis 8B. *The main components of the transferred attitudes derive from early life experiences in which one (or both) of the parents had been perceived as being responsible for the onset and termination of suffering or deprivation and typically include the following:* (a) *overestimation of the authority's personal power to increase or decrease the amount of exposure to danger;* (b) *excessive uncertainty and preoccupation as to whether the authority's intentions are benevolent or malevolent;* (c) *heightened dependency on the authority (i.e., increased need for direct or symbolic contact with the authority, combined with greater sensitivity to the authority's communications of approval and disapproval).*

Supplementary Propositions

The category "danger-control authorities" in Hypothesis 8 includes any person who is perceived as having the power either to help or to hinder one's chances of escaping exposure to external danger or of mitigating the degree of stress impact. During a crisis period, the dominant danger-control authority is most likely to be the individual from whom one most frequently receives warnings, directives, and other communications that are regarded as determining one's fate. Irrational fear of a danger-control authority in adult life may occur as a result of a tendency to attribute to the authority hostile and punitive intentions that originally were components of the child's latent attitudes toward the dominant parent, developed at times when internal or external circumstances inclined him to feel threatened by the parent's power over him. Along with the reality-oriented need to be reassured that the authorities will be available in case of emergency, there is also a strong need to counteract an irrational fear-arousing conception of a parent-surrogate. The latter need is a consequence of transference reactions and underlies an adult's efforts to develop a strong affectionate tie with a dominant danger-control authority; it might also give rise to a tendency toward defensive libidinization, which takes the form of "falling in love" with the authority figure or becoming preoccupied with fantasies of an erotic relationship.

Hypothesis 9. *At the termination of an episode of stress impact, the affective status of the person (on a continuum of euphoric versus dy-*

phoric mood) will depend upon whether the amount of perceived suffering and loss (victimization) is more or less than he had consciously expected before the onset of the stress episode: If the amount of victimization is more than had been expected, the mood will tend to be dysphoric; if less than had been expected, the mood will tend to be euphoric (provided that no further impact of severe danger or deprivation is anticipated in the near future).

Supplementary Propositions

The greater the *positive* discrepancy between the magnitude of the threat that had been expected beforehand and the amount of victimization that is subsequently perceived to have occurred ($V_e > V_o$), the greater the degree of poststress euphoria. The greater the *negative* discrepancy ($V_e < V_o$), the greater the degree of poststress dysphoria. When a biphasic stress episode occurs (as in the case of most surgical operations, severe illnesses of acute onset, injuries from industrial accidents, and large-scale community disasters), there will be an emotional sequence of euphoria followed by dysphoria if there is first a positive discrepancy ($V_e > V_o$) at the termination of the initial acute danger phase, followed by a negative discrepancy ($V_e < V_o$) during the second stress phase of prolonged deprivation. Hypothesis 9 and the above supplementary propositions pertaining to the occurrence of euphoric reactions apply only when the danger or deprivation expected in the near future (D_e) is slight or close to zero: If D_e is a substantially high value, dysphoria will tend to occur even when the discrepancy between anticipated and perceived victimization is positive ($V_e > V_o$).

Hypothesis 10. *If the degree of perceived victimization is less than had been expected and if no immediate recurrence of severe danger or deprivation is anticipated, the termination of danger impact will tend to be unconsciously assimilated to the reconciliation experiences of childhood which followed the termination of overt parental punishment; the individual's emotional state will be dominated by reduced guilt from a sense of having paid the penalty for past misbehavior and will involve a relaxation of inner superego demands, with a corresponding increase in self-indulgent behavior.*

Supplementary Propositions

The unconscious processes specified in Hypothesis 10 give rise to a reactive elation which involves genuine emotional relief, characterized by a benign mood of exhilaration, high self-esteem, warm feelings toward persons in the immediate environment, and alternations of energetic motility with calm relaxation. The reduction of superego tension which occurs in this type of reactive elation can result in a temporary remission of obsessive-compulsive behavior and related types of psychoneurotic symptoms. The reactive elation referred to in Hypothesis 10 does *not* include reactions of pseudo elation, which are motivated by a need to counteract thoughts producing depressive affect and which are characterized by inappropriateness of the affect to the external provocation, forced hyperactivity with obvious inability to relax, and momentary breakthroughs of weeping, agitation, or depressive mood. All such symptoms of pseudo elation tend to be relatively absent when a reactive elation is based on an unconscious tendency to equate the termination of an external danger episode in adult life with one's childhood experiences of reconciliation following the termination of parental punishment.

Hypothesis 11A. *If an episode of stress impact produces actual physical suffering and if the degree of perceived victimization is greater than had been expected beforehand, the episode will tend to be unconsciously assimilated to early victimization experiences which had evoked in the child feelings of intense disappointment concerning the behavior of one or both parents. The disappointments that are rearoused stem from painful episodes which had been interpreted by the child as excessive punishment caused by an angry or rejecting parent and which did not terminate in the usual degree of reconciliation.*

Hypothesis 11B. *The reactivated disappointment will be manifested as an "aggrievement" reaction (a combination of rage and grief) and will be externally directed toward danger-control authorities (resentment and retaliation against parent-surrogates) and/or inwardly directed toward the self (lowered self-esteem, self-punitive asceticism, feelings of hopelessness).*

Supplementary Propositions

Every person experiences a variety of victimization episodes during childhood and retains various emotional habits as residues of such episodes. There are at least three basic types of childhood victimization episodes, which can be differentiated according to the way they affect the cohesiveness of the child's relationship to one or both parents.

Type I. Extreme Augmentation of Cohesiveness. A punishment or deprivation episode which deviates from the norm (see Type II) in that its termination evokes in the child an exceptionally high degree of affection and amiability toward one or both parents.

Type II. The Normal Degree of Cohesiveness. The average punishment or deprivation episode during childhood, eliciting neither an exceptionally high nor low degree of cohesiveness.

Type III. Extreme Diminution of Cohesiveness. Unusually severe or unexpected victimization experiences giving rise to estrangement or withdrawal from one or both parents.

The emotional reaction patterns aroused by any one of the three types can be reactivated by any stress episode in adult life, depending upon the predispositions created by childhood relationships with the parents and the current situational factors. Hypothesis 11 specifies one major class of current situational factors which augment the probability that Type III reactions will be more likely to be reactivated than Type I or Type II in any given person (i.e., when predispositions are held constant).

Hypothesis 12A. *Given a stress episode of unexpectedly high victimization* ($V_e < V_o$), *the probability that disappointment reactions will take the form of externalized rage toward danger-control authorities (or toward other parent-surrogates) will be increased by the presence of any external cues which tend to reactivate childhood experiences of resentment against the parents for unwarranted punishment.*

Hypothesis 12B. *The effective cues which tend to reactivate childhood resentment experiences include any action or inaction on the part of a danger-control authority which is perceived as deficient behavior and which resembles the apparent deficiencies of one's parents at times when seemingly unfair, excessive, or undeserved punishment was inflicted.*

Supplementary Propositions

It is assumed that there are at least two main subtypes of childhood aggrievement situations (Type III in the discussion of Hypothesis 11 above), each of which produces low cohesiveness, but with quite different consequences for the child:

Type IIIA. Active Alienation. Unusually severe or unexpected victimization experiences which elicit indignation or animosity in the child, thus resulting in a temporary lowering of motivation for cohesiveness with the parents; the parents are felt to be unfair or blameworthy but the child remains sufficiently confident about their basic affectionate attitude to allow himself the risk of aggressively protesting or retaliating for their "bad" behavior.

Type IIIB. Passive Estrangement. Unusually severe or unexpected victimization experiences as a result of which the child perceives the parents as having withdrawn or abandoned him and he develops feelings of hopelessness ("primal grief") concerning the prospects of being reunited.

Whenever emotional reactions of Type IIIA or IIIB are reactivated by a stress episode in adult life, the person will tend to display some degree of anger against parent-surrogates and will also display some loss of self-esteem. But, in so far as the disappointment experiences involve a reactivation primarily of Type IIIA, externalized aggression will tend to be a more dominant reaction than depression. Hypothesis 12 specifies some of the conditions under which a stress episode is more likely to reactivate Type IIIA than Type IIIB. As an explanatory hypothesis, it is most directly applicable to those situations in which a person displays irrational resentment and unprovoked rage following the termination of danger or deprivation. Individual differences in sensitivity to ostensible errors and signs of misbehavior on the part of danger-control authorities are partly a consequence of exposure to idiosyncratic patterns of parental punishment, which give rise to differences in the sets of cues evoking Type IIIA reactions. Certain types of cues, however, are likely to be the product of relatively homogeneous patterns of parental punishment within our culture, based on widely shared social norms concerning "fair" or "warranted" punishment, and are therefore likely to operate as effective reactivating cues for most persons in modern society: (*a*) The danger-control authority fails to give advance warning about the magnitude of the punishment (i.e., about the danger or deprivation that actually materializes) or fails to give any prior information as to how one can avert it; (*b*) the danger-control authority misinterprets or refuses to acknowledge one's special efforts to be "good" (i.e., to conform with authoritative demands and wishes); (*c*) the danger-control authority shows little interest in observing or obtaining information about the magnitude of one's subjective suffering; (*d*) the danger-control authority, although generally continuing to act in accordance with his protective role, refuses to listen to one's protests or unsympathetically rejects one's personal plea for aid or reassurance. In so far as different subcultural, social, religious, or ethnic groups adhere to different social norms regulating parental punishment practices, there will be correspondingly different sensitivities to the apparent deficiencies of danger-control authorities during stress episodes in adult life.

Hypothesis 13A. *Given a stress episode of unexpectedly high victimization* ($V_e < V_o$), *the probability that the disappointment reaction will take the form of acute depression will be increased by any external cues which tend to reactivate childhood episodes of hopeless grief in which the child felt that it "deserved" to be punished and thought it was being physically abandoned* (*isolated*) *or psychologically abandoned* (*irrevocably rejected*) *by its parents.*

Hypothesis 13B. *The set of effective cues which tend to reactivate childhood experiences of hopeless grief includes any signs of abandonment by parent-surrogates, i.e., sustained physical isolation from affectionate persons or occurrences which are perceived as the product of their sustained rejection.*

Hypothesis 13C. *The probability of exposure to signs of abandonment, as specified in Hypothesis 13B, is a function of the temporal duration of the stress episode:* (i) *The longer the duration of a deprivational episode involving physical confinement or low mobility, the greater the degree of actual and perceived separation from most or all persons in one's prestress milieu, including those who function as affectionate parent-surrogates;* (ii) *the longer the duration of suffering and deprivation, the higher the frequency of apparent failures on the part of the danger-control authorities to mitigate discomfort and to produce the expected rewards for conforming with their demands; hence, the greater the likelihood that they will be perceived as unappeasable parental figures who have withdrawn their power to alleviate suffering.*

Supplementary Propositions

Using the same two hypothetical subtypes of childhood aggrievement experiences referred to above (Type IIIA and Type IIIB), it is assumed that, when the latter is reactivated, reactions of depression tend to be more dominant than reactions of externalized resentment. Some of the conditions under which a stress episode is more likely to reactivate Type IIIB than Type IIIA are specified by Hypothesis 13. This hypothesis is most directly applicable for explaining the seemingly disproportionate feelings of hopelessness, acute grief, and low self-esteem which persist after a stress episode even when the person intellectually acknowledges that he expects his suffering will soon be over and that he will probably experience little or no residual loss. Hypersensitivity to apparent signs of abandonment by parent-surrogates is especially likely to occur whenever guilt is stimulated by authoritative information to the effect that current suffering is attributable to one's own shortcomings or past misbehavior. Self-recriminations are augmented if the person realizes that he has recently engaged in any form of "misbehavior" which violates his own moral code. The probability of a Type IIIB reactivation during the second (deprivation) phase of a biphasic stress episode is increased if the termination of the first (acute danger) phase had elicited a temporary state of elation during which the person engaged in unconventional and self-indulgent behavior: The greater the relaxation of superego controls while celebrating the termination of the initial acute danger phase, the greater the chances of developing guilt feelings and becoming hypersensitive to apparent cues of parental abandonment during the subsequent phase of prolonged deprivation.

Hypothesis 14. *Exposure to any stress episode involving the threat of body damage will facilitate the revival of disturbing childhood memories which, up to that time, had been wholly or partially repressed. Thus, a person's early memories of danger episodes are more likely to be unrepressed under conditions where fear is strongly aroused by signs of approaching danger or deprivation than under ordinary, relatively stress-free conditions.*

Supplementary Propositions

The unrepression phenomenon specified in Hypothesis 14 does not appear to be attributable to a relaxation of superego censorship because it occurs at times when superego anxiety is relatively high, e.g., before the operation and during the depressive phase of convalescence. The phenomenon may be accounted for on the basis of one or more of the following explanatory hypotheses:

1. *The weakening of ego defenses* resulting from exposure to stress conditions may reduce the efficiency of internal censorship to the point where traumatic memories and associated screen memories can break through into consciousness.
2. The recall of disturbing past experiences that are ordinarily unavailable to consciousness may be facilitated by *the reinstatement of external (threat) cues and internal (emotional) cues* which occur during exposure to a current stress episode; the occurrence of such cues may help to overcome the usual obstacles that interfere with recall of past episodes of danger or deprivation.
3. Exposure to impending danger may increase the person's *efforts*

to mitigate anticipated punishment by confessing, and thereby renouncing, old grudges or resentments against a parental figure which had been harbored in unmodified form since childhood. The recollection and renunciation of repressed "grudge" memories may be dependent upon the momentary strength of the person's need to seek expiation.

4. *The need for reassurances about surviving or escaping from impending danger* may provide a powerful motivation to recall analogous horrifying experiences from the past, which entail the recollection of instances when the person had: (*a*) mastered the situation; (*b*) managed to survive despite exposure to extreme danger; or (*c*) experienced intense anticipatory fears which subsequently had proved to be unwarranted.

The unrepression phenomenon specified by Hypothesis 14 might contribute to therapeutic progress in the long run (if the person is undergoing psychotherapeutic treatment), but it does not necessarily lead to any abatement of psychoneurotic symptoms, nor to any immediate therapeutic progress, inasmuch as the person may be unable to assimilate and use the gain in self-insight obtained from the unrepression of childhood memories or fantasies.

Part two

Behavioral Research

18.

Scope and theoretical background

This chapter describes the purpose and general theoretical orientation of the behavioral research studies to be reported in the following seven chapters. The first part of the chapter is devoted to discussing the major reaction variables and the general hypotheses on which the studies were centered. In the second part of the chapter an attempt is made to show how the hypotheses are linked with various psychodynamic formulations derived from the psychoanalytic case material.

Major Reaction Variables

In the first part of this book a large number of hypotheses were extracted by examining psychoanalytic case data against the general background of prior research on stress behavior. A very wide range of emotional reactions, thought processes, and defense mechanisms were scrutinized in order to arrive at as comprehensive a picture as possible of adjustment to external physical dangers and deprivations. The hypotheses summarized in Chapter 17 refer to many different aspects of stress behavior and take account of a large number of variables which are assumed to affect personal adjustment during one or another stage of surgical experiences. In contrast, the behavioral research to which we now turn is of much narrower scope. It is concentrated almost entirely on two reaction variables which appear to be of fundamental importance in adjustment to stress and which can be investigated systematically with a relatively high degree of reliability and validity: (*a*) *Fear of body damage*, as manifested by verbalized attitudes of apprehensiveness, overt signs of emotional tension, and overt attempts to execute protective actions; and (*b*) *externalized anger*, as manifested by verbalized attitudes of resentment toward persons in the immediate environment, outbursts of rage, and overt acts of opposition or resistance to the demands of danger-control personnel.

These two general variables were singled out for special investigation because of their outstanding significance in current psychodynamic theory and also because of their relatively high frequency of occurrence.[1] While making observations on the surgical wards of a typical community hospital, the author noted that these two types of reaction were the most frequent forms of "problem behavior" encountered within the normal range of patients who were hospitalized for major operations. To convey the psychological significance attached to these two reaction variables in the postoperative adjustment of surgical patients, it is necessary to anticipate some of the findings which emerged from the series of case studies and from the survey research. (The methods and procedures used in those studies are described in the next chapter.) During the postoperative recovery phase, the dominant reaction in most surgical patients was found to be a relatively optimistic and generally benign emotional state. The over-all incidence of overt manifestations of depression, anger, apprehensiveness, or any other form of emotional agitation proved to be relatively low—quite remarkably so in view of the severity of the discomforts, physical assaults, and frustrations to which the patients were continually subjected.

For many days, and possibly for weeks, a convalescing patient finds himself in a world dominated by more or less impersonal caretakers who invariably fail to satisfy fully his intense need for relief from suffering and his perpetual longing for social stimulation to counteract anxiety and boredom. To make matters even worse, the caretakers repeatedly demand submission to painful, disagreeable, and embarrassing manipulations. Needles are jabbed into the patient's arms; probes, swabs, or drainage tubes are poked into sensitive wounds; stomach tubes are inserted through the nose and down into the throat; evil tasting medicine is poured into his mouth; bed pans are shoved under his buttocks and belatedly removed—these and a variety of other disagreeable demands and indignities are imposed upon him at a time when he is already in a state of general malaise, beset by incision pains, backaches, sore muscles, headaches, distended bowels, constipation, and perhaps a generous spread of angrily itching skin. Some discomforts remain for hours at a time, others are limited to excruciating moments of unnerving pain, but always there is one or another source of harassment. The series of overlapping and recurrent noxious stimuli goes on day after day, seemingly without letup, as the patient slowly regains his health. In addition, there are multiple frustrations which also contribute heavily to the patient's distressing mode of existence. Among the major sources of frustrations are lengthy periods of imposed inactivity, unappetizing meals, separation from friends and loved ones, unavailability of normal sexual gratifications, partial loss of one's status prerogatives, and almost complete loss of autonomy over one's daily activities.

Despite all the disagreeable features of the recovery period, the average surgical patient was generally found to be extraordinarily uncomplaining and in a cheerful mood most of the time. In general, the patients were warmly friendly toward their fellow convalescents, extremely grateful to physicians and nurses, and willing to adhere to almost all medical orders. In fact, they typically conformed in such a conscientious manner that their attitude could often be described as one of childlike dependency upon the danger-control authorities (see discussion of Hypothesis 8, pp. 134–138, and the descriptive material given below on pp. 305–313). The degree to which the typical convalescing surgical patient tacitly accepts the role of a docile child can hardly be appreciated until one sees what happens when a young nurse, perhaps fifteen or twenty years the patient's junior, offers a routine compliment after giving a penicillin shot. An expression of unembarrassed delight can be elicited by the nurse time and time again by her mere assertion, in a conventionalized sing-song voice, that the patient is a "good girl!" or "good boy!"

This pattern of optimism and conformity is the dominant one in that it characterizes the behavior of most postoperative patients most of the time. But there is, of course, a sizeable minority who repeatedly display negative reactions. Two outstanding deviant groups of patients were noted. One consisted of individuals who showed the dominant pattern much of the time but, superimposed on it, were disruptive outbursts of excessive fearfulness, sometimes combined with mild depression. Even though these patients were extremely docile and eager to conform with all authoritative demands, they appeared to be excessively timid and acutely upset by routine postoperative procedures, shrinking back apprehensively whenever the time came to submit to a medical or nursing treatment. Occasionally the anxiety of such a patient would become so intense as to be regarded by the hospital staff as a definite interference with the patient's physical recovery, especially when the patient's timidity made it difficult to administer essential procedures.

Among a second minority group of deviants, a different type of behavior predominated, namely, resentful anger. From the standpoint of the hospital staff, these patients were the "real problem children" on the surgical ward, their actions and words being notoriously different from those of the placidly cooperative patients who comprised the majority. The behavior of this second minority group was also quite different from that of the apprehensive group, who were likely to be regarded as idyllically passive conformists at times when no physically intrusive treatments were proffered. The resentful group included a wide range of overtly negativistic patients; the mildest cases consisted of convalescents who often complained about their treatment and, from time to time, behaved in an obviously irritable, complaining manner toward the nurses and orderlies. The more extreme cases consisted of continually morose patients, who were generally regarded as sullen, unfriendly, and liable to lose their tempers. Such patients were apt, from time to time, to become dramatically negativistic, suddenly refusing to permit routine procedures from being carried out.

Both types of deviant reactions are of considerable concern to a hospital staff, not only because of the management difficulties they create but also because of the unpredictability of their emotional behavior.[2] Out of all proportion to the apparent degree of provocation, anxiety attacks or angry resentment sometimes will unexpectedly flare up in convalescents who, prior to the operation, had been calm, cheerful and friendly.

Quite aside from the practical problems of surgical case management, important theoretical problems are posed by the two types of postoperative emotional disturbance. The main purpose of the behavioral studies to be discussed in the next seven chapters is to expand our present understanding of stress behavior by seeking to discover the factors that play a major role in augmenting or diminishing postoperative fear and anger.

General Hypotheses

The two types of acute emotional disturbances were investigated in relation to antecedent behavior tendencies that were manifested preoperatively; that is, prior to the onset of the phase of maximal physical stress. One major antecedent factor that was systematically studied was the *level of anticipatory fear.* In the course of carrying out the series of case studies on the surgical wards, the author was impressed by the fact that, following the operation, the most extreme forms of emotional disturbance appeared to be concentrated in those patients who, before the operation, had shown either an exceptionally low degree or an exceptionally high degree of anticipatory fear. This observation implies that there is a curvilinear relationship between the level of anticipatory fear and subsequent capacity to tolerate actual stress stimuli. The following general hypothesis is suggested:

Hypothesis 15. *Persons who display a moderate degree of anticipatory fear before being exposed to physical stress stimuli (pain, bodily discomforts, and severe deprivations) will be less likely to develop emotional disturbances during or after the stress exposure than those persons who display either a very high degree or a very low degree of anticipatory fear.*

It was noted that the patients who had displayed little or no fear before the operation tended to develop a different form of postoperative disturbance than those who had displayed extremely severe preoperative fear.

Absence of fear reactions during the few days preceding the surgery appeared to bear a marked relationship to subsequent reactions of anger and resentment during the postoperative period. In contrast, the patients who were extremely fearful before the operation again showed excessive fearfulness afterwards. Thus, the case observations strongly suggested the following two general hypotheses:

Hypothesis 16. *Persons who display an extremely high level of anticipatory fear or anxiety during the "threat" period will be more likely than others to display intense fear of body damage during the subsequent crisis period, when exposed to actual stress stimuli.*

Hypothesis 17. *Persons who display an extremely low degree of anticipatory fear or anxiety during the "threat" period will be more likely than others to display reactions of anger and resentment toward danger-control authorities during the subsequent crisis period, when exposed to actual stress stimuli.*

Unlike the psychodynamic hypotheses presented earlier and summarized in Chapter 17, the above three hypotheses are phenomenologically descriptive propositions. Both the antecedent and consequent variables refer to emotional states or attitudes that are readily accessible to observation (or that can be directly inferred from obvious behavioral manifestations) and no explanatory concepts are introduced into the propositions to refer to mediating psychological processes.[3] Testable predictions can be made from the three hypotheses concerning the behavioral sequelae of moderate, high, and low levels of anticipatory fear. If confirmed, the descriptive hypotheses would carry some potential implications for the dynamics of stress behavior and would help to sharpen the focus of research on certain of the mediating psychological processes discussed earlier in connection with the psychoanalytic case material.

Theoretical Background

Some of the complicated factors affecting the relationship between preoperative fear and postoperative adjustment can be inferred from several different psychodynamic hypotheses, especially those presented in Chapters 7, 10, and 15. For instance, according to Hypothesis 6, persons in whom repressed childhood fears are reactivated by slight threats of actual danger will tend to react as though they were facing an enormous danger, displaying intense emotional agitation and overt efforts to escape from the danger situation. In the discussion of this hypothesis (pp. 110–120), reference was made to a certain type of neurotic predisposition which makes for a relatively high probability that repressed childhood fears of being mutilated will be reactivated by any environmental threat of body damage encountered in adult life. Persons with such predispositions would presumably react with an exceptionally high degree of apprehensiveness during the precrisis period when the dangers of surgery are anticipated, and, again, when threatening stress stimuli occur during the postoperative crisis period itself. Moreover, Hypothesis 7 introduced the additional notion that such persons cannot gain the usual degree of emotional relief from the reassurances given by authoritative persons. Thus, from these hypotheses, one would expect to find a class of neurotically predisposed persons who react to the dangers of surgery with excessive apprehensiveness ("neurotic fear"), both before and after the operation. In such persons, the underlying source of anxiety would remain unconscious and their fear reactions would tend to persist, despite the reassurances given by physicians and nurses, as long as the danger of body damage was hanging over them.

The psychodynamic hypotheses to which reference has just been made could provide a consistent theoretical rationale to account for the relationship between exceptionally high preoperative fear and exceptionally high postoperative fear, as specified by Hypothesis 16; but, these propositions provide no cogent basis for explaining the relationship between low preoperative fear and high postoperative anger, as specified by Hypothesis 17. In fact, from what was said in the above discussion, one might be led to expect quite a different relationship, namely, the lower the degree of fear before the operation, the higher the probability of emotional equanimity after the operation. This generalization, which obviously contradicts Hypothesis 17, is *not* a necessary implication of Hypothesis 6 or 7, or of any of the supplementary hypotheses concerning the arousal of repressed fears, all of which refer only to one end of the fear continuum; they designate how persons with very extreme fear reactions (R_F) differ from those with milder degrees of fear. These hypotheses make no reference to the possible differences between persons with moderate degrees of preoperative fear (R_M) and those who are relatively unafraid (R_U); nor do they have anything to say about symptoms of postoperative emotional disturbance other than excessive apprehensiveness.

We turn now to a number of other psychodynamic hypotheses which do provide theoretical concepts pertinent to the relationship specified by Hypothesis 17. First of all, Hypothesis 3B asserts that, when a person manages to ward off anticipatory fear or anxiety by discounting the impending danger, his efforts at intellectual denial will succeed only so long as *no salient danger stimuli are present* (see pp. 74 ff.). If lack of preoperative fear is partly or wholly attributable to such defensive tendencies, one would certainly not expect those patients who are unafraid before their surgical operations to remain free from emotional disturbance when they subsequently encounter pains and other salient stress stimuli during the postoperative crisis period. But how intense is the subsequent emotional disturbance likely to be? And what forms will it take? Such questions cannot be answered from Hypothesis 3B alone. Some pertinent theoretical leads are provided, however, by the hypotheses presented in the chapter dealing with postoperative dysphoria and aggrievement reactions (see, especially, pp. 163–168). According to Hypothesis 9, the affective status of a patient during the postoperative period is partially dependent upon what his expectations were during the preoperative period: a dysphoric mood will tend to occur if one experiences *more suffering than had been expected beforehand.* Patients with very low anticipatory fear will subsequently experience more dysphoria than others if there is a marked disparity between the low amount of suffering expected and the great amount of suffering they actually undergo during the postoperative period. Furthermore, according to Hypothesis 11, a dominant consequence of this disparity will be an *aggrievement reaction* which derives its intensity from the *reactivation of childhood disappointments in one's parents.* Thus, it may be that the stage becomes set for an exceptionally dramatic crisis reaction of dysphoric aggrievement if, during the precrisis period, one successfully wards off anticipatory fear by indulging in overoptimistic beliefs and fantasies which greatly minimize the amount of suffering to be expected.

Hypothesis 12 is also of some relevance because it specifies the conditions under which externalized rage and resentment toward danger-control authorities will tend to occur. This hypothesis introduces additional considerations which might also help to explain the relationship between low preoperative fear and high postoperative anger. For example, one of the conditions to which this hypothesis refers is *absence of advance warnings from danger-control authorities.* This condition was assumed to be one of the apparent forms of deficient behavior which can become an effective cue with respect to reactivating childhood resentment experiences (see pp. 169–171). A surgical patient's low level of preoperative fear (and his failure to correct wishful, overoptimistic expectations) might sometimes be a consequence of inadequate or misleading communications from physicians or nurses. If so, the postoperative resentment might be partly explained in terms of a psychological reaction to apparently deficient behavior on the part of the danger-control authorities, as formulated in Hypothesis 12.

Finally, it should be mentioned that the formulations of Hypotheses 3, 9, 11, and 12 were influenced by Freud's theoretical comments concerning the way in which anticipatory fear or anxiety may be linked with ability to master fright-producing stimuli.

> "Anxiety" describes a particular state of expecting the danger or preparing for it, even though it may be an unknown one. . . .
>
> "Fright," however, is the name we give to the state a person gets into when he has run into danger without being prepared for it; it emphasizes the factor of surprise. . . . There is something about anxiety that protects its subject against fright and so against fright-neuroses. (S. Freud, 1950, p. 10.)

Later on, when the case study and survey results are presented, it will become apparent that the research bearing on Hypotheses 15, 16, and 17 add further substance to Freud's formulations concerning the protective value of psychological preparation for danger. It will also be seen that the findings implicate additional theoretical notions that have been introduced in the subsequent elaborations of Freud's theory of psychological trauma by other psychoanalysts. And, as has already been indicated, the research findings concerning the postoperative behavioral sequelae of different levels of preoperative fear help to elucidate the various psychodynamic hypotheses referred to in the preceding paragraphs. For the present it will suffice merely to repeat a central point of the above discussion, namely, that the three main hypotheses on which the behavioral research was focused, although formulated as phenomenologically descriptive propositions, may have direct theoretical implications for a psychodynamic analysis of stress behavior.

Notes

1. Kardiner and H. Spiegel make the following statement about the importance of fear and anger:

"... there were two features which appeared in all [observed cases of psychological trauma], either in attenuated or violent form—(1) fear and anxiety, and (2) the mobilization of organized aggression with or without the accompanying affect of rage. Fear and anxiety belong to the affects resulting from an appraisal of the threatening situation, the rage is related to the mobilization of organised mastery techniques to circumvent the danger situation and to permit the organism to continue its existence ... no situation becomes traumatic unless either of these two functions—the perception of danger or the organized combat against the threatening stimulus—fails." (Kardiner and H. Spiegel, 1947, pp. 181–182.)

Many contributors to the scientific literature on psychological stress place a similar emphasis on the importance of fear and anger in relation to a person's attempts to cope with environmental dangers (Basowitz et al., 1955; Cantril, 1940 and 1943; W. Menninger, 1946 and 1952; Rado, 1950; Titchener et al., 1956; Wilson, 1941; M. Wolfenstein, 1957; Wolff, 1953).

2. Some studies on the psychological aspects of stress behavior suggest that severe emotional upset may give rise to greater sensitivity to pain and delay a patient's recovery from somatic injuries (F. Dunbar, 1942; Lidz and Fleck, 1950; Malmo and Shagass, 1949a and 1949b; Senn, 1945).

3. Hypotheses 15, 16, and 17 can be reformulated in the following schematic way: Under conditions of direct exposure to a given set of physical stress stimuli (S_P), the occurrence of emotional equanimity (R_E) and of the two types of deviant emotional reactions, excessive fear (R_F) and excessive anger (R_A), can be predicted from antecedent behavior, viz., by observing whether during the precrisis period the person was moderately fearful (R_M), highly fearful (R_F), or relatively unfearful (R_U) in response to external signs of threat (S_T). Thus, the three hypotheses can be represented by the following formulae:

If $S_T \rightarrow R_M$, then $S_P \rightarrow R_E$.
If $S_T \rightarrow R_F$, then $S_P \rightarrow R_F$.
If $S_T \rightarrow R_U$, then $S_P \rightarrow R_A$.

For any group of people exposed to a given set of threat stimuli (S_T), the level of anticipatory fear is assumed to be a continuum ranging from extreme fearfulness (R_F) at one end to comparative absence of fearfulness (R_U) at the other. Persons who display a *moderate* degree of anticipatory fear (R_M) fall somewhere in the intermediate range of the continuum. When this assumption is made, Hypothesis 15 can be regarded as a corollary implied by Hypotheses 16 and 17. Specifically, the two hypotheses carry the following implication: The probability that $S_P \rightarrow R_F$ or R_A will be lower if, previously, $S_T \rightarrow R_M$ than if $S_T \rightarrow R_F$ or R_U.

In later chapters, and especially in Chapter 25, it will become apparent that the emotional response a person shows to S_T can sometimes be decreased or increased by exposure to auxiliary stimuli, such as communications from others that describe positive or negative aspects of the oncoming danger. A surgical patient who has been given only reassuring communications (S_X) may react quite differently when an authority figure gives him a precise description of the unpleasant features of the operation (S_Y) or if a neighbor relays frightening rumors about all the possible things that can go wrong (S_Z). Thus, it might happen that for the very same person:

$$S_T \text{ plus } S_X \rightarrow R_U$$
$$S_T \text{ plus } S_Y \rightarrow R_M$$
$$S_T \text{ plus } S_Z \rightarrow R_F$$

19.

Methods: case studies and survey research

The main purpose of this chapter is to describe the research methods and procedures used to investigate the hypotheses discussed in the preceding chapter. A detailed account is given of the way in which the intensive case studies were conducted in the surgical wards of a large community hospital, describing the main features of: (*a*) the standardized interviews conducted by the author; (*b*) the behavioral records made by nurses and physicians; and (*c*) the procedures used in assessing the data on each patient's emotional reactions and adjustment before and after the operation. In addition, this chapter includes a brief summary of the procedures used in a questionnaire survey on the surgical experiences of several hundred male adolescents who had undergone recent major or minor operations. Finally, a few statements are made to indicate how the correlations derived from the survey research were used to test the hypotheses which had emerged from the case studies data.

Intensive Case Studies

By special arrangement with the chief of the surgical service at the Grace-New Haven Community Hospital, the author was permitted to conduct intensive interviews with a series of patients hospitalized on the surgical wards. The study was conducted over a five-month period and included all interviewable patients who were hospitalized on the ward for routine surgery during that time period. It was necessary to exclude three types of patients from the sample: (*a*) patients with active tuberculosis or other contagious diseases; (*b*) patients in an abnormal mental state because of brain pathology, drug administration, or a recent traumatic accident; (*c*) patients who were unable to speak English sufficiently well to be interviewed. Only these three types of patients were left out of the series; otherwise, the sample was an unselected group of surgical ward patients.

Most patients were seen before and after undergoing the operation, thus making it possible to investigate the relationship between the preoperative level of fear and subsequent postoperative adjustment. In addition to the response variables specified in Hypotheses 15, 16, and 17, a number of related responses were also investigated, including verbalized expectations, fantasies, and cognitive judgments which are likely to be a function of the amount and type of authoritative information given to the patient during the preoperative phase. The interviews were conducted in an informal manner but a standardized interview schedule was constructed and regularly used so as to make sure that the main questions would always be worded in the same way.

The Preoperative Interview

The initial interview was generally conducted one or two days before the patient was scheduled to have the operation. Prior to the first contact with the patient, the medical case records were carefully examined. This was done for two separate purposes. First, it enabled the investigator to exclude patients with neuropathic conditions that made them unsuitable for studying normal psychological effects of surgical experiences. Second, it enabled the investigator to familiarize himself with the basic facts about the patient's medical case history which were of value in structuring the interviews.

The head nurse always introduced the interviewer to the patient as a psychologist who was on the hospital staff. The patient was further told that these interviews were a regular procedure now being conducted with practically all patients on the surgical ward. The interviewer then explained that he was already familiar with the patient's medical records and wanted to obtain some additional information.[1]

The beginning of the interview dealt with routine facts and then gradually worked into more subjective matters.

The following key questions were introduced to help assess the patient's preoperative emotional status with respect to anticipatory fear or anxiety:

QUESTION 6: When you think about having the operation, what thoughts or ideas do you have about it?

QUESTION 7: Whenever a person is going to have an operation, there are always some things about it that he or she is worried or concerned about. What are the main things that you are worried or concerned about when you think about having the operation?

QUESTION 8: Before an operation, many people experience some concern about the damage to their bodies which the operation might cause, and they sometimes imagine all sorts of things about it. What sorts of concerns and ideas do you have about the damage that the operation might cause to you?

QUESTION 9: How often during the day do you worry about the operation?

QUESTION 10: Would you say that you feel some fear or anxiety about it? (If "No": Do you have any concern about it?)

QUESTION 14: Are you at all concerned about how you will react emotionally on the day of your operation—about being able to control your emotions?

Some additional questions were designed to elicit responses bearing on the patient's defensive tendencies. Among the special questions introduced to investigate fear-reducing mechanisms were the following:

QUESTION 11: What thoughts do you have at the times when you feel fear or anxiety?

QUESTION 12: At the times when you feel some fear or concern about the operation, what things do you think about in order to get over these feelings?

QUESTION 13: Do you think of any other things which help you at times to keep from feeling too much anxiety or concern about the operation?

QUESTION 19: What do you expect the operation to accomplish for you, in your particular case? (In what particular way will you benefit from it?)

The interview also contained a series of questions concerning the patient's expectations about the nature of the surgical experience he or she was about to undergo. These included specific items concerning various sources of stress as well as a general question about the information received from the physicians and from other sources:

QUESTION 15: What do you actually expect to happen on the day of your operation? I would like you to make the best prediction or the best guess you can about the actual experiences you will have on the day of your operation.

The following questions were asked if not already covered in the spontaneous account.

A. How do you think you will feel when you are taken to the operating room?

B. What do you think you will see when you get there?

C. Do you think that you will see or hear anything that might disturb you?

D. How do you think they will give the anesthetic to you?

E. Do you think that you will be at all conscious during the operation?

F. Do you think that you will have any pain or discomfort *during* the operation? (When? How much?)

G. Where will you be when you awaken?

H. How will you feel when you awaken?

QUESTION 16: As far as you know, how will the operation be performed—what do you think is actually going to be done to you during the operation or treatment?

QUESTION 17: Do you think that you will experience some pain or discomfort after the operation? (When? How much?)

QUESTION 18: You've told me about the things that you expect to happen. Now I would like you to tell me about the things that you have actually been told about the operation. What have you been told about the experiences that you can expect to have during and immediately after the operation? (For each item: Told by whom? Do you think that will be true in your case?)

QUESTION 25: Do you feel that you have as much information about your operation as you would like to have? (If "No": What sort of additional information would you want to have?)

The above questions and several related ones proved to be of value not only for studying the way in which the patient was psychologically prepared for the stressful experiences of surgery but also for obtaining a more complete picture of the patient's preoperative emotional status. These questions were asked toward the end of the interview and occasionally evoked agitated weeping, marked trembling, flushing, sweating, or other obvious manifestations of intense emotional upset. In a few instances the patient's overt behavior while talking about these matters belied his earlier statements concerning how calm or unworried he felt. Even when there was no dramatic display of emotion, valuable information about the patient's emotional state was obtained by observing the facial expressions, motor behavior, and affective responses elicited at the time when he or she was induced to think concretely about unpleasant features of the impending surgery.

Finally, the interview ended with a few questions concerning the patient's attitudes toward the "danger-control authorities" (see pp. 134–135). One of the questions pertained to the nursing staff of the hospital:

QUESTION 24: How about the nurses here on this floor: What is your opinion about them?

It was felt to be inappropriate, however, to ask any direct questions at this time about how the patient appraised the surgeon who would perform the operation. Accordingly the following indirect questions were used:

QUESTION 20: On the basis of your own experience, what is your opinion of doctors in general?
QUESTION 21: How much confidence do you have in doctors?
QUESTION 22: When did you first talk with the doctor who is going to operate on you? How did you feel about that visit?
QUESTION 23: What things have you talked about since the first visit?

These questions regularly elicited elaborate comments about the surgeon, in which the patient expressed value judgments and personal feelings, thus providing at least a rough basis for assessing the patient's preoperative attitude toward the dominant danger-control authority.

The Postoperative Interview

The postoperative interviews were conducted about one week after the operation had been performed. In almost all cases, two postoperative sessions were held, usually on successive days, in order to cover all the questions on the lengthy interview schedule. The questions were focused primarily on five main topics:

Emotional Reactions on the Day of the Operation. An initial series of questions was designed to encourage the patient to give a detailed retrospective account of his or her subjective experiences on the crucial day when the surgery was performed. The main questions were the following:

QUESTION 27: I'd like you to tell me about the experiences you had on the day of your operation, beginning with the period when you were waiting in your room down here, then about being taken upstairs to the operating room, and so on.

After the patient had finished his story, the following questions were asked, if not already covered in the spontaneous account.

A. How did you feel when you were taken to the operating room?
B. What did you see there?
C. Did you see or hear anything that disturbed you?
D. How did they give the anesthetic to you? (Any pain or discomfort?)
E. Did you have any pain or discomfort during the operation?
F. Were you at all conscious during the operation? (If "Yes": What feelings did you have at that time?)
G. Where were you when you woke up?
H. How did you feel when you woke up?

This series was followed by a number of related questions which referred more directly to the patient's emotional reactions:

QUESTION 35: During the hour just before you were taken into the operating room, did you feel at all afraid or worried?
QUESTION 37: During the first few hours after you woke up from the anesthetic, did you feel at all afraid or worried?
QUESTION 38: Was there any other time on the day of your operation when you felt afraid or worried? (When? About what?)
QUESTION 41: Was there any time on the day of your operation when you had difficulty in controlling your emotions? (When? About what?)
QUESTION 42: On the day of the operation, did you at any time do anything or say anything which you feel may not have been the right thing to have done?
QUESTION 49: On the day of your operation did you feel annoyed at any time about anything that happened? (If "Yes": What annoyed you? Did you become angry?)

Efforts to Control Fear on the Day of Operation. Several questions, similar to the ones used in the preoperative interview, were included for the purpose of eliciting retrospective data concerning verbalizable anticipations and fantasies that may have been defensive in character.

QUESTION 31: When you knew that the operation was about to begin, what thoughts and feelings did you have?
QUESTION 32: Did you have any thoughts or ideas at that time which might have helped you from feeling too much worry or anxiety about it?
QUESTION 39: When you felt afraid (or concerned) just before the operation, what things did you think about in order to get over these feelings?
QUESTION 40: Did you think of any other things which may have helped you to keep from feeling too much anxiety or concern about the operation?

Personal Adjustment During the Recovery Phase. The interview included a few direct questions concerning the patient's postoperative mood and emotional reactions to the stresses of the postoperative period:

QUESTION 26: How are you feeling now? (What sort of mood?)
QUESTION 28: *A*. What were the most unpleasant things about the operation? *B*. What other experiences did you have that were unpleasant? (What feelings did you have at that time?)
QUESTION 50: During the last day or so how often have you thought over or repeated in your mind some of the things that happened on the day of your operation? (What things?)
QUESTION 51: *A*. Do you feel at all disturbed or upset at present? *B*. Do you feel at all disturbed when you think about the unpleasant experiences you had in connection with your operation?

These direct questions were supplemented by a number of indirect questions which also elicited pertinent information about the patient's emotional status, fantasies, and adjustment problems. Among the most useful indirect questions were the following:

QUESTION 44: As far as you know, how was the operation performed? What do you think was acutally done to you during the operation?
QUESTION 53: How did you feel about getting out of bed the first time?
QUESTION 64: *A*. Just suppose for a moment that it became necessary for you to have another operation after you recovered from this one. Would you feel at all afraid or worried about it? (More worried than about the one you just had?) *B*. What things would you want to be done differently?

Attitudes Toward Danger-Control Authorities. Included in the postoperative interview were exactly the same five questions about nurses and physicians that had been asked in the preoperative interview (see Questions 20–24, p. 227), thus making it possible to discern the changes in attitude from before to after the operation. In addition, a number of supplementary attitude questions were used. These included a few specific items about the surgeon and some indirect ones concerning the patient's appraisal of the operation, which sometimes evoked negative expressions of resentment or positive expressions of gratitude toward members of the hospital staff:

QUESTION 46: Do you feel that you made the right decision? (If "No": What caused you to change your opinion?)
QUESTION 54: What has the operation accomplished for you, in your particular case? (In what way did you benefit from it?)
QUESTION 56: How often have you seen the surgeon since your operation?
QUESTION 58: What is your opinion of him? (Do you have confidence and trust in him?)
QUESTION 66: In your opinion, how successful was the operation in improving your condition? [2]

Postoperative Dreams: At the very end of the interview, the patient was asked the following question:

QUESTION 67: Can you recall any dream—or any part of a dream—that you have had since the day of your operation?

If the patient gave a positive response, he was encouraged to relate the manifest content in detail. Then the patient was asked to give free associations to the dream elements according to a standard procedure (see pp. 328–329).

Use of Behavioral Observations in Case Records

The preoperative and postoperative interview data were supplemented by behavioral records made by independent observers, viz., the staff physicians and nurses. These records were kept in conformity with routine hospital procedures, giving not only an account of daily activities and habits pertinent to the patient's physical status but also descriptions of actions and verbalizations that appeared to the observer as being relevant to the patient's management on the ward. These descriptions included statements about the patient's sleep disturbances, manifestations of apprehensiveness, verbal complaints, and overt resistance to medical treatment (e.g., refusal to permit a drainage tube to be inserted).

The behavioral records were used primarily as an adjunct to the interview data for the purpose of assessing the two main variables in postoperative adjustment specified in Hypotheses 16 and 17, namely, fear and anger reactions. Moreover, when classifying the patients according to their preoperative level of fear, the behavioral records were also useful as a check on the interviewer's ratings based on his own observations of the patient's verbalizations and emotional behavior during the interview.[3]

Classification of Preoperative Fear Reactions

Altogether thirty surgical patients were interviewed, providing data pertinent to various psychodynamic hypotheses concerning postoperative adjustment. For eight of the ward patients, however, circumstances did not permit the investigator to obtain a complete preoperative or postoperative interview and, consequently, these cases were omitted from the part of the study dealing with the sequelae of preoperative fear or anxiety reactions.[4] The following categories, which were used for investigating Hypotheses 15, 16, and 17, were therefore applied to a total sample of 22 surgical patients:

Extremely High Preoperative Fear

There were five patients in this group, each of whom reported feeling very upset and constantly fearful of the impending operation. According to their own statements in the preoperative interview, they were extremely "worried," "jittery," or "nervous" about the operation. In addition to their own testimony, overt behavioral signs of emotional tension were noted during the preoperative interview—flushing, trembling, startle reactions, and the like. Confirmatory evidence of unusually strong preoperative anxiety was found in the case notes prepared by the staff physicians and nurses. In three of the five patients, the dread of surgery was so intense that they not only had acute anxiety symptoms but actually attempted to refuse or to postpone the operation after having been hospitalized on the surgical ward. In the other two cases, no overt escape behavior was reported but the case records described acute anxiety symptoms, such as outbursts of agitated weeping and insomnia.

Moderate Preoperative Fear

There were nine patients who displayed neither the extreme emotional reactions of the first group nor the relative absence of fear characteristic of the third group. Seven of the nine patients freely admitted feeling apprehensive prior to the operation, and reported that from time to time during the day they had felt worried and had to exert some effort to stop thinking about the fearful aspects of the impending surgery. Two patients claimed at first to be quite unworried about it but both displayed agitated emotional behavior before the interview was over; after showing obvious signs of tension, one of them reluctantly admitted feeling quite concerned about certain aspects of the operation while the other merely said that he preferred not to talk about it. For every one of the nine cases, the records by the staff personnel were consonant with the interviewer's judgment that the patient was a "part-time worrier" who was consciously afraid but was capable of a fairly high degree of emotional control. The case notes indicated that during the preoperative period signs of agitation or tension were occasionally observed in these patients but never any acute emotional outburst. Most of the time these patients had the outward appearance of being fairly calm, especially during the evening and morning hours immediately preceding the operation.

Extremely Low Preoperative Fear

There were eight patients who consistently denied feeling any apprehensiveness about the impending operation. In response to probing questions during the preoperative interview, several of these patients admitted having some slight feelings of concern about extraneous matters, such as the financial loss they would suffer from being away from their work. But all of these patients claimed to be free from worry or concern about the operation itself. As will be seen in the individual case reports presented in the next two chapters, the main attitude expressed in the preoperative interview was "I never think about it" or "There's no reason to worry about it." During the interviews, these patients showed no signs of agitation or tension which would belie their verbal testimony; they consistently spoke in a matter-of-fact manner, even when answering questions which required them to focus on the unpleasant and dangerous aspects of the anticipated operation. The physicians' and nurses' notes uniformly indicated that these patients displayed no symptoms of emotional tension before the operation: they made unusually few demands on the staff, required no sedation, slept well, and ate and drank whatever foods and fluids they were given. They kept themselves occupied during the day in "normal" activities—playing cards, reading, and conversing with visitors or fellow patients.

Within each of the above three categories, there was a fairly wide range of individual differences in age, social background, and medical status. Pertinent background data for the patients in the high, moderate, and low preoperative fear groups are presented in Table 1. There were no consistent or significant differences among the three groups with respect to: (*a*) age; (*b*) sex distribution; (*c*) occupation; (*d*) educational level; (*e*) ethnic-religious background;[5] or (*f*) type of operation. With regard to the last factor, it is noteworthy that the majority in each group underwent surgery requiring an opening in the abdominal or chest wall—operations of the type that give rise to an exceptionally high degree of postoperative pain (Keats, 1956). (This type of operation was undergone by four of the five patients in the "high" group, seven of the nine in the "moderate" group, and six of the eight in the "low" group.) In the three groups there were approximately equal numbers of patients suffering from cancer or other serious diseases requiring exceedingly drastic or dangerous operations. Additional information from the case records indicated that there were no significant group differences with respect to the following major aspects of the patients' medical status: (*a*) Diagnosis of the condition or illness for which the surgery was prescribed; (*b*) duration of the preoperative illness or impairment; (*c*) frequency and intensity of preoperative pain; (*d*) medical prognosis before the operation; (*e*) occurrence of organic complications during the postoperative recovery period; (*f*) frequency and intensity of postoperative pain; (*g*) degree of success of the surgery and general postoperative prognosis.

The fact that the three groups did not differ markedly with respect to any of the above-mentioned factors is of considerable importance

Table 1. Case Study Series: Background Information

Code No.	Level of Preoperative Fear	Age	Sex	Occupation	Ethnic and Religious Background	Educational Level	Type of Operation
				High Fear Group			
H–1	High	31	Fem.	Housewife	Amer. Protestant Negro	7th grade	Hernia repair
H–2	High	37	Fem.	Housewife	Amer. Protestant	Some H. S.	Lung lobectomy
H–3	High	46	Fem.	Housewife	Amer. Catholic	H. S. grad.	Lung lobectomy
H–4	High	43	Male	Salesman	Greek Orthodox	Some H. S.	Cholecystectomy
H–5	High	45	Male	Physician	Amer. Jewish	M.D. degree	Repair of intervertebral disc
				Moderate Fear Group			
M–1	Moderate	29	Fem.	Housewife	Amer. Protestant	Some H. S.	Lung lobectomy
M–2	Moderate	62	Fem.	Housewife	Polish Catholic	H. S. grad.	Esophageal diverticulectomy
M–3	Moderate	26	Fem.	H. S. teacher	Amer. Jewish	M.A. degree	Excision of mammary cyst
M–4	Moderate	30	Fem.	Housewife	Amer. Catholic	Some H. S.	Hernia repair
M–5	Moderate	73	Fem.	Housewife	Amer. Protestant	H.S. grad.	Subtotal gastrectomy
M–6	Moderate	50	Male	Waiter	Amer. Protestant Negro	8th grade	Colostomy
M–7	Moderate	46	Male	Transit repairman	Irish Catholic	6th grade	Evacuation of subdural hematoma
M–8	Moderate	48	Male	Factory worker	Fr. Canadian Catholic	Some H. S.	Lung lobectomy
M–9	Moderate	42	Male	Factory worker	Italian Catholic	Some H.S.	Thoracoplasty
				Low Fear Group			
L–1	Low	53	Fem.	Practical nurse	Amer. Catholic	H. S. grad.	Cholecystectomy
L–2	Low	23	Fem.	Housewife	Amer. Protestant	Some H. S.	Cholecystectomy
L–3	Low	25	Fem.	Social worker	Amer. Jewish	M.A. degree	Appendectomy
L–4	Low	65	Fem.	Housewife	Irish Catholic	Some H. S.	Repair of hip fracture
L–5	Low	44	Male	Retail salesman	Amer. Catholic	Some H. S.	Subtotal gastrectomy
L–6	Low	56	Male	Business proprietor	Amer. Protestant	H. S. grad.	Partial thyroidectomy
L–7	Low	33	Male	Mechanic	Polish Catholic	8th grade	Colostomy
L–8	Low	58	Male	Tailor	Polish Jewish	5th grade	Exploratory thoracotomy

for interpreting the findings to be presented in Chapters 20 and 21 concerning the behavioral sequelae of different levels of preoperative fear or anxiety. Specifically, the absence of any consistent group differences in medical status makes it improbable that any differences in postoperative behavior among the three groups might prove to be attributable to variations in the intensity or duration of the stress stimuli to which the patients were exposed. And the absence of any consistent group differences in the various other background factors shown in Table 1 greatly reduces the probability that any postoperative behavioral differences could be explained on the basis of extraneous differences in the social composition of the three groups. However, since the findings are based on an analysis of relationships among response variables, no definite answers can be expected to questions about the necessary and sufficient conditions which account for the observed outcome. Ultimately, all of the conclusions about causal factors which are inferred from a correlational study of this kind must be tested by more precise research, notably by controlled experiments designed to observe the behavioral effects of variables which can be systematically manipulated by the investigator. At best, by using the method of controlled comparisons in the present investigation, it is possible to preclude a number of obvious artifacts which could give rise to correlations having little or no psychological significance. It must be further emphasized that the primary purposes of the case study series were to investigate relationships among observable variables and to discover the mediating psychological processes; the data provide only very crude, preliminary results based on a very small sample. Moreover, they are subject to unconscious or preconscious distortions on the part of the observer (inasmuch as the author conducted all the pre- and postoperative interviews and then subsequently rated each patient's preoperative anxiety level and postoperative adjustment). Especially because of the latter shortcoming, it was felt to be essential to replicate the main parts of the study with a larger, independent sample of surgery cases, involving procedures that eliminate any source of observer contamination.

The Survey Research Study

The method of controlled comparisons was also used in analyzing the survey results obtained from a large sample of male adolescents. The survey was conducted in college classrooms at Yale University for the purpose of obtaining additional data with which to test the correlations predicted by Hypotheses 15, 16, and 17. A lengthy questionnaire concerning reactions to a surgical, medical, or dental experience was constructed, consisting of open-end questions combined with objective questions containing check-list answer categories.

On the basis of the factual information given by the subjects about the nature of their experience and the surgical procedures to which they had been subjected, the sample was limited to approximately 150 men, consisting of all those who gave a complete report on their preoperative and postoperative reactions to a major or minor surgical operation. (For certain comparative purposes, an analysis was also made of the responses given by an additional sample consisting of 97 men who reported on their reactions to a painful dental treatment; see pp. 284–285, Chapter 22.)

The results of the survey on reactions to surgical experiences cannot be expected to have the same degree of validity as those obtained from the intensive investigation of the smaller number of hospitalized patients in the case study series. First of all, unlike the case study research, the survey relied upon verbal reports that were retrospective rather than contemporaneous with exposure to the stress situation. Secondly, the survey results were limited entirely to the subject's own verbal statements; whereas, in the case study research, each patient's statements could be checked against at least two sources of independent behavioral observations, the interviewer's direct behavioral observations and the hospital records prepared by the physicians and nurses. Finally, the survey questionnaires were filled out in an impersonal classroom setting, which lacks the advantages of a face-to-face interview situation because it does not enable verbal misunderstandings to be cleared up through the use of extemporaneous follow-up questions and, perhaps, what is even more important, it cannot build up the subject's motivation to reveal personal details to the same degree as when there is direct interaction and rapport with an attentive listener.

Although it must be taken for granted that numerous sources of distortion enter into the verbal responses elicited by the survey questionnaire, there is certainly no reason to assume *a priori* that the results will necessarily be misleading or invalid. In the present survey research, the main working assumption was that, by using a variety of different questions concerning each of the important aspects of emotional behavior, the retrospective verbal reports obtained from fairly large groups of subjects would provide at least a crude average measure of each variable under investigation, so that fairly valid group comparisons could be made. In making this assumption as the basis for designing the survey research, the author took cognizance of one particular fact which emerged from the previously completed case study research: By and large, the surgical patients' verbal descriptions of their own emotional responses—vague feelings of anxiety, specific fears, outbursts of anger, attitudes of resentment, etc.—were generally consonant with the behavioral observations made by the interviewer and by the physicians and nurses. In only a few cases were there any marked discrepancies between what the subject said about his emotional state and his actual emotional behavior as observed by others. Thus, it seemed probable that for purposes of investigating conscious feelings of fear and resentment elicited by exposure to stressful circumstances, the questionnaire method would be adequate. Furthermore, special instructions were given in order to reduce the usual tendency to distort one's self-descriptions in order to make a good impression on other people. The subjects were told that absolute honesty was essential to achieve the scientific purposes of the research; they were assured that their answers would be kept strictly confidential, and no one would ever be allowed to examine the individual questionnaires except the trained research workers who code and tabulate the results for entire groups.

One of the advantageous features of the questionnaire used in the survey research was that all responses could be scored by independent judges in a highly reliable way, without any possibility of observer contamination. Many of the key questions provided a standard check-list of answer categories, and those questions which were open-end were scored according to a rigorously defined set of content analysis rules. Thus, the intensive interview study, which was used primarily for discovery purposes, was followed up by a systematic survey which provided objective data for testing the relationships between preoperative fear and postoperative adjustment.

Notes

1. From preliminary interview experience on the surgical wards it became clear to the investigator that this introduction was effective for establishing rapport and that there was no need to say anything more about the purpose of the interviews. The vast majority of patients were quite willing—and even eager—to talk about their personal feelings concerning the impending surgery.

For the sake of facilitating communicativeness and rapport, the interview schedule was not rigidly followed with respect to the sequence of questions. For example, if the patient spontaneously began to talk about a topic covered by several questions toward the end of the interview schedule, the interviewer simply went on to the questions pertinent to that topic and then returned to the earlier questions not yet asked.

The interviewer was also flexible with respect to duration of the interview session. If, after a short time, the patient complained that it was difficult to talk or showed obvious signs of fatigue, the session was promptly terminated; arrangements were then made to resume the interview later the same day, if possible. On the average, the preoperative interview required about one hour and was usually covered in one session. The postoperative interview, however, required about one and one-half hours and generally required two or three separate sessions, usually held on successive days.

All interviews were conducted privately at the patient's bedside or, if the patient was ambulatory, in a small private office on the surgical ward. The interviewer always tried to avoid using pressure on the patients to elicit answers to his questions. Few of the patients displayed any reluctance with respect to being interviewed.

2. There were some additional questions which also occasionally elicited expressions of positive or negative attitudes toward the hospital staff. This was especially true of the following questions which were included in the postoperative interview to help assess the degree to which the patient had been cognitively prepared for the stresses of surgery to which he was subsequently exposed. The questions were designed primarily to supplement the preoperative questions pertaining to the advance information the patient had received about his subsequent surgical experiences. (See discussion of the relationship between preoperative information and postoperative adjustment in Chapter 25, pp. 354–360.)

QUESTION 29: Let's go over the unpleasant experiences you've just told me about. Now I want you to tell me whether each experience was what you had expected to happen or not. (Interviewer records for each experience: $E =$ fully expected; $D =$ partially expected but different; or $U =$ unexpected.)

QUESTION 30: *A.* What information were you given beforehand about your operation? (When? By whom?) *B.* Where you told beforehand to expect certain unpleasant things which, as it turned out, did not actually occur? *C.* Before the operation was started were you told that it would probably cause some pain? (What were you told?)

QUESTION 33: Before the operation was about to begin, what things did the doctor talk to you about?

QUESTION 63: Do you feel that you were given as much information about your operation as you would have liked to have had?

3. The importance of the behavioral records becomes apparent when one considers the well-known errors of omission and commission that can enter into a person's verbal account of his affects, attitudes, and behavior. In addition to all the usual sources of conscious distortion that may color a subject's verbal reports, there are also likely to be unconscious motives and defense mechanisms which come into play in stress situations, with the result that the person may remain wholly unaware of what it is that is stimulating his anxieties; moreover, he may not even admit to himself that he is experiencing anxiety or other emotional reactions. (See statements about rationalization and displacement of fear in the discussion of Hypothesis 4, pp. 80–82.)

It was because of the above considerations that the investigator made careful efforts to obtain detailed behavioral observations of the emotional behavior displayed in each interview, thus providing a check on the patient's self-description of his or her emotional reactions. The behavioral records made by physicians and nurses were also used for the same purpose.

4. The omitted group of eight surgical patients had been given incomplete interviews because of fortuitous circumstances. For example, on certain days of the month, the investigator's academic duties prevented him from spending any time on the surgical ward. Since most patients were admitted only one or two days before the operation was scheduled, the investigator's absence occasionally coincided with the entire preoperative hospitalization period for some of the surgical ward patients. The available background data concerning the type of operation and the age, sex, education, and occupation of the eight omitted patients were compared with the corresponding data for the group of patients with whom both preoperative and postoperative interviews had been conducted. No consistent or significant differences were noted and, hence, it appears that the omission of the eight cases from the investigation of Hypotheses 15, 16, and 17 did not introduce any obvious selective factor that could affect the representativeness of the sample.

Among the 22 patients included in the systematic investigation were three special cases who were not in the original surgical ward sample. (In Table 1, the background information for the three patients is shown in the rows designated by the following code numbers: H–5, M–3, and L–3.) These three had undergone major surgical operations similar to those of the other cases but had been hospitalized as private patients and were not interviewed until shortly after they had left the hospital. Although no preoperative interview had been conducted with these three patients, the investigator decided to add them to the case study series for the following three reasons. First, they were well-educated professional persons who were generally aware of the values of scientific research and who gave exceptionally frank accounts of their subjective overt responses, including a considerable amount of rich detail concerning preoperative as well as postoperative emotional reactions. Second, it was possible to check on some of the important details, especially those pertinent for categorizing their preoperative level of fear, by obtaining information from one or more independent observers. Third, after categorizing the three cases according to their preoperative level of fear, the investigator noted that each case happened to fall into a different one of the three categories of "high," "moderate," and "low" preoperative fear. Consequently, even though the three cases differ in various respects from the other 19 cases, their inclusion could not introduce any substantial source of bias into the basic findings relevant to investigating the relationships specified by Hypotheses 15, 16, and 17.

5. The possibility that ethnic differences may be related to emotional reactions to surgery and hospitalization has been suggested by Zborowski (1952). Although he gave no systematic evidence, this author reported having noticed marked differences in manifestations of emotional tension and attitudes toward the hospital staff among hospitalized patients from different ethnic groups—Irish, Italian, European Jews, and "old" Americans.

In the present study, there were very few cases in each of the various ethnic categories. Accordingly, no attempt was made to test Zborowski's hypotheses. Rather, the data on ethnic and religious background in Table 1 were used simply to make sure that there were no marked ethnic differences with respect to level of preoperative fear.

20.

Behavioral sequelae of high anticipatory fear

This chapter is devoted to the case material pertaining to the postoperative behavior of the five patients who displayed acute fear and anxiety symptoms before the operation. In all five cases, overt manifestations of emotional disturbance occurred during convalescence. The dominant form of postoperative disturbance was acute apprehensiveness, characterized by excessive concern about the ordinary aches and pains caused by surgery, coupled with extreme timidity and exaggerated fears of unpleasant procedures.

The five patients displayed varying degrees of elation immediately after the operation but, within a short time, all of them developed postoperative anxiety symptoms combined with mild depression. Despite their excessive apprehensiveness, however, these patients rarely displayed actual refusals or interferences with postoperative treatments. Moreover, their postoperative attitudes toward the surgeon and the hospital staff were generally favorable.

The brief case study summaries which follow describe the outstanding deviant characteristics of their postoperative behavior.

Case Summaries

INTERVIEW CASE H–1

Mrs. C., a 31-year-old housewife, was in a chronic state of fear before the operation. On two occasions she became so agitated that she attempted to leave the hospital in order to avoid having the operation (hernia repair). She consented to remain only after considerable coaxing and reassurance on the part of the nursing staff.

Throughout the week following the operation she expressed a high degree of relief about the fact that everything had worked out well and she felt that her fears had been unjustified. Nevertheless she continued to display symptoms of acute emotional disturbance. On her first postoperative day she felt elated for a few hours but, later on, began to feel extremely worried and wept frequently because, as she put it, "I felt like a tractor had run into me and made chopped meat of me." During the following five days her uncontrollable crying spells persisted, occurring mainly when she was alone in her room, thinking about the operation. Each night she felt very tense and suffered from insomnia:

> I can't sleep nights. I've seen and heard so many things here, it bothers me. I get upset when the other patients shriek. I'd be more calm at home.

This patient was generally cooperative, extremely grateful, and warmly affectionate toward all the nurses and physicians; but she became very apprehensive whenever any of them came into her room to administer routine treatments. She was reluctant to conform with demands that might result in pain or discomfort. For example, when the nurses asked her to stand up for the first time (on the second postoperative day), she managed to conform, but she described her subjective experience as follows:

> I felt terrified. I had a cold sweat all over my body. I didn't think I could stand it. I thought my stomach would fall on the floor. . . . But I did what they told me; I just tried to stand it.

INTERVIEW CASE H–2

Mrs. S., a 37-year-old housewife, displayed marked anxiety reactions before a chest operation (a partial lobectomy). During the preoperative interview, she became extremely agitated, trembled, sweated profusely, and complained that she felt "terribly nervous." She was especially concerned about the possibility of heart failure, even though the physicians had repeatedly assured her that there was no danger in this respect: "I'm afraid I'll go under and not wake up again."

After the operation, she felt temporarily relieved but complained about her pains in a rather depressed way:

> At the time I awoke from my operation I was disgusted, I didn't care if I died or not, and I feel the same way now because there is nothing else to do but think. . . . Sometimes I think I'm sorry I had it done. I'm suffering now like the devil.

One main source of postoperative distress was the drainage tube procedure which the patient had great difficulty in tolerating:

> When the doctor said I had to swallow the tube I let him do it but I was mad. I knew it was for my own good but still I couldn't stand it. . . . It was over pretty quick but the second time I made another fuss about it before I let them do it.

According to the nurses' records, on one occasion this patient became so apprehensive that she almost prevented the insertion of a rectal tube, and on several other occasions she reacted in a similar way to the drainage tubes. The nurses also noted that this patient complained about having nightmares on several nights following the operation.

INTERVIEW CASE H–3

Mrs. M., a 46-year-old housewife, was hospitalized for chest surgery (partial lobectomy). Before the operation, she repeatedly expressed her fears to the nurses and physicians. In the preoperative interview she reported feeling constantly worried about the operation and she exhibited tremor, flushing, fidgeting, and other behavioral signs of extreme emotional tension.

Postoperatively, she reported feeling much relieved that the surgery was over and she was somewhat elated for several days. But when interviewed five days after the operation, she said that she was "scared" every time a nurse or doctor came into her room to administer any form of examination or treatment: "I'm always afraid I'll be hurt." She also asserted that frequently, when left alone in her room, she felt "panicky about being all choked up." Also, several times when her lung was irrigated, she felt "terribly frightened because I thought I might strangle." According to the case records, this patient was unusually apprehensive about routine postoperative procedures. Her fearfulness was particularly noteworthy in connection with the daily requests to cough up mucus; she required prolonged urging almost every time. Excessive anxiety about her general physical condition was often observed by the staff physicians during daily rounds since she generally expressed considerable concern about the usual postoperative discomforts or complained about vague aches and pains.

INTERVIEW CASE H–4

Mr. L., a 43-year-old salesman, was extremely fearful and agitated while in the hospital awaiting his abdominal operation (cholecystectomy). Earlier, against the advice of his physician, he had postponed coming to the hospital. Following the operation, he asserted that he was glad he had allowed it to be done and was proud of his courage. But throughout the entire convalescent period he felt continually "worried" about his physical condition. At times he displayed an unusually low ability to tolerate pain or discomfort. On the second postoperative day, he made a loud outcry and begged the physician to stop while he was being turned over on his side. When asked to get out of bed later that day, he conformed to the nurse's demands, but felt at first that he was not ready for it because there might be unbearable pain if he stood up. For several days, despite repeated prodding by the physician, he would not try coughing up the mucus in his throat, complaining that it "hurts too much." This patient made several complaints about the nurses which apparently arose from an exaggerated notion of how people should respond to the suffering he was experiencing during the convalescent period; his critical comments were centered almost entirely upon the alleged failure of the nurses to express the appropriate degree of sympathy:

> Nurses should take account of how people feel, if a man is worried or not. The profession shouldn't use an organization by remote control without human feeling. Some people like to be babied and some like to be treated other ways. I feel I'd like to have someone take care of me when I am in pain and not when I feel O.K. . . . When in pain I don't like to be told, "Oh, just wait a minute!"

INTERVIEW CASE H–5

Dr. N., who was hospitalized for surgical repair of an intervertebral disc, reported that he experienced considerable fear beforehand. He knew from his own experience as a physician that the particular operation was occasionally unsuccessful and that there was some real danger of serious complications. Keenly aware of these possibilities, this physician felt extremely anxious and postponed having the operation as long as possible.

The operation proved to be completely successful and the postoperative course was medically uneventful. Nevertheless, this highly sophisticated patient was inordinately apprehensive during the convalescent period. He evidently became agitated and obsessively pessimistic about the potentially crippling effects of the operation.

> I really felt that I'd be a cripple and all my concern was centered upon being dependent upon my wife for the rest of my life. . . . I had been through combat during the war and was able to stand that O.K., but the thought of being a cripple—and requiring constant care as an invalid and having to have my wife support me—was an emotional obsession I couldn't get rid of all through that first week. [A week after the operation] . . . I was still worried about it but no longer obsessed. . . . I could tell you I went through it fine, but the truth is that I didn't. I was like a child after the operation and I really learned what intense anxiety is from that experience.

Because of excessive concern about his physical condition, this patient was reluctant about conforming to certain of the routine postoperative procedures. On the second postoperative day, when the surgeon asked him to get up on his feet, he was extremely afraid that doing so might aggravate his condition or even result in permanent crippling. He resisted the request at first but, under persistent pressure from the surgeon, he finally got up. The same sort of reluctance occurred on subsequent days and apparently contributed to the development of an attitude of distrust and resentment toward the hospital staff:

> The food they served must have been bad because a lot of the patients, including myself, got diarrhea. I had to get up 15 times a day to go to the bathroom. I felt that they shouldn't have me do this, that it was very harmful and would tend to make me a cripple.

Personality Predispositions as Causal Factors

All five patients who were highly anxious before the operation displayed clear-cut postoperative emotional disturbances. Common to all five patients are hypochondriacal concerns and excessive timidity about convalescent treatments, both of which can be regarded as manifestations of postoperative anxiety. Such postoperative reactions very rarely occurred among the other 14 patients, who had displayed a moderate or low level of preoperative fear. Thus, the five patients who reacted to the threat of the impending operation with exceedingly high anticipatory fear displayed anxiety reactions again after the operation, when confronted with the uncertainties, discomforts, and pains of the convalescent period.[1] It was these case observations which led to the formulation of Hypothesis 16 (see p. 217).

Perhaps the simplest explanation of the postoperative behavior of the hyperanxious patients is that they suffer from a special form of neurotic disorder that strongly predisposes them to react with high anxiety to any environmental situation in which there is a threat of body harm or actual physical suffering. The causal role of neurotic personality predispositions is definitely suggested by some of the information obtained in the interviews. Four of the five patients in the high preoperative fear group described earlier operations, childbirth experiences, or medical treatments to which they had also reacted with extremely high anxiety (Cases H–1, H–2, H–3, and H–4). Three of these patients stated that they had been suffering for many years from persistent neurotic symptoms. For example, Mrs. C. (Case H–1) described herself as a "nervous person," constantly worried about her own health, her children's welfare, and her family finances. She reported that ever since the experience of protracted labor in giving birth to her first child eleven years earlier, she had been afraid of coming to a hospital for any sort of treatment and had avoided doctors as much as possible. Throughout her entire adult life she had experienced intense fear in connection with crossing streets, which seemed to be linked with strong self-punitive impulses. This phobic reaction originated, according to the patient, at the age of ten when she made a suicide attempt on the street in front of her house:

> I was badly beaten by my mother one day and I felt there was no use going on living. So I threw myself under a car and I was run over but not badly hurt. . . . I've been afraid of crossing streets ever since then, and I worry about my children crossing streets because of it.

It appears likely that a special type of neurotic predisposition plays a critical role as a determinant of high preoperative and postoperative anxiety.[2] Some of these patients are probably similar to the ones described in the psychiatric literature as suffering from excessive fear of mutilation or annihilation (Blanton and Kirk, 1947; Fenichel, 1945, pp. 194–198).

The inner stimulus which gives rise to exaggerated fears of surgery may be a fantasy of personal destruction mobilized by the threat of having to submit to the anesthetic and the surgeon's knife. This type of fantasy was illustrated in the psychoanalytic case material from Mrs. Blake. After the initial period when she had denied feeling worried about it, came a period when her anticipatory fear was very high, as a result of psychoanalytic interventions which temporarily broke down her denial defenses. During this latter period, she made repeated attempts at developing reality-based reassurances, but her high level of fear nevertheless persisted. Her failure to gain normal reassurance was linked, as we saw, to powerful masochistic tendencies and to other unconscious neurotic motives which represented *internal dangers* that were stimulated by the external danger. These observations led to the formulation of Hypotheses 6 and 7, which refer to the effects of repressed fears.

In this connection, it is noteworthy that the apprehensions expressed by the five patients who displayed extremely high preoperative fear were much more vague than those expressed by the group of nine patients who had displayed a moderate degree of preoperative fear. The verbalized fears of the latter patients tended to concentrate on *specific* sources of danger of a fairly realistic character—not being able to breathe during administration of the anesthetic, experiencing acute postoperative pain, failure of the operation to alleviate the original illness or disability, etc. (See the examples cited in the case study summaries in Chapter 23, pp. 314–322.) The patients who were most fearful before the operation spoke about some of the same dangers but also made many comments concerning vague or remote dangers that appeared to be the product of neurotic fantasies—the surgeon's knife might make a fatal slip; too much anesthesia might be given; heart failure might occur; something awful might happen which the doctors could not prevent.

It seems probable that a neurotic inability to dispel fantasies of being damaged by surgery might implicate a number of different internal dangers, including those which give rise to unconscious self-punitive wishes or a need to project one's own hostility onto authority figures.[3] In any case, whatever unconscious processes might provide the explanation for the type of disturbance displayed by the hyperanxious convalescent patients, their intensive preoperative anxiety seems to be a direct consequence of a generalized personality weakness such that they fail to mobilize reassuring thoughts in the face of anticipated danger. Unable to rid themselves of the recurrent image of being mutilated or killed by the operation, they seem helpless to dispel the internal symbolic stimuli which evoke persistent anxiety feelings and which arouse strong escape tendencies.

The intense relief and gratitude toward the staff after the operation may arise from reduced guilt as well as from the temporary realization that the punishment was far less than had been feared. During the convalescent period, after the main dangers were over, several of the patients displayed a marked reaction of elation. A major basis for feelings of satisfaction and emotional relief may well have been the great disparity between the dire expectations they had built up beforehand and the limited amount of suffering they actually experienced. (See the discussion of Hypothesis 9, pp. 143–145.) However, it seems that this disparity provides, at best, only temporary emotional relief, without producing any substantial modification of the basic emotional habit of overreacting to threats of danger. In other words, the neurotic personality structure of the four patients remained unaffected by the opportunity for emotional learning provided by their successful operation experience. When new threats were encountered during the convalescent period, these patients again reacted with exaggerated fears.

The lack of change in these patients can be partly accounted for by the explanatory concepts derived from the psychoanalytic case study (see, especially those presented in the discussion of Hypotheses 6 and 7, pp. 116–124). Presumably, when a hyperanxious patient is required to undergo routine postoperative medical treatments, such as having stitches removed, swallowing a gastric tube, getting out of bed the first time, etc., he will again react with fantasies of personal destruction, just as before the operation. If the underlying source of neurotic anxiety is repressed, the patient will continue to be dominated by such fantasies, which are undoubtedly facilitated by the fact that, for the average patient, there are no clear-cut reality signs showing that he is out of danger, and the clues pertaining to the permanency of his suffering and disability are somewhat ambiguous. Thus, the repressed tendencies which underlie exaggerated preoperative anxiety might again come into play during the convalescent period, giving rise to (*a*) excessive anxiety feelings, (*b*) overt escape efforts in the face of routine medical treatments, and (*c*) a low degree of responsiveness to the reassuring communications given by the hospital staff. Speculatively, we might assume that behind the hyperanxious patient's excessive timidity about undergoing new procedures is a latent attitude to the effect that: "The operation came out well but maybe the worst isn't over, maybe it is *now* that I really will have to undergo terrible suffering." Anxiety reactions in the form of hypochondriacal concern evoked by incision pains or other distressing occurrences after the operation might be mediated by the same type of irrational expectation.

More intensive personality investigations of anxiety-ridden surgery patients will be necessary in order to test and sharpen the formulation of the above tentative hypotheses concerning the latent personality factors which are singled out as determinants of excessive anxiety reactions. The one conclusion which is most strongly suggested by the case study material is that some form of neurotic personality predisposition is the key factor which explains the emotional reactions of the hyperanxious group. Thus, the empirical finding that patients with very high preoperative anxiety tend to differ markedly from other patients in their postoperative emotional reactions is interpreted as a noncausal (static) relationship. That is to say, the preoperative anxiety state does not seem to play any role in *producing* the subsequent postoperative anxiety reaction. The preoperative and postoperative anxiety reactions apparently occur in certain patients simply because they have a chronically low anxiety threshold that makes them regularly overreact to any environmental situation which signifies or actualizes a threat of body damage.

We have noted that in several patients with extreme apprehensiveness, the low anxiety threshold was part of a more general neurotic predisposition which can be regarded as a chronic personality disorder. However, as previously stated, it is probably erroneous to assume that for all cases who display anxiety symptoms before and after an operation, the low anxiety threshold is necessarily symptomatic of chronic neurosis. A person may be relatively free from neurotic anxiety symptoms in normal everyday life but may develop temporary (nonpathological) symptoms of exaggerated fear in connection with an isolated surgical episode. Because of unique past experiences, there are some clinically normal individuals who are especially vulnerable to a specific kind of external threat, such as being anesthetized or cut open with a knife; conversely, there are some severe neurotics (e.g., obsessive-compulsive personalities) whose symptoms do not ordinarily take the form of excessive apprehensiveness in the face of environmental dangers. (See discussion of chronic neurotics who use extreme denial defenses and remain relatively free from manifest feelings of fear, pp. 262–266.)

Although the life history materials concerning Cases H–4 and H–5 were rather meager, it seems likely that one or both were of the nonpathological type. For Case H–4, there is definite information that the anxiety symptoms and mild depression he displayed before and after his operation were linked associatively with a mutilation experience which had occurred several years earlier and which may have sensitized him to certain types of symbolic or real external threats (see pp. 249–250). The earlier experience, which involved mutilation of the patient's nose as a result of an auto accident, had been followed by a temporary loss of self-esteem; he regarded the injury as equivalent to a self-inflicted wound. It is conceivable that the accident mobilized a latent fear of a masochistic tendency which, under ordinary conditions of daily life, had remained fairly well sublimated or had been so effectively controlled that it exerted relatively little influence on the patient's emotional behavior. Thus, the patient's latent vulnerability may be such that it gives rise to emotional disturbances only in an extremely circumscribed area, e.g., the unique circumstances of a surgical operation, which requires passive submission to body mutilation. In such a case, the predispositional factor would be characterized as a *special vulnera-*

bility, which does not necessarily imply any general form of neurotic disorder.

Perhaps a similar type of limited, nonpathological predisposition was present in Case H–5, the physician who before and after a spinal operation was extremely fearful of becoming a helpless cripple. In this case, the patient's detailed medical knowledge about the potential risks of the operation contributed to the intensity of his anxiety reaction. In addition, the special status accorded to him as a physician, together with his trained ability to notice subtle deficiencies of the hospital staff, apparently had the effect of preventing him from obtaining the usual degree of reassurance that the average patient can derive by relying upon the danger-control authorities. (See Chapter 24, pp. 371–373, for further discussion of this patient's dilemma as an illustrative example of the conditions under which expert knowledge and detailed information about potential risks can have unfavorable psychological effects.) But even if the various factors arising directly from the patient's professional role and training were assumed to be major causal factors in accounting for his intense fears, the relationship between his preoperative and postoperative emotional reactions would still be regarded as an essentially noncausal one, just as in the case of the other four patients. The emphasis would not be placed exclusively on the causal role of *neurotic vulnerability* to threats of body damage, but also on predispositions of a somewhat different type, which are a more direct product of the person's recent social interactions and are much more modifiable via social communication (i.e., his *cognitive expectations* concerning the danger of being crippled and his *attitudes* toward the surgeon, the hospital staff, etc.). In this case as well as in the others, therefore, the postoperative fear reactions appear to be consequences of one or another predispositional factor which accounts for the high level of anticipatory fear.

Thus, so far as the available case evidence goes, the relationship between preoperative and postoperative fear specified by Hypothesis 16 seems to be explicable in terms of *consistent individual differences* in predispositional factors. This point is emphasized here because it is a strongly contrasting alternative to the explanatory concept which will be introduced in the next chapter in the discussion of the causes of postoperative resentment.

Notes

1. A similar relationship was noted *within* the moderate preoperative fear group. The nine patients in this group seemed to vary considerably with respect to the frequency and intensity of preoperative fear, ranging from cases who reported only slight twinges of apprehension to patients who were frequently distressed by fairly severe fear symptoms (though not as severe as in the high fear group). If we select from this group the three patients who were most fearful *before* the operation, we find that after the operation they turned out to be somewhat more fearful than the remaining patients in the same group.

2. Cases H–1, H–2, and H–3 were the most manifestly disturbed personalities in the entire group of 22 surgical patients. In these cases it appears to be a chronically neurotic fear of body damage that underlies both the high level of anxiety prior to the operation and the excessive timidity and hypochondriacal concern after the operation. Some indications of a long-standing neurotic disturbance were also noted in case H–4. The pertinent information for Cases H–2, H–3, and H–4 is as follows:

Case H–2 reported that over the past few years, whenever she experienced pain or became ill, she would become "terribly worried" because she thought she was going to die. One of the salient reasons for her intense preoperative anxiety was the fact that for some time she had an apparently irrational hypochondriacal concern about the condition of her heart:

"My heart sometimes feels like it's not strong—a funny feeling like it stops. Now I'm afraid I'll go under and not wake up again. . . .

"I really shouldn't worry about my heart because the doctors should know if it's O.K. and they told me it was."

Case H–3 reported having had a "nervous breakdown" nine years earlier, following the death of her mother. Her acute symptoms at that time included insomnia, constipation, and a variety of interrelated phobias: fear of sudden death, of being alone, of being in an enclosed room, and of seeing sick people. The latter phobia, according to the patient's own account, had persisted over the past nine years: "Since my mother's death I can't stand seeing sick people because I feel their pain and suffer from it." This patient described yet another persistent phobic attitude.

"I've always had a horror of doctors—whenever I see one, I have a shaky feeling and I'm so frightened I sweat all over. I have every confidence in the world in doctors but I just can't help fearing them when I see them."

This morbid fear, which undoubtedly played an important role in her entire hospital adjustment, began, according to the patient, at the age of five, when one of her playmates died and she developed the belief that her family doctor had killed the child.

Case H–4, although manifesting nothing comparable to the long-standing anxiety symptoms of the first three cases, reported nevertheless that, following an auto accident ten years ago, he had reacted in a highly neurotic way. He had been extremely upset about the fact that in an effort to save the driver's wife he had swerved in such a way that he failed to protect himself when the car crashed: "Why did I have to save someone else and injure myself?" He asserted that, "Because I was mad at myself," he refused a local anesthetic while receiving emergency treatment on his face; for many weeks afterward he was extremely worried about the scar on his nose. From the way this patient described his feelings about the effects of the present operation, explaining them by referring to his self-punitive reactions to the earlier accident, it appears likely that he, like the first three, also was predisposed to overreact to certain types of body damage. The following statements from his preoperative interview suggest that his current fears were rooted in deep-seated anxieties.

"An operation has an important effect on a person's mind. . . . I feel it's a cut; my flesh has been cut. When a person is cut, it's there; you can't eliminate it. Sometimes I say to myself, it's not on my face or eyes, it's on my tummy; no one can see it so it's not so bad. . . . You feel you are cut up—something is missing, something in you is scarred, like after the auto accident when I worried so much about the scar on my nose."

The above statements, together with the patient's self-critical comments about the causes of the earlier mutilating accident, suggest that the present surgical operation took on a special symbolic significance for this patient, probably because it mobilized repressed fears associated with dangerous inner impulses of masochistic submission. (See pp. 247–248, for a more specific hypothetical construction of the predisposing factor in this patient.)

For Case H–5, there was no information available concerning previous neurotic symptoms.

3. Inability to provide reassurances to oneself may sometimes be linked with a neurotic superego reaction: "I deserve to be punished." This tendency is suggested by certain of the depressive features noted in the highly fearful patients together with specific bits of their life history data: (*a*) the suicide attempt made during early puberty by Case H–1, and her persistent phobic reaction to the site where she made the attempt; (*b*) the chronic hypochondriacal concern about heart failure in Case H–2; (*c*) the persistent fear of death in Case H–3 which developed following the death of her mother, and (*d*) the intrapunitive attitudes and behavior noted in Case H–4 who had earlier reacted self-punitively following an auto accident. Perhaps, too, the excessive anxiety reactions were based in part on a fantasy of being maltreated by authority figures, as is suggested by the history of a chronic irrational fear of physicians in Cases H–1 and H–3.

21.

Behavioral sequelae of low anticipatory fear

Perhaps the most outstanding findings derived from the entire case study series are those bearing on the relationship between anticipatory fear and subsequent aggressive behavior. Postoperative resentment and noncompliant actions were rarely observed except among the patients who beforehand had been consistently unconcerned and relatively free from any apparent symptoms of anticipatory fear, as stated in Hypothesis 17.

Among the five hyperanxious patients discussed in the preceding chapter, there were no clear-cut instances of postoperative rage or hostile, negativistic behavior. Even when their fears mounted to the point where they were momentarily unable to accept the demands made upon them by the physicians or nurses, they were nevertheless respectful and relatively nonaggressive, if not obsequiously apologetic. Although occasionally angry and resentful, these patients generally felt grateful toward the hospital staff; all of them made great efforts to conform, despite their apprehensive timidity. Similarly, the nine patients who had displayed a *moderate* level of fear before the operation were relatively free from aggressive and noncomplaint behavior.

Throughout their convalescence these people were highly cooperative, and accepted without protest the numerous injections, postoperative examinations, stomach tubes, removal of stitches, and other uncomfortable procedures which all surgical patients are required to undergo.

That the same cannot be said about the third group of patients, those who displayed a low degree of preoperative fear, is apparent from the case material presented in this chapter. First, a case description is given which serves to illustrate some of the typical manifestations of aggrievement, low frustration tolerance, and overt resistance noted in this group of patients. This is followed by a brief summary of the postoperative behavioral disturbances observed in the other 7 patients in the low fear group, together with comparative statements about the relative incidence of such disturbances among the 14 patients in the other two groups. Finally, a series of detailed case studies are presented which help to answer some general theoretical questions concerning personality predispositions and alternative causal sequences that may account for the relationship specified in Hypothesis 17.

An Illustrative Case Summary

INTERVIEW CASE L–7

Mr. R., a 33-year-old mechanic, was hospitalized for exploratory surgery after his symptoms—a growing abdominal lump, cramps and constipation—were diagnosed as indicating an abdominal tumor. Before the operation, he complained of some acute pains but was extremely optimistic, asserting that he felt no concern about any aspect of the impending surgery. Following the operation (a colostomy), he displayed the characteristic sequelae of resentment and overtly resistant behavior.

In the preoperative interview, when asked whether he felt worried or concerned about the operation, he responded:

> I don't worry about it—I don't think about it at all. . . . I figure it's not a serious operation. I don't worry because I just figure they'll get what's troubling me out of there.

He expected that when he awoke from the anesthetic he would experience *no pain at all.* He thought there would be some postoperative pain "when it starts healing" a day or two after the operation, but it would be less than the pain he was currently experiencing. In fact, he was looking forward to the operation because "it should make things all right and I'll have no more pain." He supposed he would be "back in shape in a couple of weeks, just like with my appendix operation." In general, he thought that his postoperative experiences would be similar to those of his appendix operation, which had occurred five months earlier. All his comments about the hospital staff during the preoperative interview were favorable.

During the week following the operation, the nurses noted that, despite an excellent physical recovery, this patient became irritable and very difficult to manage. The hospital records stated that shortly after the operation he put up a struggle when his leg was being bound for a routine blood transfusion. Also, on the fourth postoperative day, he objected to the application of hot compresses and actually removed them when the nurse left the room. During the next three days, according to the hospital records, he continued to refuse the hot compresses. Time and again, the nurses attempted to carry out the treatment, sometimes offering to compromise by using only a hot water bottle, but the patient would not permit it. In addition, he would not get out of bed to sit up in a chair when a nurse informed him that his physician said he was ready to do so.

At the time of the postoperative interview (seven days after the operation), the patient again reported that he had had no fear or concern about the operation during the preoperative period, right up to the time he had been brought to the operating room. But he told about numerous unpleasant aspects of the operation which turned out to be very disturbing to him. When asked whether during the last day or so he had thought about any of the things that happened on the day of the operation, he spoke about how surprised he had felt at the time when he was brought into the operating room, indicating that he frequently ruminated about the unfamiliar, fear-evoking situation.

> I think about it a lot. I keep thinking about how those guys looked, running around with their gowns on. I always thought they wore white. It surprised me to see them wearing green. It made me feel funny and I just kept on wondering "why green?"

The experience of awakening from the anesthetic also proved to be unexpectedly disturbing. Whereas he had anticipated having little or no distress, it turned out that he had been in a state of acute pain and, in addition, he had felt like he was "dying of thirst." He reported that for an entire day and a half he constantly asked for water but was given only small pieces of cracked ice:

> They kept telling me that it wasn't good for me to have water or to use a lot of ice; every time they gave me some, it just relieved my thirst a little bit—I still wanted more but couldn't have it.

Intense anger was this patient's dominant affective reaction during the initial postoperative period of pain and deprivation. He gave a vivid account of how he felt when, upon awakening after the operation, he had found himself suffering from severe pain, and with his aching left leg firmly restrained.

> I was mad as hell because they had my leg tied down, giving me a blood transfusion. I didn't know what it was they were doing and it made me mad. I didn't know I was going to get a transfusion. [What thoughts did you have at that time?] I don't know what I was thinking about—I just didn't like the idea of having my leg tied down. I hollered and I guess I struggled to get out, but it didn't do no good. The nurses held me down and told me to take it easy, that it was a blood transfusion and that I needed it. I guess I took it easy after that.

This incident furnishes a good example of the readiness with which persons in the immediate environment are blamed when the unexpected distressing sequelae of the operation are first experienced. But, in addition, there is evidence that this initial episode contributed to a general attitude of distrust and resentment toward the nurses which persisted throughout the entire convalescent period.

During the postoperative interview, the patient reported that the most unpleasant feature of the entire postoperative period was the continual sensation of pain in his leg (which evidently was a physical consequence of the surgical procedure). He spoke about his leg so frequently and so elaborately during the interview that it became apparent that the painful leg had, for the moment at least, become the central focus of preoccupying interest in his life. He also elaborated on the refusal incidents mentioned in the hospital records. He admitted that, on the one hand, he had repeatedly complained about his leg pains to the staff physicians but, on the other hand, he would not permit the nurses to apply hot compresses to the leg in accordance with his physician's orders. He was reluctant to talk about his resistant behavior, but he made several critical comments about the nurses and complained about their lack of solicitude: "They always make you feel you're giving them too much trouble, bothering them too much." (For additional material concerning the latent attitude underlying this patient's distrust of the nurses, see pp. 341–345.)

The behavioral disturbances described in the above case study were by no means the most extreme ones observed among the eight patients who had displayed low anticipatory fear. As will be seen shortly, several others showed as much or more postoperative anger, aggrievement, and negativism.

Table 2. Postoperative Aggressive Behavior

Qualitative summary of data from intensive case studies

Cases*	Resistant Behavior	Anger Reactions	Complaints Against Staff
High fear group			
H–1 (p. 240	On the second postoperative day was reluctant to stand up when nurse told her to, but conformed to the demand.	None	None
H–2 (pp. 240–241)	On the first three postoperative days was somewhat reluctant to have drainage tubes and rectal tubes inserted but, nevertheless, permitted the insertions to be made.	Was angry during initial insertion of drainage tube.	None
H–3 (pp. 241–242)	On first three postoperative days was reluctant to cough up mucus when asked to do so but, nevertheless, conformed with the demand.	None	None
H–4 (p. 242)	On the second postoperative day, while being turned over on his side for a routine medical examination, asked physician to stop because of pain; on second, third and fourth postoperative days refused to cough up mucus.	None	Complained that nurses were unsympathetic.
H–5 (pp. 242–243)	On second postoperative day, was reluctant to get out of bed when asked to do so, but conformed.	None	Complained about poor food and reported feeling "somewhat resentful" about having diarrhea.
Moderate fear group			
M–1 (pp. 361–363)	On second postoperative day verbally expressed some reluctance about swallowing stomach tube but conformed in response to physician's urging.	None	None
M–2 (pp. 314–318)	None	None	None
M–3 (pp. 364–366)	None	None	None
M–4 (pp. 318–324)	None	None	None
M–5 (pp. 366–367)	None	None	None
M–6	None	None	None
M–7	On the fourth postoperative day, walked from bed to the hall lavatory despite having been told by nurse to remain in room and to use bed pan.	None	None
M–8	None	None	None
M–9 (pp. 363–364)	None	None	None

* The page references given in parentheses refer to the places in the text where a more detailed account of the patient's pre- and postoperative behavior can be found.

Table 2. Postoperative Aggressive Behavior (Cont.)

Cases	Resistant Behavior	Anger Reactions	Complaints Against Staff
Low fear group			
L–1 (pp. 264–266)	Refused aspirin on fourth postoperative day; resisted swallowing stomach tube on fifth postoperative day; refused to swallow it on twelfth postoperative day.	None	Complained that staff physicians contributed to her nervousness by withholding information.
L–2 (pp. 267–268)	Refused to get out of bed when asked to do so on the third postoperative day.	None	Made numerous complaints, asserting that nurses were lax, untidy, undependable.
L–3 (pp. 345–348)	None	Became angry in O.R. and again when awakening from the anesthetic; ruminated about possibility that surgeon had "sadistic" motives or might have performed a hysterectomy.	Complained that nurses were to blame for causing or failing to alleviate various discomforts.
L–4 (pp. 258–259)	Refused to eat solid foods when prescribed on the tenth postoperative day.	None	None
L–5 (pp. 262–264)	Struggled violently in O.R. when anesthesia was administered; on first postoperative day resisted having gastric drainage tube inserted and pulled it out when physician left the room; on second postoperative day again refused to have drainage tube inserted despite repeated attempts by several physicians. On second postoperative day refused to sit up when asked.	Became outraged about discomfort of gastric drainage tube; expressed an openly hostile, belligerent attitude toward nurses on several occasions.	Blamed the "god-damn doctors," as well as nurses, for causing unnecessary postoperative pains.
L–6 (pp. 268–270)	On first postoperative day refused to permit nurses to give hypodermic injection prescribed by his physician.	On fourth postoperative day became angry and threatened to assault nurse and ward supervisor when his wife was asked to leave at the end of visiting hours. On several other occasions "lost temper"; repeatedly quarreled with nurses.	Complained that the nursing staff was grossly negligent and fed him the wrong diet; charged the doctors with laxity because they ignored his repeated complaints about the incompetence and misbehavior of the nurses.
L–7 (pp. 252–254)	On first postoperative day struggled against routine blood transfusion and had to be physically restrained; on fourth postoperative day removed a hot compress prescribed by staff physician; on fourth through seventh postoperative days consistently refused hot compresses and also refused a hot water bottle.	Became enraged while being given blood transfusion.	Complained that nurses were unavailable when needed and unwilling to help him.
L–8 (pp. 259–261)	None	None	None

Comparative Data on Aggressive Behavior

For the purpose of obtaining comparative data, brief case summaries were prepared which include all the documented instances of postoperative aggressive behavior among the 22 patients in the case study series. The pertinent case material is presented in Table 2, which is based on a systematic examination of the interview data together with the behavioral reports from the hospital staff.

Since the table presents an exhaustive list of all known items of aggressive postoperative behavior, the findings can be readily summarized in terms of relative frequency of occurrence. For each group, the number of cases displaying three main types of aggressive behavior is shown in Table 3. Although the total number of cases in each group is very small, the low fear group differs significantly from the moderate fear group on all three types of aggressive behavior. The probability-values based on Fisher's exact probability test are as follows: .025, .05, and $<.01$, respectively, for the proportion of cases who: (*a*) perform one or more acts of *extreme resistance* (refusal to conform with a demand made by a nurse or physician as part of prescribed postoperative

Table 3. Anticipatory Fear in Relation to Postoperative Aggressive Behavior

Quantitative summary of data from intensive case studies

Type of Postoperative Aggressive Behavior	Level of Preoperative Fear: Low (8 cases)	Moderate (9 cases)	High (5 cases)
1. Overtly resistant to medical demands			
a. Extreme: refused to conform	6	1	1
b. Mild: reluctant conformity	0	1	4
c. No resistant behavior	2	7	0
Total	8	9	5
2. Anger reactions toward staff			
a. Occurred once or more	4	0	1
b. Never occurred	4	9	4
Total	8	9	5
3. Complaints against the staff:			
a. Made one or more complaints	6	0	2
b. Made no complaints	2	9	3
Total	8	9	5

medical care); (*b*) display one or more episodes of *anger* (overtly enraged, loss of temper, outburst of hostile or belligerent behavior, etc.); and (*c*) express serious *complaints* against the hospital staff in the postoperative interview (alleged maltreatment, incompetency, or negligence). The differences between the low and high fear groups are in the same direction but are not large enough to be statistically significant. It is noteworthy that the resistant behavior displayed by the five cases in the high fear group differs qualitatively from that in the low fear group. The former group tended to display a *mild* form of resistance—hesitation and reluctant conformity to medical demands, usually accompanied by manifestations of extreme apprehensiveness; the low fear group, however, tended to display much more extreme resistance in the form of outright refusal to conform, often accompanied by a display of anger or resentful complaints.

The findings in Table 3 contribute to the plausibility of Hypothesis 17. They also lend some support to the conception that patients with a moderate degree of anticipatory fear are less likely than others to display postoperative disturbances, as stated in Hypothesis 15. The proportion displaying *no* overt resistant behavior in the moderate group is not only significantly larger than in the low fear group ($p =$ .05) but is also significantly larger than in the high fear group ($p =$ .025).[1]

Two Exceptional Cases

For the purpose of obtaining some clues to the necessary conditions for the occurrence of aggressive reactions to stress, it is instructive to examine the case material concerning the two patients in the low fear group who did *not* share the general pattern of postoperative resentment that occurred among the other six.

INTERVIEW CASE L–4

With the exception of a single isolated instance of postoperative resistance (refusal of prescribed solid foods), this 65-year-old woman was generally cheerful, affable, and cooperative after, as well as before, the operation. She had suffered intense pain for three weeks from a fractured hip following a fall on an icy sidewalk, and was hospitalized for corrective orthopedic surgery. Preoperatively, this patient was kept in continual traction, which contributed to her distress. At this time she expressed no fear or concern about the impending surgery, consistently asserting that she looked forward to it because it would relieve her pain. Such expectations were, of course, expressed by other patients in the low fear group, but this case was unique in that her expectation was very promptly confirmed. In contrast to all the other patients in the entire series of 22 cases, this woman experienced *a marked diminution in pain during the first few days after the operation*, which consisted of repairing the shaft of her broken femur (Smith-Peterson nailing procedure). The only new sources of pain or discomfort produced by this particular type of surgery were of a minor character, as compared with the severe hip pains which had been alleviated.

In this particular case, both the degree of victimization expected (V_e) and the degree obtained (V_o) seemed to be close to zero and, hence, there was no discrepancy. The discrepancy factor ($V_e - V_o$) has been singled out as a necessary condition for aggrievement reactions in certain of the hypotheses derived from the psychoanalytic case study. (See discussion of Hypothesis 9, pp. 143–144 and Hypothesis 11, pp. 163–167.) According to these hypotheses, unless there is a negative discrepancy ($V_e - V_o < 0$), the stresses of the postoperative period are not likely to elicit dysphoria or give rise to any marked disappointment experiences of the type which reactivate childhood rage or grief.

The lack of any sizeable discrepancy between expected and obtained victimization may have also been a factor in the absence of aggression in another patient in the low fear group. In this particular case, however, the surgery revealed an inoperable cancer, and the postoperative picture was complicated by the patient's pseudo elation defense, which was apparently motivated by an effort to deny the hopeless prognosis.

INTERVIEW CASE L–8

Mr. H., a 58-year-old tailor, was hospitalized for an exploratory chest operation after many months of illness. For over a year the patient had suffered from recurrent coughs with occasional bloody expectoration, but he regularly ignored his symptoms and refused to heed the urgent advice of his relatives to see a doctor. Finally, when his symptoms became so acute as to alarm several members of his family, he underwent a medical examination and was informed by the physician that he needed an operation. For several weeks this man refused to believe that the operation was necessary, until the physician, at the request of the family, told him that he had a serious tumor in his lungs and that if he waited any longer it might be too late for surgery to help.

In the preoperative interview, the patient repeatedly denied being at all concerned about his physical condition or about the operation. He doubted that his illness was serious, asserting that he could probably get along quite well without the operation but that, since everyone said he should have it, he was willing to give it a try. During the interview, the patient made many joking, facetious remarks, and behaved in such a way as to give the interviewer an impression of forced gaiety. When asked the standard series of questions about his expectations and feelings concerning the impending operation, he responded in a stereotyped manner, mechanically shrugged his shoulders, grinned, and remarked: "What's the use of worrying? I've got nothing to worry about." When asked what his doctor had told him, he again grinned, gave an accurate account, but concluded with the statement that he felt sure the doctor was exaggerating.

As it turned out, the exploratory operation revealed that his lung cancer had already metastisized into the pleura and was too widespread to be operable. Consequently, the surgical incision was promptly closed without any excision of lung tissue. Before closure, however, he was given an intercostal nerve block to minimize postoperative pain.

According to the medical records, this patient experienced relatively mild physiological effects as a result of the surgical procedure used: he had only a slight degree of intercostal neuralgia, felt very little incision pain, had no special difficulties with his bowels, required no nasal tubes, etc. During the postoperative period he maintained the same type of gay exterior that had characterized his preoperative behavior. He was friendly and cooperative, and displayed no resistant behavior. In the postoperative interview, he maintained that he was in fine shape, and it became obvious that he had obtained no medical information about what his operation revealed, and was not interested in finding out.

For this patient, the postoperative stresses produced by the surgery itself were mild and brought about no essential change in his physical or psychological situation. The major source of emotional disturbance —the seriousness of his illness—remained the same as before the operation, and was dealt with in the same defensive fashion.

According to the surgeon's note, surgery could have been successful in arresting the patient's slowly growing tumor mass if it had been performed when his symptoms first became apparent; but, because of the long delay, even a palliative resection was out of the question. The patient was not expected to live for more than a year and, in fact, died eleven months later. Thus, the patient's denial tendency, which had been continually dominant during the lengthy period when he refused to see a physician and during the preoperative period when he refused to believe that an operation was necessary, did not lead to any new behavioral disturbances after the operation; but, in a very real sense, his denial reactions cost him his life.

In the light of the foregoing case material, it becomes obvious that Hypothesis 17 requires a proviso which specifies something about the *intensity* of the stress stimuli to which the person is actually exposed. Both patients who displayed low anticipatory fear without developing postoperative aggression had experienced an unusually low degree of postoperative pain and discomfort, in fact, less than that of any of the other twenty patients in the case study series. For the six patients who displayed low anticipatory fear followed by high resentment, the degree of postoperative suffering was comparatively high (although not any more so than that for the average patient in the moderate fear group).

Predispositional Determinants

So far the discussion in this chapter has been concerned solely with the empirical question of whether or not the relative absence of anticipatory fear is related to subsequent behavioral disturbances. The main conclusion suggested by the small sample of intensive case studies has been stated as a general descriptive hypothesis (17) which predicts that during the crisis phase of a stress episode, reactions of anger and resentment are most likely to be seen in persons who had displayed a very low degree of anticipatory fear during the threat phase. From the few case studies examined so far, one obviously cannot assess the validity and generality of this hypothesis, but some confirmatory correlational evidence from a larger sample of surgical patients will be presented in the next chapter.[2] If the present findings continue to be confirmed by other studies of persons exposed to surgery or to other types of physical danger, it will be possible to apply Hypothesis 17 to a variety of practical problems, such as those involving the assessment of military personnel who might subsequently be exposed to wartime dangers and the prediction of civilian behavior under conditions of large-scale disaster. But, quite aside from whatever practical applications may subsequently be made on the basis of such empirical findings, the next step in the inquiry consists of the important theoretical task of ferreting out the psychological factors that help to explain the observed relationship.

The first type of explanation to be considered is one which assumes that the relationship between low preoperative fear and high postoperative resentment is essentially a noncausal one, reflecting individual differences in responsiveness to threat and stress stimuli. As was seen in the preceding chapter, an explanation solely in terms of fixed predispositional factors appears to be a very promising one to account for the observed behavior of the high fear group. A corresponding hypothesis remains to be considered as a possible explanation of the postoperative reactions of the patients in the low fear group. The latter group might consist predominantly of personalities who characteristically react to environmental threats with little or no fear but with a high degree of aggressiveness. In the clinical literature we find descriptions of personalities who typically defend themselves against fear or anxiety by responding in a highly aggressive way. In the face of environmental danger, such persons apparently manage to suppress or repress any feelings of apprehensiveness and, instead, experience feelings of anger or hostility toward some object in the immediate environment. These individuals are sometimes described as "extrapunitive" personalities (Murray, 1938; Rosenzweig, 1944). Conceivably, a personality predisposition of this type could provide an explanation of the finding that those patients who experience little or no preoperative fear tend also to display marked aggressive behavior. Nevertheless, from the available case study observations, it will be seen that this type of explanation is, at best, an incomplete one and, therefore, inadequate.

We shall first examine the case material from two patients for whom it seems quite plausible to assume that some such personality predisposition may have been present. Then we shall examine several additional cases for whom such an explanation seems wholly implausible. Pertinent evidence will be cited which suggests that at least for some of the patients in the low fear group—and perhaps for some or all in the moderate fear group as well—the relationship between the level of anticipatory fear and subsequent emotional reactions to stress is a modifiable one, implying a causal sequence of intervening processes that can be directly influenced by social communication or by other environmental events during the threat phase.

The following case study deals with a patient in the low fear group who showed a marked tendency to ward off fear by reacting in a belligerent manner.

INTERVIEW CASE L–5

Mr. J., a 44-year-old salesman, was hospitalized because of a stomach ulcer for a routine subtotal gastrectomy. Before the operation, he completely denied having any feelings of fear and seemed to be going out of his way to express an unsentimental "hard-boiled" attitude concerning all aspects of the operation. Following the operation, he became highly agitated, resisted routine hospital treatments, and developed an attitude of extreme hostility toward the hospital staff.

When interviewed on the day before his operation, Mr. J. stated in a very casual manner that he expected the operation to relieve his stomach aches and to prevent his stomach ulcer from eventually turning into a cancer. He asserted that he had no feelings of worry whatsoever. As far as the operation itself was concerned, he repeatedly stated: "I don't think about it at all." Throughout the interview he spoke in a very self-confident manner (e.g., "I feel that I can 'take' almost anything") and expressed a high degree of optimism: "I have all the confidence in the world that everything will be O.K." He made a few minor complaints about the "poor service" he was getting from "the help around here," referring to the nurses and attendants. He also expressed a mild degree of annoyance about the fact that his operation had been postponed for 24 hours. Nevertheless, he expressed confidence in and respect for the staff physicians and surgeons; none of his complaints or criticisms were directed against them.

In the operating room, the first of a series of overtly resistant acts occurred. While the anesthetic was being administered, he struggled so violently that it was necessary to have several nurses restrain him. On the day after the operation, he resisted the routine procedure of having a drainage tube inserted and actually pulled the tube out after the physician left his room. The tube was reinserted, but the patient continued to resist the treatment. On the second day after the operation, according to the physician's case notes, it was necessary to abandon the drainage treatment because the patient adamantly refused to have it.

The patient was also uncooperative in connection with other, less important, procedures. For example, when asked to sit up for the first time, he refused at first and then, after considerable coaxing, conformed reluctantly, complaining all the while that he was not feeling well enough and ought to be left alone.

During the interview conducted five days after the operation, the patient expressed extremely derogatory attitudes toward the hospital staff. In contrast to his former favorable attitude toward the physicians and surgeons, he now felt extremely hostile toward them.

> The god-damn doctors around here are always coming around to stick needles in you. They take your blood all the time for no reason. I don't want any of these things—they're not for my own good. I've answered questions to all the doctors and I've had enough of it. All these treatments are useless around here. I just want my own [private] doctor; he's the only one that can really take care of my condition.

This patient's aggressive manner prior to the operation seemed to form part of his defense against anticipatory fear. The clinical impression derived from the preoperative interview was that of a rigid character who was strongly motivated to maintain a "tough" exterior and who rejected feelings of anxiety as intolerable signs of weakness. He seemed to be making great efforts to run things his own way, to "stage his own operation," so to speak—in protest against the passivity and dependency implicit in the role of being a hospitalized surgical patient.

After the operation, he became much more hostile toward the hospital staff and overtly belligerent, but the roots of these hyperaggressive reactions could be detected in the milder forms of aggressive comments and complaints he expressed before the operation. Thus, in this particular case, it seems quite plausible to assume that both the low level of anticipatory fear and the aggressive reactions to the actual stresses of surgery stemmed from a defensive personality structure which predisposed him to react to any fear-arousing circumstances in a characteristically aggressive way.

The combination of preoperative denial and postoperative aggression might have been linked with a personality predisposition in one other patient who displayed a marked aggrievement reaction.

INTERVIEW CASE L-1

Mrs. Y., a 53-year-old housewife, was hospitalized at a time when she was suffering spasmodically from gall stones. Prior to the operation (cholecystectomy), she was aware of the risks involved but was completely unperturbed about the operation. After the operation she became overtly resistant to routine postoperative treatments. She developed negative attitudes toward the hospital staff, lost some of her former self-confidence, and became a serious management problem because she refused to undergo routine treatments that were an essential part of her medical care.

In the preoperative interview she asserted: "I never worry about the operation at all—that's God's honest truth." In discussing the impending operation, she said that she deliberately avoided thinking about it, and minimized its importance: "A gall bladder operation today is becoming like having your appendix out or a tooth pulled, it's so simple." She acknowledged the fact that there would be some postoperative discomfort, but she felt certain that the risks were negligible compared with the gains to be derived from having the operation: "I can't live like this . . . if I don't have the operation I'm going to die sooner or later anyhow. . . . I know that after the operation I'll be right here on earth to finish up my work." Coupled with her fatalistic attitude was a strong affirmation of her own ability to meet whatever contingencies might conceivably arise: "As long as I feel I have a fighting chance, I'll fight; I'm not going to lie there and say, 'I'm sick, I'm going to die, I give up.' " Although she alluded indirectly to the possibility of death several times, it was in a detached, affectless manner. This patient completely denied having any feelings of worry or concern about her various physical disorders or about the outcome of the operation.

Following the operation, Mrs. Y. displayed overtly resistant behavior on several different occasions, beginning with a trivial incident on the first postoperative day, when she refused to take an aspirin. On the fifth postoperative day, she refused to swallow a stomach tube. After much coaxing, she allowed it to be inserted but was still unable to swallow it:

> I had exactly the same thing before the operation without any trouble, but after the operation I felt fed up with it and I just couldn't stand the idea of having it in for a long period of time.

A week later, after almost complete recovery from the operation, she refused to permit a routine diagnostic test which again required swallowing a stomach tube:

> I couldn't swallow another tube; I told them, "Please don't hold it against me but I just can't take it"; I felt it wasn't absolutely necessary and I felt I could get along without it.

Unlike her preoperative attitude of self-confidence, Mrs. Y.'s postoperative self-appraisals were harshly deprecatory: "I'm just turning into a sissy; I just can't take it any more." She asserted that this change was due to the fact that the operation left her in a "weakened and nervous condition." She also expressed a lack of confidence in the staff physicians and blamed them for some of her nervousness: "They told me I have nothing to worry about, but they haven't really told me what's wrong and that just keeps me guessing." This attitude, too, was in marked contrast to the unequivocally positive attitude of trust and confidence she had expressed preoperatively.

In seeking to understand this patient's emotional reactions, we must take account of the following statements from her preoperative interview which suggest that this woman regularly tended to ward off feelings of fear:

> I've never had any fear in connection with any of my illnesses. . . . I've never been concerned about my emotional reactions. I keep all my emotions inside. All I ever feel is the butterflies I get in my stomach, and I just work hard to work it off. I have felt upset at times in the past but I never express it—I don't know why, but I can't cry for more than a few

minutes. It's all inside of me like a big lump and I can't let it out. I must keep occupied. I haven't thought about this operation and so I haven't been upset in any way. I didn't want to be upset because you are tense and it's hard to take care of you—the nurses and doctors have a more difficult job when the patient is tense. . . . I have never had any fear. It's a peculiar feeling, I imagine, because I've never experienced it.

The patient's preoperative reaction can be readily explained as simply another instance of her general tendency to repress feelings of fear in the face of any environmental threats. Nevertheless, it should be borne in mind that this patient, like most other patients in the low fear group, did *not* exhibit any apparent aggressive or depressive reactions until *after* the operation. During the preoperative period, she appeared to be extremely calm, affable, and cooperative. Therefore, we cannot assume that the personality predisposition of this patient consists of a general tendency to react to the environmental *threats* of danger with aggression rather than anxiety. In this case, the role played by personality factors in determining aggrievement reactions after the operation seems to be more complicated than in Case L–5.

Alternative Causal Sequences

There are two main causal sequences to be considered which can be regarded as alternative ways of explaining the postoperative aggressive reactions displayed by most of the patients in the "low" fear group. First, the personality predisposition may be limited to influencing the preoperative emotional response (repression or suppression of fear); once this response (or lack of response) occurs, it may play a causal role in increasing the subsequent vulnerability of the patient when postoperative stress is encountered. For instance, the absence of preoperative fear may result in inadequate psychological preparation for postoperative stress, and this may somehow increase the chances of severe disappointment reactions during the postoperative period, with a consequent increase in the probability of developing aggrievement reactions. This type of explanation has been referred to earlier as a "modifiable" causal sequence. The alternative approach is to postulate a noncausal or static relationship, that is, to assume that both the postoperative aggression and the preoperative fear are attributable to a common, relatively unmodified, predisposition. For example, the assumption might be that the patient has some special type of motive, attitude, emotional bias, or character structure which causes the two types of reaction tendencies to be manifested sequentially or at different times, such that: (*a*) when signs of the *threat* of approaching danger occur, the person habitually displays a pseudocalm exterior by suppressing or repressing thoughts that would give rise to anticipatory fear, and (*b*) when actual *stress stimuli* occur (e.g., pain and impairment of body functions), the person tends to react aggressively.

The evidence from the last case discussed (L–1) is entirely equivocal in that it could be equally well interpreted according to either a dynamic or static explanatory concept. But additional case material, to which the remainder of this chapter is devoted, suggests a modifiable causal sequence.

INTERVIEW CASE L–2

Mrs. A., a 23-year-old housewife, was hospitalized for a cholecystectomy. She denied experiencing any anxiety or concern about the operation beforehand. After the operation, she became somewhat agitated and occasionally resisted the demands made by the nurses. For example, on the third postoperative day, when asked to get out of bed for the first time, she refused: "I just didn't want to; I was kind of leary about it." In the postoperative interview she made several complaints about the nurses, claiming that they were lax about bringing her the bed pan when she needed it, that she was not washed promptly when she awoke each morning, that her bed was never made up until very late in the day. In addition to these complaints, she expressed a definitely negative evaluation of nurses in general: "I don't have any confidence in them any more, like I did before the operation; they don't do anything for you when you need them."

Additional evidence indicates that the very low degree of anticipatory fear before this particular operation cannot be regarded as a typical or habitual type of reaction for the patient. Hospital records show that the patient had been confined for childbirth six months earlier and, at that time, had displayed a high degree of apprehensiveness beforehand. Moreover, since the birth of her child she had been continually worried about her own health and about the baby's nocturnal crying. Furthermore, this patient reported, in both her preoperative and postoperative interviews, that she had felt extremely afraid before an appendectomy, which had taken place a few years earlier. After stating that she had felt enormously relieved once that operation had been over, she went on to say: "I don't know why I felt so afraid that time and not at all this time." According to the hospital records as well as the patient's retrospective account, the patient had been cooperative and uncomplaining throughout the postoperative convalescence following the appendectomy, with no instances of resistant behavior.

In this case, the relative absence of preoperative fear does not seem to be attributable to a fixed predisposition but rather appears to be the outcome of the preceding operation experience together with the current circumstances. With respect to the latter, the patient's statements clearly indicate that the present operation offered a welcomed opportunity to escape, for a time, from her home situation which had been creating considerable inner tension and with which she apparently felt unable to cope. Her memory of the emotional relief experienced during the earlier operation might have contributed to the tendency to perceive this operation more as an opportunity for emotional relief than as a dangerous threat.

A similar history of earlier episodes of high anticipatory fear occurs in the next case to be considered.

INTERVIEW CASE L–6

Mr. G., a 56-year-old business man, consistently impressed the hospital staff as one of the most cheerful, carefree, and cooperative patients who had ever been hospitalized for surgery. Following his operation (partial thyroidectomy), this man became so resistant, tense, and hostile that he was scarcely recognizable as the same person.[4]

In a very relaxed, sociable mood during the preoperative interview, the patient denied having any feelings of fear:

> When they told me last night that the operation was definitely scheduled, I had no reaction, no fear at all. . . . I feel the same way about it now. . . . Having this operation is like a vacation for me.

Detailed questioning about his feelings revealed only that he felt a slight degree of concern about the possible long-range effects of having too much thyroid tissue removed, but he maintained that he had no "real" concern about this because of his absolute confidence in the doctor's ability to take proper care of him. Throughout the interview, he expressed extremely optimistic expectations, not only in connection with the outcome of the operation but also with respect to any temporary pain or discomfort it might produce. As the basis for his optimism, he repeatedly referred to an operation of the same type he had undergone less than a year before, from which he had recovered rapidly, without any marked discomfort.

Enthusiastically, he praised the hospital staff several times during the preoperative interview. His comment about the nurses, for example, was:

> The nurses? They're 100 percent good. . . . Of course, they could stand another nurse on this floor when they have a full house like this. But those girls really do a wonderful job—busy every minute, always on the job.

Following the operation, those who were in daily contact with him were surprised to discover that he had become very quarrelsome and irritable. On a number of occasions, he displayed extreme anger and overt resistance to routine postoperative treatments. The day after his operation, for example, he aggressively refused to take a hypodermic injection ordered by his physician, despite repeated urging by the nurses.

In the postoperative interview, five days after the operation, the patient recounted, with much heated affect, one grievance after another against the nurses and ward attendants. The following is a sample of the innumerable incidents which he reported as having enraged him:

> Instead of fresh orange juice, they gave me canned juices and broth that tasted like a mixture of piss and quinine. . . . When the nurses tried to kick my wife and son out last night, I argued with them and with the supervisor so much that it made me sick, I got so excited and upset. . . . The nurses give me all kinds of god-damn excuses about not keeping my diet, always saying "it's not on the chart." . . . If I wasn't knocked out from my operation yesterday [when the nurse sassed me], I would have knocked her down on the floor, I really mean it!

Before the operation he had asserted "this is one of the very best hospitals in the world," but after the operation his attitude was markedly changed, colored by the alleged mistreatment he had suffered: "If any of my friends said they were going to come here I'd tell them not to—I'd warn them about the nurses here." Even his attitude toward the staff doctors, which he claimed was as favorable as ever, appeared to be affected to some degree by his hostility toward the nurses: "I told some of these things [about the negligence of the nurses] to the doctors yesterday, but—you know how they are—they just defended them." Similarly, his statement that "the operation was 100 percent successful" was contradicted by other statements in the same postoperative session: "I think that all that worry [caused by the nurses] has given me a terrific setback."

In one way or another, he also blamed the nurses and the ward attendants for the unpleasant experiences he had from gas pains, muscular aches, urination difficulties, and other postoperative discomforts which, before the operation, he had so optimistically excluded from his expectations. (See pp. 339–340 below for further details about the content of this patient's complaints.)

Although he freely admitted having experienced apprehensiveness about his physical condition since the operation, the patient consistently maintained that prior to the operation he had felt no concern whatsoever. Of particular interest for the present discussion is the fact that this patient readily admitted having been worried about his health and about medical treatment at various times in the past. Approximately eight months earlier, he had undergone an operation similar to the present one. At that time, however, he had experienced considerable fear beforehand, and he was deeply impressed by the fact that after the operation he had experienced very little pain and had actually enjoyed the indulgent care, attention, and sociability that characterized the convalescent period, which he referred to as a "real vacation." As mentioned earlier, he made constant reference to this earlier gratifying surgical experience in his preoperative interviews, particularly when describing his expectations with respect to the present operation. Apparently the favorable memory of the antecedent operation played a major role in determining the low level of anticipatory fear before the present operation. The contrasting preoperative emotional reactions to the two very similar operations, only eight months apart, show quite clearly that such reactions can be extremely variable. After the first operation, he had been friendly with the entire staff of his ward; whereas after the second operation, his hostility was so overt that he became exceptionally disliked by essentially the same personnel.

From the two cases just described, it seems that the occurrence of a low degree of anticipatory fear cannot be explained in all cases as a simple manifestation of a personality predisposition. Unlike the patient described earlier (Case L–5), who appeared to be chronically motivated to maintain a tough, hypermasculine attitude toward external dangers, these two patients did not characteristically repress or suppress their apprehensiveness. In fact, both patients had actually reacted with moderate or relatively high fear in the recent past when confronted with a physical threat situation similar to the present operation. The fact that these patients reacted at this particular time with very low preoperative fear appears to be due largely to specific events and situational factors—favorable experiences after a recent operation, desire for relief from the tensions of the present job or home situation, etc. Similar factors also appear to play a substantial role in determining the level of preoperative fear in other patients as well. For example, Case L–3 (whose preoperative and postoperative reactions will be described in considerable detail in a later chapter, pp. 345–348) was highly influenced by communications from others concerning the nonseriousness of the appendectomy she was about to have. This woman had not undergone any previous operations, but the author had the opportunity to obtain detailed information about her personality charateristics and behavior in a variety of minor stress situations. In this case, neither the low level of anticipatory fear nor the subsequent aggression appeared to be characteristic of her responses to environmental stress. In general, she was an emotionally labile person who displayed a moderate or high level of anticipatory fear in objective threat situations and who rarely displayed any reactions of externalized aggression. The extraordinarily low level of anticipatory fear she experienced prior to the appendectomy seemed to have been fostered by two situational factors. First, the operation came at a time when it seriously interrupted her professional work, and her efforts to minimize the disruption evidently furnished an excellent opportunity for distraction. Second, she knew that the operation was a very minor one, as far as medical risks were concerned, and she was told by her physician and others that there was "no need to worry about it." She reported that everyone to whom she mentioned the impending operation shared the view that "there is really nothing to it." These situational conditions seemed to have played a major role in determining her low level of anticipatory fear, enabling her to focus all of her concern upon problems connected with her work and to avoid thinking about the threat represented by the operation itself.

The case history material from the three patients just discussed suggests that postoperative aggressive reactions are likely to occur if, for *any* reason (whether due to personality factors or situational factors), the patient experiences a very low degree of anticipatory fear. This inference is consistent with the assumption that the preoperative emotional reaction plays a dynamic or causal role in producing the postoperative aggressive reactions.

There are other considerations which also suggest that, if a unitary explanation is to be given, a modifiable causal sequence is more plausible than a static predispositional concept.[3] One of the testable implications pertains to the effects of preparatory communications. Let us assume that a sizeable proportion of surgical patients spontaneously will have low anticipatory fear before entering the operating room because, like several of the cases observed in the "low" anticipatory fear group, they sincerely believe that there is "nothing to worry about." The emotional status of such patients should be markedly influenced by preparatory communications which point up the unpleasant or dangerous aspects of the impending surgical experience. In Chapter 25, we shall examine correlational evidence which provides tentative support for the prediction that advance information about postoperative pains and discomforts *raises the level of anticipatory fear* and subsequently makes for a *decrease in the incidence of postoperative resentment.* The next few chapters will furnish some additional evidence which also favors an interpretation in terms of a dynamic process such that the suppression or repression of fear before the operation is a causal factor in the development of postoperative anger and resentment. Chapter 22 will present quantitative data from the survey research bearing on the relationship between anticipatory fear and postoperative emotional disturbances. Then, in Chapters 23 and 24, additional case study evidence will be analyzed for the purpose of arriving at a more specific conception of the role of anticipatory fear in the psychological processes which mediate postoperative adjustment.

Notes

1. The probability values were determined by using the tables given by Siegel (1956) for Fisher's exact probability test. All probability values are one-tailed, since the hypotheses under discussion specify the direction of the group differences.

2. A search of the literature on reactions to surgery and to other danger situations failed to turn up any systematic findings bearing directly upon Hypothesis 17. However, some incidental observations reported by several clinical investigators seem to be compatible with this hypothesis and with Hypothesis 15. For example, H. Deutsch (1945), on the basis of her psychoanalytic work with patients who gave retrospective accounts of their past surgical experiences, noted that those who had reacted with manifest anxiety before the operation had not necessarily become emotionally disturbed after the operation. Similarly, Lindemann (1941, p. 146) reported that, in a series of 38 surgical patients, ". . . we could not confirm certain plausible assumptions, for instance, that the display of anxiety before the operation is an indication of probable later psychiatric difficulties."

In studies of psychological stress that deal with danger situations other than surgery, there are some suggestive indications along the same lines. Redlich et al. (1946), in their observations of reactions to lumbar punctures, noted that some patients who were extremely calm beforehand became upset when the procedure was under way. Margolin and Kubie (1943), in a study of traumatic reactions among torpedoed seamen, reported that intense emotional disturbances frequently occurred among those who had been quite unafraid before they were shipwrecked. I. Romalis (1942) gave an account of the emotional problems of the wives of American service men in which she asserts that those women who remained unworried about the prospects of their husbands being drafted subsequently became extraordinarily upset and resentful when the separation entailed by military service became an actuality.

3. An explanation in terms of a modifiable causal sequence seems much more promising, if one is attempting to develop a unitary theoretical explanation of the differences between the low fear group and the moderate fear group—an explanation in terms of a *single* explanatory concept which could give a satisfactory account of the postoperative behavior of all patients in both groups. A unitary explanation would be one which assumes that whenever a very low degree of anticipatory fear occurs, whether due primarily to personality predispositions or to situational factors, the *same* mediating process will occur (or the *same* essential

adjustive process will *fail* to occur), as a result of which the person will somehow become sensitized to react to subsequent stress stimuli with intense resentment.

For the high anticipatory fear group, I concluded that the relationship between the postoperative and the preoperative emotional disturbances was probably a static one, attributable to a predispositional tendency. Before the operation, the patients in that group manifested high fear and, again, after the operation, they showed the same sort of reaction. Hence, there was no evidence that any sort of psychological *change* had occurred during the hospital experience; this, together with other evidence, contributed to the conclusion that the reactions could best be explained in terms of stable predispositions.

But for the group with which the present chapter is concerned, it should be noted that very low preoperative fear is predictive of *changes* in attitudes and behavior. In addition to developing aggressive attitudes toward the hospital staff during the course of their postoperative hospital experience, most of the patients in the low anticipatory fear group also showed a change in their overt aggressive behavior. For instance, none of the patients were resentful, uncooperative, or resistant in their overt behavior *before* the operation, but many of them became so *after* the operation. The fact that low preoperative fear precedes and is predictive of such changes in affect, attitude, and behavior suggests that some dynamic process is involved whereby the patient's preoperative affective responses somehow condition or influence his reactions to subsequent environmental events. (See pp. 340 ff. for hypotheses concerning mediating processes.)

4. It was considered possible that the temporary personality change in this particular case might have been attributable to an organic factor, as a result of alterations in thyroid functioning. But neither the surgeon nor the staff endocrinologist felt that there was much likelihood of this possibility, especially since the standard postoperative endocrinological regime was followed, just as after the patient's earlier thyroid operation, which had produced no apparent behavioral changes.

22.

Survey findings: preoperative fear and postoperative adjustment

The interview evidence presented in the preceding chapters indicates that there may be a curvilinear relationship between the level of preoperative fear and postoperative emotional disturbance: (*a*) High preoperative fear tends to be followed by high postoperative fear and other forms of emotional upset; (*b*) low preoperative fear also tends to be followed by various forms of emotional disturbance (mainly taking the form of rage reactions and resentment toward the hospital staff); (*c*) a moderate degree of preoperative fear tends to be followed by a relative absence of postoperative emotional disturbance. However, the case study results are merely suggestive rather than definitive. So few cases are involved that one cannot feel confident about the trends noted. Moreover, as has been repeatedly mentioned, there is the possibility of *contamination* since the same observer conducted the pre- and post-interviews and did the assessment of pre- and postoperative emotional status.

The same relationships between preoperative fear and postoperative reactions, as specified by Hypotheses 15, 16, and 17, were reinvestigated with a much larger sample, using questionnaire survey data obtained from college students. In analyzing the survey data, it was possible to test the three hypotheses in such a way as to eliminate the possibility of contamination. But the findings, of course, have their own limitations, inasmuch as they are based on the patients' written reports obtained in questionnaires which were filled out after the surgical experience was over. Such reports are obviously subject to many more distortions than those obtained from contemporaneous interviews, not only because there is much greater opportunity for memory errors but also because it is much easier to withhold embarrassing details when filling out a questionnaire. Accordingly, the questionnaire survey cannot be regarded as a completely valid source of information, and the findings are carefully evaluated in terms of their consistency with the intensive case study findings. By using a combination of quantitative survey results and intensive case study observations, one can feel much more confident about the conclusions than if one were to use either method alone.

This chapter presents the main findings from the survey research. First, the procedure used in sorting subjects into the high, moderate, and low preoperative fear groups is described, and some evidence is presented concerning the reliability of the sorting criterion. Then some data are given bearing on the way in which emotional reactions are related to the severity of objective threat. That is, the level of preoperative fear is examined in relation to the amount of *pain*, the type of *anesthetic*, the nature of the *surgical procedure* to which the individual was about to be exposed, and other objective features of the stress situation. The evidence concerning such relationships is important because it provides background information about the potential sources of fear. It also enables one to assess the likelihood that the main survey findings, all of which are based on retrospective reports, might be seriously affected by the subjects' memory distortions. The men who were confronted with the most postoperative pain, for example, might remember and report more fear reactions when asked to describe how they had felt before and after the operation, thereby yielding a correlation which seems to support Hypothesis 16 but which merely reflects the effects of a postoperative stimulus variable. A variety of factors associated with the magnitude of the threat or the intensity of the stress stimuli were investigated, primarily for the purpose of identifying those factors which were relatively constant for the different levels of preoperative fear and those which were not. The latter require special analytic procedures of controlled comparisons in order to hold them constant. Once these methodological considerations become clear, we turn to the main findings bearing on Hypotheses 15, 16, and 17. Comparisons are made of surgical patients in the high, moderate and low preoperative fear groups with respect to the following aspects of postoperative adjustment: (*a*) fear reactions during convalescence; (*b*) symptoms of sustained emotional disturbance; and (*c*) attitudes of resentment and hostility toward the hospital staff.

Selection of Subjects

A survey questionnaire which asked each subject to describe a recent medical or dental experience was submitted to over 1000 male undergraduate students at Yale University.[1] The first step in the analysis was to select those men who reported specifically on a surgical procedure, whether major or minor. There were over 200 such cases but a sizeable minority (51 cases) reported that they had not known about the operation until the day it took place. The latter subjects were excluded from the present results because they include a heterogeneous variety of deviant cases, including: (*a*) a few major surgery cases brought to the hospital in an unconscious state because of a sudden traumatic injury; (*b*) a number of major and minor surgery cases who were given an emergency operation because of acute symptoms or suspected malignancy; (*c*) a number of minor surgery cases who were subjected to such a simple and rapid procedure that it could be done in the examining physician's office and on the spur of the moment. These cases were also exposed to a miscellaneous assortment of atypical situational factors which would make it extremely difficult to interpret behavioral comparisons between this heterogeneous group and any group of surgical patients who knew about the operation beforehand. It appeared best, therefore, to eliminate from the present analysis anyone who reported that he had *not known* about the prospective operation on the day before it took place.[2] The remaining 149 cases comprised the survey sample.

The social composition of the sample was relatively homogeneous. Since all 149 subjects were Yale undergraduate students, there was a narrow range of age (17–21) and of educational level. Although the social origins of the men varied somewhat, almost all were from American middle- or upper-class families; there were practically no men who adhered to the social norms or mores of a foreign ethnic group. The advantage of having a sample with a restricted range of social variation is that, when the subjects are sorted into different subgroups (e.g., high, moderate, low fear), the investigator is not so likely to encounter any marked subgroup differences in national or ethnic origins that could account for the behavioral differences. Personality characteristics, on the other hand, may vary widely in such a sample.

Self-Ratings on Level of Preoperative Fear

The key question used for assessing degree of preoperative fear was as follows:

QUESTION A: *On the day before* the actual day it was performed, how much of the time altogether did you worry about the operation (or treatment) or feel concerned about it?

____Was worried or concerned about it *during most of the day before.*
____Was worried or concerned about it *during a good part of the day before.*
____Was worried or concerned about it *occasionally throughout the day before.*
____Was worried or concerned about it for *a short time during the day before.*
____Was worried or concerned about it for *only a few minutes altogether on the day before.*
____Was *not at all* worried or concerned about it during the day before.
____Didn't know about the operation or treatment on the day before it was performed.

As previously stated, all subjects who gave the last answer ("Didn't know"), as well as those who gave no answer to this question, were eliminated from the sample. The remaining 149 subjects, all of whom gave a usable self-rating on level of fear on the day before the operation, were sorted into "low," "moderate," and "high" fear groups in the following way. First it was noted that almost one-fourth of the cases (35 cases, which constituted 23½% of the total sample) had answered "Was *not at all* worried." This sizeable minority was classified as low preoperative fear. An effort was then made to select the upper one-fourth of the sample as the high fear cases. The closest approximation that could be obtained was provided by using the top three answer categories, which gave a group of 47 cases, or 31½% of the total sample. The remaining 67 cases (or 45% of the total sample) were classified as moderate fear cases.

Thus, the three groups were obtained by selecting roughly the upper and lower quartiles and were defined as follows:

1. The high fear group consisted of those who reported having been worried "occasionally throughout the day before," or "during a good part of the day before," or "during most of the day before."

2. The moderate fear group consisted of those who reported having been worried for "only a few minutes" or "for a short time."

3. The low fear group consisted of those who reported having been "not at all worried or concerned."

Although no precise data were available for assessing the reliability and validity of the above three categories, a rough indication of the consistency of the self-ratings was obtained by taking account of the relationship between these ratings and those obtained from two other questions which also dealt with preoperative fears. One question asked about the *intensity* of anticipatory fear and referred to the same time period as the key sorting question:

QUESTION B: *On the day before* the actual day of the operation or treatment, how intense was the *most severe* fear or anxiety that you experienced when you thought about the fact that you were going to have the operation or treatment?

____ Extremely intense fear or anxiety.
____ Very intense.
____ Fairly intense.
____ Moderate.
____ Slight.
____ Very slight.
____ None at all.
____ Didn't know about the operation or treatment on the day before it was performed.

The following categories were used in order to obtain a percentage distribution comparable to that obtained on the key question.

Severe fear (first four categories)—39 cases or 26% of the sample.
Slight fear (the next two categories)—78 cases or 52% of the sample.
No fear (seventh category)—32 cases or 22% of the sample.

The relationship between the self-ratings on intensity and those obtained from the key question is shown in the upper half of Chart 1. The bar chart shows that there is a very marked positive correlation between responses to the two questions (the probability value based on a Chi-square test is well beyond the 1% significance level).

The lower half of Chart 1 shows the relationship between the key question and another question which also dealt with the intensity of preoperative fear, but for a different time period.

QUESTION C: *During the hour immediately before the operation or treatment was started* (before you were given the anesthetic, if any), how intense was the *most severe* fear or anxiety that you experienced?

The answer categories were the same as for Question B, and were trichotomized in the same way to obtain the three categories, "severe," "slight," and "none." This trichotomy yielded a percentage distribution similar to Questions A and B, but with a somewhat higher incidence of "severe" reactions, presumably attributable to the closer proximity of the threat (see Chart 2 and the discussion of the temporal course of fear reactions, pp. 284–285). Again, the bar chart shows a strong positive relationship between this measure of intensity of fear and the key sorting question. (The probability value based on a Chi-square test is well beyond the 1% significance level.)

Chart 1. Consistency of Self-Ratings on Preoperative Fear*

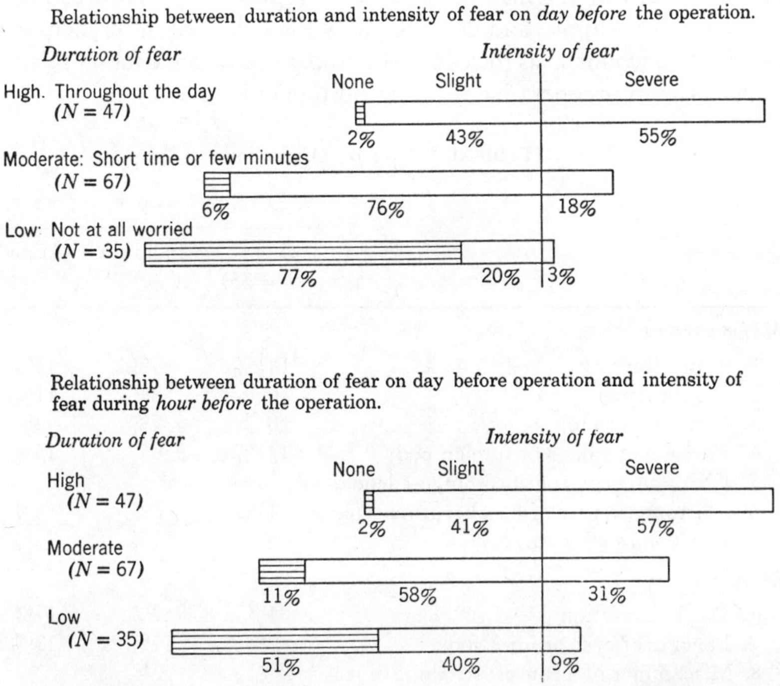

* *Note:* All cases who reported that they did *not* know about impending operation on the day before it took place were excluded from this study.

In summary, the results in Chart 1 show that those men who reported high, moderate, and low fear on the key sorting question (dealing with *duration* of fear on the day before the operation) tended to give similar responses on the other two questions dealing with the *intensity* of their preoperative fears. Since the subjects were found to be fairly consistent in their self-ratings of preoperative fear, the likelihood is increased that the criterion used to assess preoperative fear is fairly reliable.

Magnitude of Stress

It is generally recognized that high anticipatory fear is much more likely to be elicited when an objective threat is severe rather than mild, or when the anticipated stress stimuli are of high rather than low magnitude. One expects to find, therefore, that anticipatory fear is highest in those surgical patients who face the most serious surgical operations —those involving the greatest risk of body damage, the greatest amount of pain, and the most severe deprivations. This section presents evidence concerning the magnitude of stress reported by the three groups in the surgical sample, and describes how the observed differences were taken into account so as to reduce the ambiguity of the data on relationships between preoperative fear and postoperative reactions.

Table 4. Type of Operation

	Level of Preoperative Fear		
	Low ($N = 35$)	Moderate ($N = 67$)	High ($N = 47$)
Major surgery			
1. Appendectomy	14⅓%	9%	11%
2. Hernia repair	0	3%	11%
3. Hemorrhoidectomy	0	2%	4%
4. Excision of tumor or foreign body	14⅓%	9%	15%
5. ENT surgery: tonsillectomy, adenoidectomy, repair of nasal septum, etc.	14⅓%	8%	16%
Total major surgery	43%	31%	57%
Minor surgery			
6. Tooth extraction	34%	42%	17%
7. Lancing of cyst or infection	9%	12%	13%
8. Misc. minor procedures: stitching of laceration, repair of ingrown nails, etc.	14%	15%	13%
Total minor surgery	57%	69%	43%
Total	100%	100%	100%

Table 4 shows the type of operation undergone by patients in the high, moderate, and low fear groups. The results are based on the subjects' answers to the following question:

QUESTION D: Give the name of the operation or treatment (or describe briefly the nature of it).

The distinction between "major" and "minor" operations used in Table 4 is based on current medical terminology and pertains to the usual level of physiological stress produced by the given type of surgical intervention. "Major" operations generally require the use of hospital operating room facilities, usually involve the administration of a general or spinal anesthetic, and carry the risk of physiological shock and other postoperative complications. "Minor" operations, on the other hand, are generally performed in the office of a physician (or dental surgeon), typically involve the use of either a local anesthetic or no anesthetic, and ordinarily carry such little risk of physiological distress that the patient is not given any special nursing care following the operation.

As expected, the patients in the high preoperative fear group were more likely to be facing major surgical operations than those in the other two groups. The difference between the high and moderate groups shown in the subtotals of Table 4 is statistically significant beyond the 1% level. Thus, a reaction of high preoperative fear appears to be more likely if a person is facing a major rather than a minor surgical operation.

The low group, however, does not differ significantly from the moderate group. This finding suggests that a low level of anticipatory fear, as compared with a moderate level, is not associated with a lower degree of objective threat or stress. In fact, the results in Table 4 show that a slightly higher percentage of the low fear group was facing the more serious type of surgery than of the moderate group. A pertinent assumption, stated earlier, is that psychological variables—such as personality predispositions, attitudes concerning one's vulnerability to the stress stimuli, and the degree to which one has been informed about the consequences of the threat—are the main factors which determine whether a person will react to a given external threat with moderate fear or with a relative absence of fear. The results in Table 4 are consistent with this assumption, though they obviously cannot be considered as proving it.

Additional comparative data on objective features of the surgery experience, presented in Table 5, show essentially the same picture as Table 4. The comparisons are based on questions dealing with the following four characteristics, all of which may be expected to make some difference with respect to severity of stress: (1) the time interval between the day when the patient was informed that the operation was definitely necessary and the day of the operation; (2) the type of anesthetic; (3) the number of days the patient was kept in bed after the operation; and (4) the number of weeks before the patient was able to resume work and engage in usual daily activities. The results in

Table 5. Objective Features of the Operation Related to Level of Preoperative Fear

Self-Ratings on Objective Features of the Operation	Level of Preoperative Fear Low ($N = 35$)	Moderate ($N = 67$)	High ($N = 47$)
1. Informed that operation was definitely necessary:			
More than one week before	52%	52%	49%
Two to seven days before	28%	24%	28%
One day before	20%	24%	23%
Total	100%	100%	100%
2. Type of anesthetic:			
General (completely unconscious)	26%	21%	38%
Spinal	9%	9%	11%
Local	57%	61%	45%
Don't know or none	8%	9%	6%
Total	100%	100%	100%
3. Number of days kept in bed after operation:			
More than fourteen days	14%	8%	11%
Three to fourteen days	29%	20%	30%
One to two days	11%	17%	23%
Less than one day	46%	55%	36%
Total	100%	100%	100%
4. Number of weeks before able to resume work and usual activities:			
More than four weeks	12%	11%	19%
Two to four weeks	20%	13%	21%
One to two weeks	11%	13%	13%
Less than one week	57%	63%	47%
Total	100%	100%	100%

Table 5 again indicate that there is little difference between the low fear group and the moderate group. The percentage differences are very slight and nonsignificant on all four items. The high fear group, on the other hand, differs from the moderate group in that a significantly higher percentage ($p < .05$) reported: (1) having received a general anesthetic; (2) having been kept in bed for one day or more; and (3) having been unable to resume work and normal activities until two weeks or more after the operation. These findings bear the same implications as those in Table 4, since major surgery usually differs from minor surgery in these three respects. Thus, the findings in Table 5, like those in Table 4, provide evidence which indicates that (*a*) the high fear group contained proportionately more cases facing severe danger and deprivation than the moderate group; but (*b*) there was no essential difference in this respect between the moderate and low fear groups (or between the high and low fear groups).

Table 6. Incapacitation and Pain

Self-Ratings on Incapacitation and Pain:	Level of Preoperative Fear		
	Low ($N = 35$)	Moderate ($N = 67$)	High ($N = 47$)
1. *Incapacitation* from preoperative illness or injury:			
Severe: stayed in bed	9%	8%	0%
Moderate: restricted activities	9%	10%	11%
Slight: performed normal daily activities	82%	82%	89%
Total	100%	100%	100%
2. Duration of *physical pain* on day before operation:			
During most of day	17%	12%	11%
Occasionally	14%	22%	32%
Only a few minutes or not at all	69%	66%	57%
Total	100%	100%	100%
3. Intensity of the *most severe pain* on day before operation:			
Very or extremely intense	12%	8%	11%
Slight or moderate	31%	36%	42%
No pain at all	57%	56%	47%
Total	100%	100%	100%
4. Number of days before *postoperative pains subsided:*			
More than seven days	21%	23%	28%
Two to seven days	46%	48%	33%
One day or less	33%	29%	39%
Total	100%	100%	100%

Additional data obtained from a series of questions bearing on incapacitation and pain are shown in Table 6. A slightly higher percentage of the "high" fear group reported experiencing preoperative and postoperative pain, but none of the differences are statistically significant. The "moderate" and "low" fear groups report almost exactly the same incidence of preoperative and postoperative pain, which again supports the conclusion that these two groups did not differ significantly in severity of stress stimuli.

The latter conclusion obviously does not necessarily imply that the presence or absence of fear is wholly unrelated to the severity of threat or stress stimuli. That the occurrence of fear reactions depends to a considerable extent upon objective characteristics of the danger or deprivation is clearly shown by Chart 2, in which major surgery patients

Chart 2. Temporal Course of Fear Responses Reported by Three Groups Exposed to Different Degrees of Stress: Major Surgery, Minor Surgery, and Dental Treatment

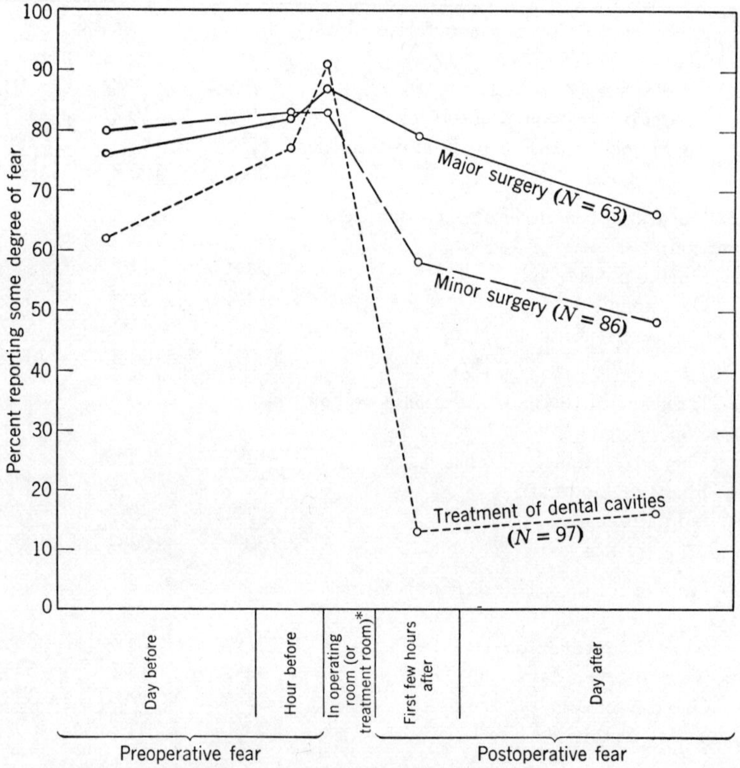

are compared with minor surgery patients and with patients who were subjected to routine dental drilling. This chart shows the percentage of each group reporting slight or severe fear (100% minus the percentage reporting no fear) in response to each of a series of questions about the intensity of fear at various stages of the stress episode.[3]

The incidence of fear reactions on the *day before* the operation (or treatment) is significantly lower among the dental patients than among the major or minor surgery patients ($p > .05$). During the hour before the operation or treatment and when the patients were actually in the operating or treatment room, the vast majority in each group reported having been fearful; at these time points, the differences among the three "stress" groups are very small and nonsignificant. During the period following the operation or treatment (during the first few hours after and during the day after) there is an extremely marked difference between the dental patients and the surgery patients ($p < .001$), and there is also a sizeable difference between major and minor surgery patients ($p > .05$). If we were to take the self-rating results at face value, Chart 2 would be interpreted as indicating that immediately after *dental treatment*, fear reactions drop down so markedly that the vast majority of dental patients experience no fear at all; immediately after a *minor operation*, fear reactions subside somewhat, but about half the cases still experience some degree of fear during the first and second postoperative days; immediately after a *major operation*, however, fear reactions subside only very slightly, if at all, and the vast majority of patients continue to experience fear during the first two postoperative days (and perhaps much longer). The differences among the groups shown in Chart 2 undoubtedly reflect the differential stress stimuli to which the dental and surgical patients were exposed.

The above results, as well as additional questionnaire data for the dental and surgical cases, consistently bear out the general assumption that a less severe type of stress episode will evoke a lower incidence of emotional disturbance.[4] The fact that the findings conform with this assumption can be regarded as a rough indicator of the validity of the measures used to assess emotional disturbance. In so far as the retrospective questionnaire items on postoperative emotional reactions discriminate successfully between patients exposed to mild degrees of stress stimulation (dental treatment) and those exposed to a much greater degree of stress stimulation (surgery), they can be expected to be useful for investigation of relationships with other factors as well. The main antecedent factor with which we are concerned, of course, is the level of preoperative fear. The central problem for which the questionnaire items were used can be formulated in the following way: When the type of stress epsiode is held relatively constant, do postoperative emotional disturbances vary as a function of the level of preoperative fear? The main forms of disturbance investigated were those specified by Hypotheses 16 and 17, i.e., postoperative fear and resentment.

In view of the findings presented in Chart 2 and in Tables 4 and 5, it is of particular importance to take account of the fact that individual differences in level of fear, to some extent, will tend to reflect objective differences in the actual amount of stress stimulation to which different individuals are exposed. We have seen that when we sort surgical patients into high, moderate, and low preoperative fear groups, we find a disproportionately large number of subjects who had major surgical operations in the high fear group. To take account of differences in magnitude of stress, additional analyses were carried out which make use of the method of controlled comparisons. Supplementary tables were constructed in which the correlational data are given separately for "major" and "minor" surgery subgroups. (See Tables 7, 8, and 9.) These data enable one to determine whether the over-all relationships obtained for the *total* sample are replicated *when the magnitude of stress is held relatively constant.* Thus, with this control procedure, one can ascertain the likelihood that the results bearing on Hypotheses 15 and 16 are affected by the stress factors that differentiate the high group from the other two groups.[5] Nevertheless, even with this control procedure, there is always the possibility that some unknown differences in stress stimulation remain which may conceivably account for a higher level of postoperative fear. Therefore, the correlational data should be regarded as relevant but not definitive evidence for testing the hypotheses.

The evidence bearing on Hypothesis 17, although subject to the usual limitations that apply to any correlational findings based on retrospective self-ratings, is much less ambiguous than that bearing on the other two hypotheses, because the available data (Tables 4, 5, and 6) indicate no differences between the low and moderate groups with respect to any factor that may be indicative of differential degrees of stress. In other words, the findings in the foregoing tables and charts increase the weight that can be given to the evidence bearing on Hypothesis 17, since they consistently indicate that the low fear group suffered just as much pain, experienced just as much incapacitation, and was exposed to essentially the same type of surgical procedures as the moderate group.

In the following sections, the evidence on postoperative anxiety is examined first, in order to assess Hypothesis 16. Then the evidence on postoperative aggressiveness is considered, which bears on Hypothesis 17. Finally, both sets of evidence are re-examined to determine whether the curvilinear relationship specified by Hypothesis 15 is substantiated.

Postoperative Anxiety

According to Hypothesis 16, persons who display relatively high fear during the threat phase (preoperatively) will tend to show relatively high fear and anxiety symptoms during the phase of actual exposure to stress (postoperatively). Pertinent data are presented in Chart 3, which shows the temporal course of fear responses for patients in the high, moderate, and low preoperative fear groups.

Chart 3. Temporal Course of Fear Responses Among Surgical Patients in the High, Moderate, and Low Preoperative Fear Groups

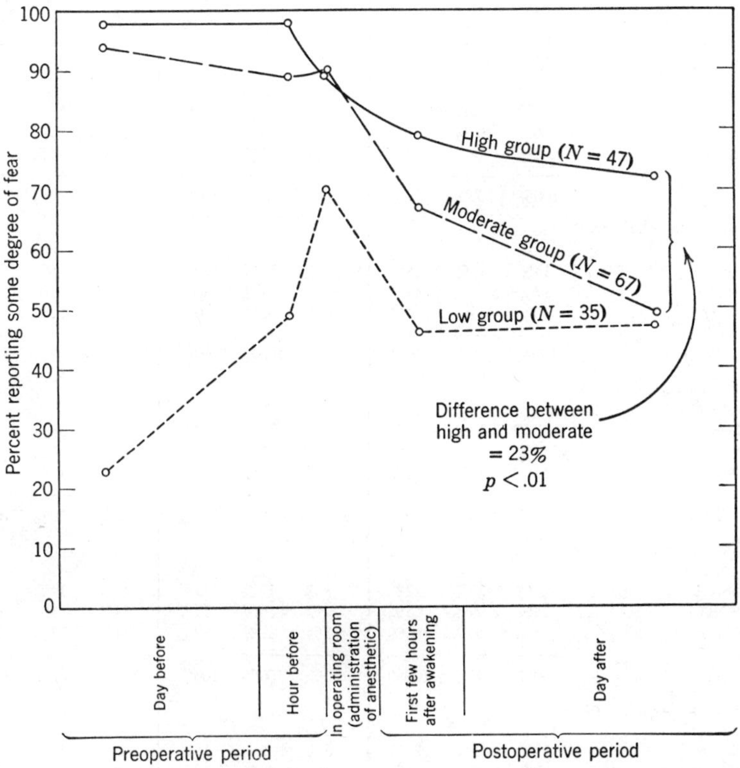

This chart is based on the same series of questions used for Chart 2. The subjects were asked to recall and rate the intensity of their fear at various stages of the operation experience. Each curve shows the percentage of subjects who reported some degree of fear at each time point. It is readily seen that the curve for the high preoperative fear group remains consistently higher than that for the moderate and low preoperative fear groups, during the postoperative period. For the day after the operation, the difference between the high and moderate group is 72% − 49% = 23%, which is significant at beyond the 1% level. This finding, which obviously supports Hypothesis 16, does not

Table 7. Fear Responses Among Major and Minor Surgery Cases

	Major Surgery Cases			Minor Surgery Cases			Total Surgery Cases		
	Preoperative Fear			Preoperative Fear			Preoperative Fear		
Self-Ratings on Intensity of Fear	Low (*N* = 15)	Moderate (*N* = 21)	High (*N* = 27)	Low (*N* = 20)	Moderate (*N* = 46)	High (*N* = 20)	Low (*N* = 35)	Moderate (*N* = 67)	High (*N* = 47)
1. During day before operation:									
Severe	7%	19%	48%	0%	17%	65%	3%	18%	55%
Slight	20%	67%	48%	20%	81%	35%	20%	76%	43%
None	73%	14%	4%	80%	2%	0%	77%	6%	2%
Total	100%	100%	100%	100%	100%	100%	100%	100%	100%
2. During hour before operation:									
Severe	13%	19%	48%	5%	37%	70%	9%	31%	57%
Slight	47%	62%	48%	35%	57%	30%	40%	58%	41%
None	40%	19%	4%	60%	6%	0%	51%	11%	2%
Total	100%	100%	100%	100%	100%	100%	100%	100%	100%
3. During administration of anesthetic:									
Severe	33%	19%	52%	22%	41%	82%	27%	34%	64%
Slight	54%	71%	33%	33%	49%	12%	43%	56%	25%
None	13%	10%	15%	45%	10%	6%	30%	10%	11%
Total	100%	100%	100%	100%	100%	100%	100%	100%	100%
4. During first few hours after operation:									
Severe	21%	20%	22%	5%	11%	15%	12%	14%	19%
Slight	36%	60%	63%	32%	50%	55%	34%	53%	60%
None	43%	20%	15%	63%	39%	30%	54%	33%	21%
Total	100%	100%	100%	100%	100%	100%	100%	100%	100%
5. During day after operation:									
Severe	15%	15%	27%	5%	9%	15%	9%	11%	22%
Slight	39%	35%	58%	37%	39%	40%	38%	38%	50%
None	46%	50%	15%	58%	52%	45%	53%	51%	28%
Total	100%	100%	100%	100%	100%	100%	100%	100%	100%

Note: Cases of "no answer" responses were rare; a sizeable number of such cases occurred only on the third question but constituted, nevertheless, only about 7% of the sample. Whenever "no answer" responses occurred, they were omitted from the computation of the percentages.

appear to be attributable to differences in type of operation, since it is fairly well substantiated when the comparisons are limited solely to major surgery cases (see Table 7).[6]

Additional evidence bearing on Hypothesis 16 is presented in Chart 4, which makes use of three different measures that were obtained for the purpose of assessing *sustained emotional disturbances.* One measure was based on responses to the following question, which was designed to determine whether the patient was preoccupied with disturbing reminiscences during the week following the operation:

QUESTION E: During the *week after* the operation or treatment, how often did you think over or repeat in your thoughts some of the *unpleasant* experiences that had occurred on the actual day of the operation or treatment?

____Many times.
____Occasionally.
____A few times.
____Once.
____Not at all.

A second measure was based on answers to the following question concerning current emotional disturbances:

QUESTION F: *At the present time* do you feel at all disturbed emotionally when you think about the unpleasant experiences you had in connection with the operation or treatment you have been describing?

____Feel *very disturbed* when I think about it.
____Feel *somewhat disturbed.*
____Feel *slightly* disturbed.
____Feel *very slightly* disturbed.
____Feel *not at all* disturbed.

Chart 4. Relationship Between Level of Preoperative Fear and Postoperative Emotional Disturbances

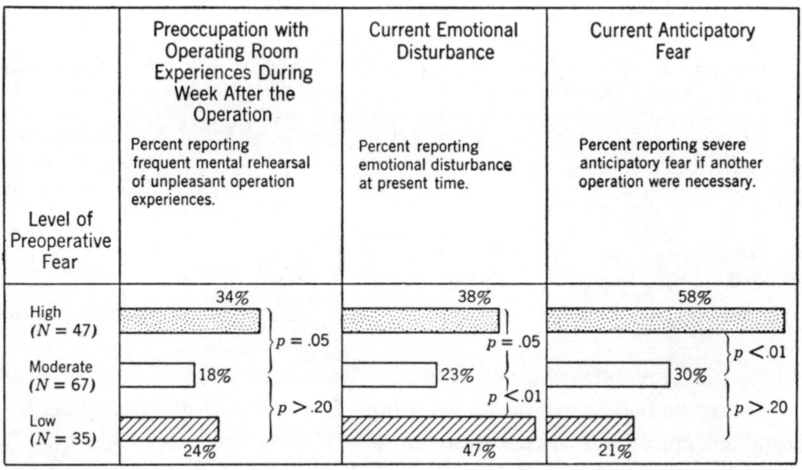

The third measure was based on responses to the following question concerning current anticipatory fear:

QUESTION G: Suppose that it were necessary for you to have another very similar operation *several days* from now. How much fear or anxiety would you probably experience when you thought about it? (Same check list as Question B.)

On all three measures, the percentage reporting reactions indicative of sustained emotional disturbance was significantly greater in the high preoperative fear group than in the moderate group. These findings, which give additional support to Hypothesis 16, are well substantiated when the type of operation is held relatively constant by limiting the comparisons to major surgery cases (see Table 8).

Table 8. Postoperative Emotional Disturbances Among Major and Minor Surgery Cases

	Major Surgery Cases			Minor Surgery Cases			Total Surgery Cases		
	Preoperative Fear			Preoperative Fear			Preoperative Fear		
Type of Disturbance	Low ($N = 15$)	Moderate ($N = 21$)	High ($N = 27$)	Low ($N = 20$)	Moderate ($N = 46$)	High ($N = 20$)	Low ($N = 35$)	Moderate ($N = 67$)	High ($N = 47$)
1. Preoccupation with operating room experiences during week after operation:									
Frequent	33⅓%	15%	41%	17%	20%	25%	24%	18%	34%
Seldom	33⅓%	50%	41%	44%	56%	45%	40%	55%	43%
None	33⅓%	35%	18%	39%	24%	30%	36%	27%	23%
Total	100%	100%	100%	100%	100%	100%	100%	100%	100%
2. Current emotional disturbance when recalling operation:									
Disturbed	53%	5%	26%	40%	30%	55%	47%	23%	38%
Not disturbed	47%	95%	74%	60%	70%	45%	53%	77%	62%
Total	100%	100%	100%	100%	100%	100%	100%	100%	100%
3. Current anticipatory fear, if another operation were necessary:									
Severe	21½%	19%	63%	20%	35%	50%	21%	30%	58%
Slight	21½%	76%	30%	55%	52%	45%	41%	60%	36%
None	57%	5%	7%	25%	13%	5%	38%	10%	6%
Total	100%	100%	100%	100%	100%	100%	100%	100%	100%

Thus, the available evidence consistently indicates that a high level of preoperative fear is predictive of a high level of postoperative fear and sustained emotional disturbance. Some of the measures (e.g., self-ratings on current emotional disturbance when recalling the operation) presumably refer to residual symptoms of anxiety that had continued for many months, or in some cases even for years, after the surgery episode was over.

Postoperative Aggressiveness

Before examining the results which compare the postoperative aggressive responses of the low group with the moderate group, there are some incidental findings on fear and other emotional disturbances in the preceding charts which should be taken into consideration. In Chart 3, the low group, as expected, shows a markedly lower incidence of fear reactions during the preoperative period; but the difference disappears entirely on the day after the operation. In Chart 4, we note further that the percentage of cases reporting current emotional disturbance is significantly *greater* for the low group than for the moderate group.[7] In the light of these findings, it seems highly improbable that the men in the low group had greater reluctance than the others to admit feelings of emotional disturbance. When describing their feelings during the postoperative period and at the time of reporting, the low group showed as much willingness, if not more, to admit emotional disturbance. These findings decrease the likelihood that the self-ratings of the low group might possibly be the product of a current motivation to deny or minimize emotional responses, as a result of

Chart 5. Relationship Between Level of Preoperative Fear and Subsequent Aggressive Reactions

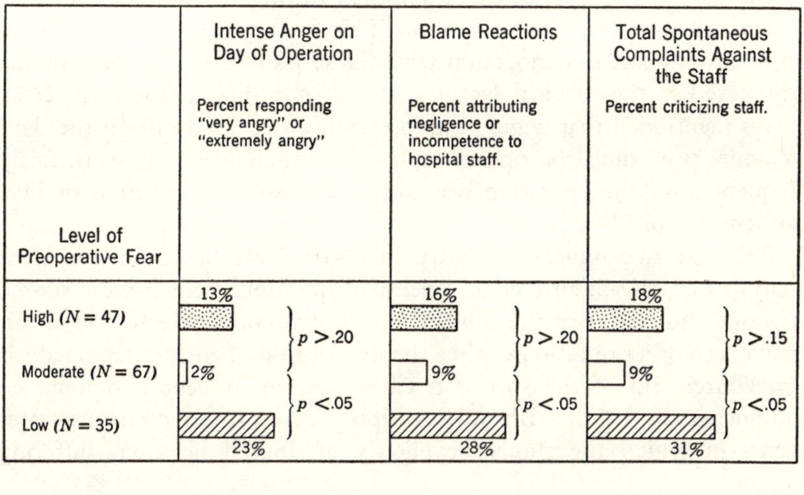

which the self-ratings might be less genuine or accurate than those given by the other groups. The available evidence tends to substantiate the working assumption that the self-ratings of the low group are likely to be just as genuine and accurate as those of the other groups.

The findings most pertinent for testing Hypothesis 17 are shown in Chart 5. Three main indicators of postoperative aggressiveness were used. The first was based on the following question:

QUESTION H: On the day of your operation or treatment, did you feel *angry or annoyed at any time* about anything that happened in connection with the operation or treatment?

____Felt *extremely angry*.
____Felt *very angry*.
____Felt *fairly angry*.
____Felt *slightly angry* or annoyed.
____*Did not feel at all angry or annoyed* at any time.

Although the wording of this question does not specifically refer to the period *after* the operation, it was possible to ascertain the approximate period during which anger reactions occurred by analyzing the write-in responses to the following supplementary question, which followed immediately after Question H in the questionnaire:

QUESTION I: What was it that made you feel angry or annoyed? (Describe the specific circumstances or events that caused you to feel angry or annoyed.)

The answers to this open-end question showed that in almost every instance the reported anger reaction occurred *in the operating room* when the operation had actually begun or *during the postoperative period* of the day of the operation, rather than during the period while the patient was awaiting the operation. This finding is consonant with an observation made in connection with the series of intensive case studies conducted in the surgical wards. In the preceding chapter (p. 266), it was mentioned that anger reactions rarely occurred during the days or hours preceding the operation, whereas such reactions were fairly frequent after the operation was over (see also the discussion of Hypothesis 1, pp. 54–58).

The next two indicators shown in Chart 5 are based on a content analysis of write-in answers to open-end questions, which were scored without knowledge of the subject's level of preoperative fear or of his answers to other questions. (See the description of the content analysis procedures and of the special devices used to prevent contaminated judgments, p. 297). "Blame Reactions" refer to spontaneous statements in which the subject explicitly attributed his own suffering or annoyance to the *negligence or incompetence of the surgeon, the nurses, or some other member of the hospital staff.* The statements examined were those contained in the subject's answers to the following question:

QUESTION J: Before answering this question, take a few moments to review in your mind the whole operation or treatment and think of the unpleasant things that occurred. What were the major unpleasant aspects of it? Make a list of the *five most unpleasant things* that occurred. Write a brief sentence describing each of the five, stating the *specific* experience you had which was unpleasant. (For example, "I felt a sharp pain in my back for a few seconds when the needle was stuck into my spine to give me the spinal anesthetic.") You can include any experience that occurred during the actual operation (or treatment), or during the hours immediately preceding it, or during the hours that followed it.

Four specific subcategories were included in the category of "Blame Reactions." The four subcategories consisted of explicit complaints against the staff (physicians, nurses, orderlies, or the staff in general) for: (*a*) inflicting *unnecessary* pain or discomfort because of *carelessness, lack of interest, or sadism;* (*b*) causing humiliation or embarrassment because of *crude, ill-mannered,* or *inconsiderate behavior;* (*c*) *failing to administer* the anesthetic properly or *poorly executing* any other aspect of the surgical procedure; (*d*) *making errors* or *performing ineptly* when executing any postoperative treatment or procedure.

The third indicator, "Total Spontaneous Complaints Against the Staff," was based on a content analysis of all pertinent open-end questions, including Question J. There were numerous other questions in response to which some subjects spontaneously expressed clear-cut criticisms of the staff. Each of the questions which asked for self-ratings on postoperative emotional reactions was followed by a supplementary question which asked the subject to explain his answer or to tell what it was that evoked the reaction. The answers to these supplementary questions sometimes contained sharp criticisms of the staff and, hence, were taken into account in determining the total incidence of "spontaneous complaints."

The categories used for "spontaneous complaints" included the four subcategories listed above for attributions of incompetence and negligence and, in addition, critical comments about impersonal treatment, poor food, inadequate toilet facilities, and unnecessary rules or restrictions imposed during the postoperative period.

The results on all three indicators in Chart 5 show that aggressive reactions occurred significantly more often in the low group than in the moderate group. This over-all outcome is almost exactly replicated when the data are broken down into major and minor surgery subsamples (see Table 9). These results consistently support Hypothesis 17.[8]

Table 9. Postoperative Anger and Resentment Among Major and Minor Surgery Cases

	Major Surgery Cases			Minor Surgery Cases			Total Surgery Cases		
	Preoperative Fear			Preoperative Fear			Preoperative Fear		
Type of Response	Low (*N* = 15)	Moderate (*N* = 21)	High (*N* = 27)	Low (*N* = 20)	Moderate (*N* = 46)	High (*N* = 20)	Low (*N* = 35)	Moderate (*N* = 67)	High (*N* = 47)
1. Self-ratings on *degree* of anger during the day of the operation:									
High	27%	0%	7%	20%	2%	20%	23%	2%	13%
Moderate	6%	10%	15%	0%	2%	10%	3%	4%	13%
Low	67%	90%	78%	80%	96%	70%	74%	94%	74%
Total	100%	100%	100%	100%	100%	100%	100%	100%	100%
2. Blame reactions: Content analysis of description of *unpleasant occurrences*.									
Physician or others on staff blamed (for negligence or incompetence)	33%	19%	18%	24%	6%	12%	28%	9%	16%
No one blamed	67%	81%	82%	76%	94%	88%	72%	91%	84%
Total	100%	100%	100%	100%	100%	100%	100%	100%	100%
3. Total complaints against the staff: Content analysis of answers to all open-end questions:									
Explicit complaints	47%	10%	18%	19%	8%	17%	31%	9%	18%
Implicit complaints	6%	14%	8%	14%	8%	8%	11%	10%	8%
No complaints	47%	76%	74%	67%	84%	75%	58%	81%	74%
Total	100%	100%	100%	100%	100%	100%	100%	100%	100%

Postoperative Adjustment

To determine whether there is a curvilinear relationship between preoperative fear and postoperative emotional adjustment, as predicted by Hypothesis 15, all the pertinent survey results must be re-examined. Altogether nine different items have been used as indicators of various types of postoperative emotional disturbance in connection with assessing Hypotheses 16 and 17. The main question which must now be considered is the following: Does the moderate fear group consistently show a lower incidence of emotional disturbance than the other two groups?

Table 10 presents an over-all summary of the findings, showing for each indicator of emotional disturbance whether the answer is "Yes" or "No" when one examines the data to see if the percentage of disturbed responses is lower for the moderate group than for (1) the high fear group and (2) the low fear group. If Hypothesis 15 predicts correctly, the answers should be "Yes" for both sets of comparisons.

Table 10. Summary of Survey Findings Bearing on Adjustment of Moderate Fear Group (Major and Minor Surgery Cases Combined)

Table in which Data Appear	Item No.	Content	Does the Moderate Fear Group Show a Lower Incidence of Disturbance than: 1. The Low Fear Group?	2. The High Fear Group?
7	4	Fear during first few hours after operation.	No*	Yes
7	5	Fear during day after operation.	No	Yes*
8	3	Fear at present time if another operation is necessary.	No*	Yes*
8	1	Frequent preoccupation (mental repetition of operation) during first postoperative week.	Yes	Yes*
8	2	Current emotional disturbance when recalling operation.	Yes*	Yes*
9	1	Anger during day of operation.	Yes*	Yes*
9	2	Blame reactions: physicians or staff accused of negligence or incompetence.	Yes*	Yes
9	3	Total complaints against staff.	Yes*	Yes
†		Does *not* now have "high" confidence in surgeon.	Yes	Yes

* The difference is large enough to be statistically significant at the .05 level or better.
† See p. 300

The results, shown in Table 10, are in the predicted direction on six of the nine indicators, and there are two significant reversals. It will be noted that the low fear group does *not* show a higher incidence of disturbed responses than the moderate fear group on any of the three items which explicitly refer to postoperative feelings of "fear," and it is for two of these items that the significant reversals occur. But then we find that for all six other indicators of postoperative emotional disturbances, the results turn out to be in the predicted direction. For two of these indicators, the predicted curvilinear relationship is extremely clear-cut inasmuch as the moderate fear group differs significantly from both the high fear group and the low fear group. Thus, some tentative support for Hypothesis 15 is provided by certain of the findings, namely, *for those items which do not refer to manifest fear.* The fact that the low fear group does not show a higher incidence of disturbed response than the moderate fear group for any of the three items dealing with manifest fear could be interpreted in a number of different ways. For example, the low fear cases might be persons, who are:

1. Consciously unwilling to admit feelings of fear but willing to admit other forms of emotional disturbance.
2. Partially successful in suppressing or unconsciously denying their subjective feelings of fear by displacing or rationalizing their disturbing emotional reactions (see discussion of Hypothesis 4, pp. 80–82).
3. Actually free from fear but subject to other types of emotional disturbance (i.e., the data summarized in Table 10 might be taken at face value as an accurate description of the postoperative emotional status of the patients).

From the evidence presented so far, there is no way of deciding among such possibilities; but there are some supplementary findings, to be presented in later chapters, which suggest that for many cases the second alternative may be most applicable. (See especially pages 341–350). In any case, the general conclusion from Table 10 is that the predictions which follow from Hypothesis 15 are partially confirmed, the positive results coming from those self-ratings which refer to postoperative emotional disturbances other than manifest feelings of fear.

Notes

1. After qualitative and quantitative pretesting, ambiguous items were revised and unreliable or inconsistent items were eliminated on the basis of an analysis of the internal consistency among each set of questions. The final revised questionnaire was then administered to about ten large undergraduate classes. The subjects were given the following general instructions:

"A. The purpose of this study is to obtain information about how people react to surgical operations or to other painful medical or dental treatments. In filling out the questionnaire which follows you should report about one particular operation or treatment that you have personally experienced.

B. If you had an operation *within the last five years* and if you can remember the experience quite clearly, that is what you should report about in this questionnaire. If you have had more than one such operation, choose the most recent one. . . ."

Although more than a 1000 men filled out the questionnaire, over 700 cases could not be used in the present study because they reported on routine medical treatments, such as injections and ENT examinations. Approximately 100 men reported on dental drilling, and this subsample was used for certain comparisons with the 150 cases who reported on surgical experiences. (See Chart 2, p. 284.)

2. In selecting and eliminating questionnaires for this study, the only information used was that on the cover sheet (type of operation or treatment), and the answer to the question as to whether the man knew about the operation on the day before. No other basis was used for excluding cases from the sample, and it is unlikely that any source of bias could enter in.

Once selected for inclusion in the sample, the subject's questionnaire was routinely coded by research assistants who were unfamiliar with the hypotheses to be tested. The coded data from all objective questions were put on IBM punch cards and all correlations derived from these questions were based on tables obtained from IBM cross tabulations.

Open-end questions were handled in a similar way. A clerk-typist went through each questionnaire and typed each answer on a separate card, using a code number to identify the case. The cards for each question were scored by the author on the basis of a detailed content analysis procedure (developed especially for this purpose), without knowledge of the answers given to any other question. Thus, any possibility of contamination of content scoring was eliminated. The content analysis scores were entered in the margin of the card next to the typed excerpt and, after the scoring was completed, a clerical assistant sorted the cards according to the code numbers into the high, moderate, and low preoperative fear groups, and carried out the necessary talleys for subgroup comparisons of the content categories.

3. The same questions were asked of all three groups concerning degree of fear on the day before, the hour before, the first few hours after, and the day after. In addition to Questions B and C, the following two standard questions were used:

"During the first few hours after the operation or treatment was over (or during the first hours after you *awoke* from the anesthetic), how intense was *the most severe* fear or anxiety that you experienced?" (Same check-list as Question B.)

"During the day after the actual day of the operation or treatment, how intense was *the most severe* fear or anxiety that you experienced when you thought about your operation or treatment?" (Same check-list as Question B.)

The question dealing with fear in the operating room (or treatment room) was not worded in the same way, however, for the dental patients as for the surgical patients. The following question was asked of the surgical patients:

"When you were being given the anesthetic, how intense was *the most severe* fear or anxiety that you experienced?" (Same check-list as Question B.)

This question could not be used with the dental cases because less than 20% of them had a local anesthetic and the rest had none. Therefore, a different question was used for the dental sample:

"How intense was the *most severe* fear or anxiety that you experienced while the actual operation or treatment was being performed?" (Same check-list as Question B).

Because this question refers to the *most* severe fear experienced during the entire dental procedure, it may have elicited answers which give an overestimate of the comparative incidence of fear reactions in the treatment room among the dental sample. It will be noted that for all other time points, where identical questions were used, the dental patients consistently show a lower incidence of fear reactions than the major and the minor surgery cases.

4. On five other self-rating items concerning emotional reactions, *the dental patients consistently showed a lower incidence of emotional disturbance than the major and minor surgery patients.*

In response to a question about being preoccupied with disturbing thoughts during the week after the operation (or treatment), only 2% of the dental patients reported frequent mental repetition of unpleasant experiences, as against 20% of the minor surgery cases and 32% of the major surgery cases. On this item the dental patients differ significantly from both the minor and major surgery cases.

Similar results were obtained from the following four items bearing on postoperative emotional effects: (*a*) self-ratings of current emotional disturbance when recalling the operation (or treatment); (*b*) current anticipatory fear if another similar operation (or treatment) were necessary; (*c*) degree of anger during the day of the operation; and (*d*) spontaneous complaints about alleged negligence or incompetence on the part of danger-control personnel—dentist, physician, or hospital staff (based on a content analysis of the patients' answers to a question which asked them to write a description of their unpleasant experiences.) On each of these items, the *dental* patients gave a significantly lower percentage of self-ratings on emotional disturbance than did the *major surgery* cases. On the same three items, the *minor surgery* cases showed more disturbance than the *dental* patients, but the differences were significant only for item (*a*).

As was expected, the minor surgery cases occupied an intermediate position between the major surgery cases and the dental cases on all the items. In no instance, however, were the differences between the major and minor surgery cases sufficiently large to approach statistical significance.

5. The results in Table 6 imply that no special control procedures need be introduced to equate the groups on degree of pain. Therefore, the only control procedure used is the breakdown of all correlational findings into major versus minor surgery cases so as to make sure that the differences are not attributable to type of operation or degree of postoperative incapacitation.

When one limits comparisons to the major surgery patients (Table 11), there are no marked differences with respect to specific type of operation. The one category in Table 11 which yields a statistically significant result is the difference between the high and low groups on "Hernia repair." This difference is irrelevant, however, for testing the three hypotheses under investigation. Hypothesis 15 involves comparing both the high group and the low group with the moderate group, but in Table 11 there are no differences that approach statistical significance involving the moderate group. Hypotheses 16 and 17 can be tested by comparing the moderate group with each of the other two groups, and the type of operation is held fairly constant whenever such comparisons are limited to major surgery cases.

Table 11. Type of Major Surgery

Type of Major Surgical Procedure	Level of Preoperative Fear: High (N = 27)	Moderate (N = 21)	Low (N = 15)
Appendectomy	19%	28½%	33⅓%
Hernia repair	19%	9½%	0%
Hemorrhoidectomy	7%	5%	0%
Excision of tumor or foreign object	26%	28½%	33⅓%
ENT surgery: tonsilectomy, etc.	29%	28½%	33⅓%
Total	100 %	100 %	100 %

For the distribution obtained within the *minor* surgery category (Table 12), the difference between the high group and the moderate group is statistically significant on tooth extraction. It appears that the patients with high preoperative fear were less likely to be facing a tooth extraction and more likely to be facing a lancing procedure, or some other type of minor surgery (e.g., repair of an ingrown nail). Hence, comparisons between the high and moderate group may reflect, to some extent, the difference in specific types of surgery. For this reason, the data bearing on Hypotheses 15 and 16 derived from the minor surgery cases cannot be given as much weight as those derived from the major surgery cases. The low group and moderate group, however, are fairly well equated on type of minor surgery and, consequently, for purposes of testing Hypothesis 17, the comparisons based on the minor surgery cases can be given as much weight as those based on the major surgery cases.

Table 12. Type of Minor Surgery

Type of Minor Surgical Procedure	Level of Preoperative Fear: High (N = 20)	Moderate (N = 46)	Low (N = 20)
Tooth extraction	40%	61%	60%
Lancing of cyst or infection	30%	17%	16%
Miscellaneous: stitching of laceration, nail repair, etc.	30%	22%	24%
Total	100%	100%	100%

Of incidental interest is the fact that the data in Tables 11 and 12 suggest that to some extent, the level of preoperative fear depends upon the specific nature of the major or minor surgery. With respect to the various types of major surgery represented in our sample, a high level of preoperative fear appears to be especially likely if one faces hernia repair or hemorrhoidectomy and less likely if one faces an appendectomy. These survey findings are in line with the widely reported observation that a person's level of preoperative fear will depend partly on the site of the operation, with maximal fear being elicited by the threat of being cut in the anal region or in the lower abdominal region near the genital area. (H. Deutsch, 1942; Lindemann, 1941; Titchener et al., 1956.) Another factor involved may be the person's expectations about the risks of the operation. Less preoperative fear may be evoked by appendectomies because this type is popularly thought to be a "safe" operation, as compared with other types of major operations. The same factor may account for the tendency for tooth extractions to elicit relatively less preoperative fear than lancing procedures and other minor operations.

6. The case studies suggested that immediately after the operation there was a temporary period of elation (relief about having survived) among high-anxiety cases. This was followed by some sharp rises in fear later on, especially when postoperative procedures were introduced. By the second or third day, the high-anxiety patients no longer displayed elation and, instead, began to express considerable worry about their lack of recovery and about the possibility of being permanently maimed. This sequence is fairly well borne out by the data in Chart 3 and Table 7 for the major surgery cases: for item 4 of Table 7 (p. 288), the high fear group shows almost the same incidence of (slight or severe) fear as the moderate fear group; whereas, for items 1, 2, 3, and 5, the high group differs significantly from the moderate group. The fact that on the day after the operation the high group again exceeds the moderate and low group provides some support for Hypothesis 16.

7. It should be noted that a sizeable second-order difference occurs for the item dealing with "current emotional disturbance" (see item 2 of Table 8, p. 290). For the *major* surgery subsample, the difference in percentage between the low and moderate group is 53% − 5% = 48%; for the *minor* surgery subsample, the corresponding difference is 40% − 30% = 10%; the second-order difference of 38% is statistically significant at beyond the .10 level. This is consistent with the following *interaction* hypothesis (see pp. 259–261): If a stress episode is relatively severe (e.g., as in most cases of major surgery), then a low level of anticipatory fear predisposes the person to develop *sustained emotional disturbances* which persist long after the stress episode is over; if, however, the stress episode is relatively mild (e.g., as in most cases of minor surgery), a low level of anticipatory fear will make much less difference, if any, with respect to the development of sustained emotional disturbances.

8. Of some pertinence to Hypothesis 17 are the results obtained from the following additional question which was included for the purpose of studying sustained attitudes toward the physician:

QUESTION K: *At the present time,* how much confidence and trust would you have in that same doctor or surgeon (if it were necessary for you to have another, similar operation or treatment)?

— Absolutely complete confidence and trust in him.
— Almost complete confidence and trust in him.
— Fair amount of confidence and trust in him.
— Slight amount of confidence and trust in him.
— Very little confidence and trust in him.

Unfavorable answers to this question can be regarded as a rough indication of *sustained* aggressive attitudes, but they do not necessarily provide a direct test of Hypothesis 17, which refers only to aggressive reactions occurring *during the period when the individual is being exposed to actual stress stimuli* (i.e., in the case of surgery, during the period of postoperative pain and deprivation).

The results show that the low preoperative group expressed somewhat less confidence than the moderate group, but the differences are not large enough to be regarded as statistically significant. Among the major surgery cases, 100% of the moderate group ($N = 21$) expressed high confidence ("almost complete" or "absolutely complete" confidence) in the surgeon, as compared with 73% of the low group ($N = 15$). For the minor surgery cases, the corresponding percentages were 83% and 75% respectively; for the total sample, the percentages were 88% and 74% respectively. Although these findings are inconclusive, they suggest that in future investigations it may be worthwhile to check on the possibility that one of the sequelae of low anticipatory fear (especially before a major surgical operation) may be the development of a persistent derogatory or critical attitude toward the physician which continues long after the surgical episode is over. (See p. 358 for additional findings based on answers to Question K.)

23.

Effective and ineffective reassurances

In the preceding chapters the description of postoperative reactions of patients with low, moderate, and high preoperative fear was largely restricted to verbal and overt behavior for which objective data were available. Thus the discussion so far has dealt almost exclusively with those emotional and adjustive aspects of behavior that are readily amenable to self-observation or to the observation of others. No attempt has been made, as yet, to specify the inner processes which might account for the observed correlations between preoperative fear and postoperative adjustment.

The present chapter will attempt to provide a theoretical explanation for one of the main conclusions which emerged from the case studies and the survey research, namely, that patients who manifested a *moderate* level of anticipatory fear, as compared with those who manifested either very high or very low anticipatory fear, tended to adjust most adequately to the stresses of the postoperative period. The patients in the moderate fear group were able to maintain high morale despite severe deprivations and they showed comparatively little overt resistance to medical demands, made few complaints, and were relatively free from excessive fear, anger, or depression.

In order to seek for an explanation of these findings, it is necessary to examine carefully the available information concerning the cognitive processes and the emotional states that occurred before and during exposure to intense stress stimuli. Although the data at hand provide only fragmentary indications of the patient's subjective responses during moments of crisis, it is worth while to take account of whatever clues are contained in the available material because such clues can help us to identify mediating internal processes and, thereby, increase our insight into the psychological determinants of different modes of adjustment to stress.

At the end of Chapter 21, we considered the question of whether the relationship between preoperative fear and postoperative resentment is static or modifiable in character. Case study evidence was cited showing that, at least for some of the patients in the low fear group, if not for all of them, it is plausible to assume that the relative absence of anticipatory fear plays a causal role in producing the subsequent reactions of anger and hostility toward the danger-control authorities. The main evidence consisted of fairly well-documented instances of intrapersonal variability in emotional response, indicating that certain patients who displayed a relative absence of preoperative fear at the time of the present study had reacted in a markedly different fashion to a comparable stress episode in the recent past. In each such instance, the patient can be regarded as his own control with respect to representing the key variables in the following proposition: *If circumstances are such that an individual's anticipatory fear is not stimulated prior to a stressful event (e.g., when there is a lack of warning), the person will tend to react to the stress stimuli with anger and resentment; whereas, if the same person is exposed to precrisis threat stimuli which arouse some degree of anticipatory fear, the probability of developing such reactions is markedly less.*

If we assume tentatively that there is such a causal relationship between the arousal of preoperative fear and the subsequent occurrence of resentment, the next step in our inquiry is to attempt to discern the *mediating psychological factors.* What happens psychologically to a person when his anticipatory fear is stimulated as against when it is not? Why is it that the arousal of some degree of anticipatory fear has what appears to be a psychological *inoculation* effect such that the individual is better able to meet the adversity of a stress episode without becoming hostile or resentful? These are the main questions with which we are concerned in this chapter and the next chapter. First we shall scrutinize the content of the "reassurances" reported by major surgery cases in the survey research sample, concentrating especially on the difference between the moderate and low fear groups. Then we shall turn to a detailed examination of emotional and cognitive processes revealed by intensive interviews of several patients who displayed a moderate level of preoperative fear. The latter case material enables us to gain some further insights into the reassurance mechanisms that facilitate stress tolerance.

Survey Results: Manifest Content of "Reassurances"

In order to obtain some data bearing on the ways in which surgical patients attempt to reassure themselves during the time when anticipatory fear is aroused, the following two open-end questions were included in the survey questionnaire:

QUESTION L: Whenever a person expects to have an operation or a painful treatment he is likely to try to think about things which help him to keep from feeling too worried about it. During the period *before* you had your operation or treatment, what thoughts or ideas did you have that may have helped you to keep from feeling too much concern or anxiety about it?

QUESTION M: When the operation or treatment was about to begin or while it was being performed, what thoughts or ideas did you have that may have helped you to keep from feeling too much worry or anxiety about it?

Following the same general procedures used to obtain the data in Table 9, a systematic content analysis procedure was applied to the written responses given by each subject who had undergone *major* surgery. The results, broken down into low, moderate, and high levels of anticipatory fear, are shown in Table 13. The first two categories, which involve the most extreme forms of minimization, occur predominantly among the patients in the low fear group. Typical examples of their reports about adopting a joking or facetious attitude are the following: "I mainly did a lot of laughing and joking with the doctors and nurses"; "I was lighthearted about it, facetious, joking about the operation, flirting with the nurses, etc." For this category, the percentage difference between the low and high groups is statistically significant at beyond the 10% level; the difference between the low and the moderate groups is in the same direction but is not statistically significant. The second category refers to minimizing notions such as the following, which were reported by patients in the low fear group:

Table 13. "Reassuring" Beliefs and Activities Reported by Patients with Low, Moderate, and High Anticipatory Fear*

	Level of Preoperative Fear		
	Low ($N = 15$)	Moderate ($N = 21$)	High ($N = 27$)
1. Adopted a joking or facetious attitude.	40%	10%	0%
2. Thought that operation would be of a very minor or trivial nature.	27%	10%	15%
3. Felt confident in surgeon or gained reassurance from talking with him.	27%	48%	26%
4. Made effort to learn about the operative procedure or its effects.	13%	29%	11%
5. Thought that pains and discomforts would be of short duration or free from medical complications.	7%	19%	4%
6. Concentrated on anticipated gains from the operation.	13%	14%	33%
7. Plunged into distracting games or fantasies.	7%	5%	22%
8. Adopted an attitude of resignation, fatalism, or trust in God.	0%	5%	15%
9. Miscellaneous contents.	7%	10%	7%

* The data are based on a content analysis of written answers obtained in a questionnaire survey of 63 major surgery cases.

Note: The percentages add up to more than 100% because some subjects mentioned more than one type of reassurance.

"I thought that there is nothing to it"; "I felt that the operation was a very minor one, and I thought there would be absolutely no unfavorable residual effects from the operation"; "I felt that the operation was of such a mild variety that I had no reason to feel concerned—no more than going down on an elevator or crossing streets." For this category, the differences are again in the expected direction, but are not statistically significant.

Relatively few patients in the moderate fear group reported the first two types of reassurances, the predominant ones in this group being categories 3, 4, and 5.

There seems to be a fairly consistent pattern with respect to the way the moderate fear group differs from the low fear group on the first five categories, even though no single category yields a significant difference. What is tentatively suggested by this pattern is that patients with a moderate level of fear may be more likely than those with low fear to develop reassuring concepts that take account of: (*a*) the dominant threats to which they will subsequently be exposed, and (*b*) the danger-reducing aspects of the stress situation, such as the availability of help from protective authority figures. Instead of dismissing the impending operation as a trivial or joking matter, they may be inclined to *seek information* about the threat and to think in terms of *mitigating factors* (e.g., "there will be pain but it will not last long and I will be in good medical hands"). The descriptive comments made by a few subjects suggest that the latter type of reassurance requires a "working through" process in advance of being exposed to the danger situation. For example, one of the students in the moderate fear group described how his fear of having his body cut open was gradually overcome during the day before he was brought into the operating room:

> I didn't like the idea of having my body opened up by some guy I'd never seen before, and in such strange surroundings. This feeling was assuaged, however. . . . I was greatly reassured when I met the doctor, who appeared to be extremely efficient and spoke to me in a way that inspired confidence. He told me that the operation was a simple procedure and that he appreciated the fact that I might be more anxious since he was a complete stranger. After that I lost most of my anxiety.

When *not* concerned about the impending dangers, most people probably remain unmotivated to seek the type of reassurance described in the foregoing excerpt. There are some indications that if a man has low motivation to obtain reassurance from the surgeon, he is less likely to develop an attitude of trust and confidence, even when there is a good deal of direct interaction between him and the surgeon beforehand. For example, a student in the low fear group who reported having talked frequently with the surgeon before the operation gave the following subjective account of his experience in the operating room:

> I realized that it isn't every day that one undergoes an operation. A trauma is bound to take place when you feel a part of your body is being removed. The helplessness, and the realization that your body is at the mercy of another human being's skill, was one of the most disturbing things that I ever experienced.

It seems plausible to assume that the mental rehearsal of being "helpless" and "at the mercy of" an authority figure was one of the major characteristics of the anticipatory fear reactions of patients in the moderate fear group; this source of fear may have motivated their relatively high degree of reliance on the surgeon (category 3, Table 13). Many patients in the low fear group may have been unable to develop such an attitude because, by the time they accepted the fact that the operation was no joking matter, the danger was already at hand. Later in this chapter, and in the next chapter, we shall encounter numerous bits of case study evidence which clearly suggest that, unless a strongly positive attitude toward the surgeon is built up in advance, the patient's relationship with him may become drastically impaired at the moment when the patient is brought to the operating room and realizes that it is the surgeon who is the agent responsible for inflicting the hazardous procedures that are about to begin.

The over-all pattern of reassurance reported by the high fear group is somewhat different from that of the low fear group. The former group shows a slightly greater preference than the other groups for category 6 (anticipated gains) and for category 7 (distracting games and fantasies). These differences, however, are not large enough to be statistically significant. The most outstanding feature of the high fear group is that many patients apparently were quite unsuccessful in warding off certain types of exaggerated fears of surgery. This is suggested by the following findings which emerged when a content analysis was made of all open-end questions in the survey questionnaire: Thirteen of the twenty-seven patients in the high fear group (48%) reported that their preoperative concerns were centered on the possibility of being mutilated or killed by the operation, whereas only three of the twenty-one patients in the moderate fear group (14%) and two of the fifteen in the low fear group (13%) mentioned any such thoughts.[1] (The percentage difference between the high fear group and each of the other two groups is statistically significant at beyond the 10% level.)

The exceptionally high frequency of preoperative fears concerning body damage and death reported by the patients in the high fear group tends to be consistent with one of the main explanatory hypotheses suggested on the basis of the case evidence presented in Chapter 20, namely, that patients with high preoperative fear are unable to provide effective reassurances to themselves or to gain reassurance from optimistic communications from others, because their fantasies of mutilation or annihilation stem from unconscious neurotic conflicts that are aroused by the external threat.

During the preoperative period, both the moderate fear group and the low fear group were presumably much more successful than the high fear group in reducing anticipatory fear by means of one or another type of reassurance. But, although the moderate and low groups may have been equally successful in warding off exaggerated notions about the dangers of surgery beforehand, they may have used different adjustment mechanisms to control their fears. The content of the reassurances which predominate in the two groups suggests that the patients in the low fear group may have been overoptimistically indifferent toward the potential dangers that were in store for them, whereas the patients in the moderate fear group may have been undergoing a process of imaginative fantasying or mental rehearsal which enabled them to "work through" some of the impending unpleasant experiences in advance.

Before attempting to delineate the implications of this statement, it will be useful to examine some case evidence first, which enables us to see rather clearly the way in which a patient's mental set is altered when anticipatory fear is stimulated.

A Patient's Reassurance Efforts

The following case material deals with the reassurance efforts of a woman who was intensively interviewed before her operation. (Because of administrative difficulties, this patient was not seen after her operation and hence could not be included in the regular sample.)[2]

INTERVIEW CASE X–1

The patient, a 50-year-old woman of German descent, had spent her entire adult life working together with her husband on a small farm which they owned. She was hospitalized for orthopedic surgery on her right leg and was interviewed on the day preceding the operation. At the beginning of the interview, one of her first statements was that she wished she could have the operation right away so that she would be able to return home as soon as possible. She explained that it was now the fall harvest season, and her husband needed her help badly; that was why she hoped to be able to go home by the third day after the operation. When asked a series of questions about her thoughts and feelings concerning the impending operation, she claimed that she felt no concern about the surgery itself:

> I don't want to get no stiff leg. That's what worries my husband. People say you can get a stiff leg from what I've got. . . . The only thing that ever worries me is getting a stiff leg. I don't want that to happen so that's why I'm here. I just feel I want to get well and I'll do anything to get well.

In addition to denying being worried about undergoing the operation, this patient made several statements in which she optimistically minimized the unpleasant effects; e.g., "Everyone tells me it's nothing to it so I just take it as being nothing."

However, the patient began to show increasing signs of emotional disturbance as the interviewer went through the sequence of questions which asked the patient to state her expectations as to what would actually happen during and after the operation (see the questions listed in Chapter 19, pages 226–227). The patient began to fidget in her chair, her face became more and more flushed, and she gradually began to admit feeling fearful. Her first admission was: "I know it's *not* nothing like people say; it's *my* leg, not theirs." Then, when asked whether she expected any pain or discomfort during the operation, she said:

> They say you don't feel nothing. But I don't really know. I think I will feel a little bit uncomfortable. I don't want to have it said I'm scared and a sissy. . . . I'm more scared right this minute than I ever was before. I'm just thinking about the operation for the first time.

While saying this, the patient's movements and facial expressions showed marked agitation and, as she made the last statement, she broke out into overt weeping and trembling. With much apparent effort she composed herself and then began to speak at some length about *reassuring aspects* of the impending event—introducing a number of mitigating considerations which she had not mentioned at all during the earlier part of the interview:

> I heard they might take out a piece of bone but they say you can get along without that. . . . I know surgery is tremendously improved nowadays, they can do all kinds of wonderful things. . . . They say Dr. L. [the surgeon] is the best one there is and my husband says he is the only one he will let operate on me.

Toward the end of the interview, she began to emphasize more and more the specific compensatory gains which she hoped to derive from the operation:

> I just want to do what's right. I don't say I want the operation done or not, I just want it to make me better and I want help. I want to run around again like I did before, to milk the cows, to pick strawberries, to do everything on our farm. That's why I want to have it done. That's what I'm looking for, that day when I can run around again. Before I couldn't go no place, to church or no place; I just stay home all the time and only go out to go to a doctor.

When the interview was over, she spontaneously spoke about the effect the interview had upon her and described a markedly different conception of the consequences of the operation:

> I felt so scared while I was talking to you because I hadn't thought the operation was anything until you asked me all those questions. I never thought about it before, that's why those questions made me so scared. . . . I hope all my leg troubles will be cured; sometimes good things hap-

pen out of going through bad. . . . I hope I won't have to be here too long, but maybe it will be a long time; maybe it will be Christmas [five weeks away] before I get home. But I wouldn't stay that long, they'd have to tie me down to keep me!

The outstanding feature of the interview was the marked shift in verbalized defensive attitudes that occurred after the patient's anticipatory fear was stimulated by the interviewer's questions, which had forced her to think about the consequences the operation would have for her.[3] During the early part of the interview, she calmly maintained that the only thing she worried about was being away from home. Her expectations were extremely optimistic—there would be nothing to the operation and she would go home in about three days. Once her attention became focused on the concrete details of the impending experience, she gradually began to realize what it would mean—surgical cutting, loss of part of her body, the possibility of prolonged hospitalization, pain, etc. And, correspondingly, her emotional reactions gradually mounted to the point where she momentarily experienced, evidently for the first time, acute anticipatory fear. Once this occurred, she could no longer feel reassured by the old optimistic formula that there would be *nothing to it.* Her initial conception of *blanket* immunity from danger was replaced by much more *differentiated* set of reassurances which took account of some of the contingencies and specific unpleasant events that might be in store for her. Thus, as she thought about certain specific dangers of surgery, she began to develop a new set of reassurances in which she emphasized the skill of modern surgery and the wonderful reputation of her own surgeon. Moreover, she began to concretize the ultimate reward to which she could look forward. At the end of the interview, she was contemplating not merely the prevention of lameness, which she had mentioned at the beginning of the interview, but also the restoration of certain locomotor abilities which would enable her to engage in desirable activities from which she had had to abstain for over a year as a result of her illness.

Consequences of Different Modes of Reassurance

The transformation of vague over-all reassurances to concrete ones, as illustrated in the foregoing case study, might make a considerable difference with respect to the individual's capacity for coping with subsequent stress. At a time when a surgical patient finds himself suffering from severe pain and sustaining the loss of important bodily functions, he will obviously find himself unable to use a blanket immunity type of reassurance to the effect that "there will be nothing to it." Although such reassurances may be successful during the threat phase, they are apt to be falsified once the stress stimuli are actually encountered. The differentiated types of reassurances, however, are more likely to be keyed to the specific sources of stress, in so far as they have been realistically anticipated beforehand; thus they are more likely to continue to function as *effective self-delivered reassurances in the crisis situation.*

By a "self-delivered reassurance" is meant any symbolic response (e.g., a fantasy, slogan, or thought sequence) which is in the person's response repertoire and which, upon being silently verbalized to himself in the presence of threat or stress stimuli, is promptly followed by a momentary or sustained reduction in emotional tension (fear, guilt, or anger). It seems plausible to assume that, as a consequence of the arousal of preoperative fear, the average surgical patient will be stimulated to build up his repertoire of reality-tested reassurances. *Before exposure* to the crisis situation of the operating room and before exposure to the stress stimuli of the postoperative phase, he is likely to assuage his fear by developing concepts and anticipations concerning the limited duration of pain, the protective features of the environment, and the compensatory gains to be derived as recompense for undergoing the suffering. We assume further, that in order to develop differentiated concepts which will function effectively as reassurances in the actual stress situation, it is necessary for the person to go through a more or less prolonged learning process, which involves a considerable amount of reality-testing in the form of: (*a*) obtaining information about the sources of potential danger, how these dangers can be surmounted, the mitigating or protective features of the environment, etc., and (*b*) mentally rehearsing or fantasying what the danger situation will be like, vicariously trying out various reassuring concepts, and then accepting, rejecting, or modifying them after thinking about their truth value. Thus, the assumption is that unless a person experiences anticipatory fear, he lacks motivation to undergo this rather unpleasant learning process in advance; and, unless he undergoes this learning process, he is unlikely to have available in his response repertoire a set of reality-based reassurances that can be effectively used in a moment of crisis.

In any danger situation people are quite capable of spontaneously trying out a variety of self-delivered reassurances. For example, interviews of disaster victims indicate that, at the moment when people unexpectedly perceive the onset of grave danger, their thoughts tend to be concentrated on attempts at reassurance, such as: "God will protect me"; "Our part of town won't be affected" (M. Wolfenstein, 1957).

But if disaster actually strikes, such spontaneous attempts at reassurance are much less likely to be effective in lowering emotional tension than those differentiated ones which have been reality-tested in advance.

Perhaps the most serious psychological consequence of a very low degree of anticipatory fear is that the individual relies upon grossly overoptimistic expectations and blanket immunity concepts which are likely to be shattered at the time when he is exposed to actual danger and deprivation. According to this explanatory concept, one of the essential differences between patients in the low fear group and those in the moderate fear group is that the latter, by virtue of their anticipatory fear reactions, were strongly motivated to develop reality-oriented reassurances. The same tendency is assumed for the high fear group, since the high level of fear is a powerful motivating factor. In such cases, however, the differentiated reassurances evidently fail to reduce anticipatory fear. According to Hypothesis 7, the inability to gain reassurance from authoritative statements about the low risks entailed by an impending operation is attributable to the influence of repressed fears linked with unconscious conflicts. The latter, in turn, are assumed to be predominant among persons who suffer from certain forms of neurotic disorder. The available case evidence concerning the high fear patients (pp. 240–250) as well as the survey data on the patients' fear of being mutilated or killed in the operating room (p. 307 and pp. 326–328) are consistent with this explanation.

In summary, then, the following assumptions seem plausible concerning the reassurance mechanisms that accompany different levels of anticipatory fear:

High Anticipatory Fear: These patients are strongly motivated to develop reality-oriented reassurances but fail to gain much emotional relief from them because repressed sources of fear remain active and dominant; few effective self-delivered reassurances are available when stress stimuli are subsequently encountered.

Moderate Anticipatory Fear: These patients are motivated to varying degrees to develop reality-oriented reassurances and they gain considerable relief from them; such reassurances are then in the person's repertoire and available when stress stimuli are subsequently encountered.

Low Anticipatory Fear: These patients are relatively unmotivated to develop reality-oriented reassurances because they are either unaware of the threat or they succeed in eliminating anticipatory fear by means of blanket denials of personal vulnerability; these denials then remain as the dominant self-delivered reassurances in the person's response repertoire. The latter defenses are not effective when stress stimuli are subsequently encountered, and emotional tension is unrelieved because there are relatively few reality-oriented reassurances available in the person's response repertoire.

Illustrative Case Studies of Successful Reassurance

We return now to some of the interview observations which contain suggestive evidence bearing on the foregoing theoretical assumptions. The interview data from Case X-1 have already provided a clear-cut illustration of the impetus toward trying out new and more differentiated types of reassurance responses when anticipatory fear is stimulated. But this case material does not provide any information about postoperative behavioral sequelae. Unfortunately, there were no follow-up observations available for this case that would enable us to assess whether the development of such reassurances played any role in the patient's subsequent postoperative adjustment. However, from an examination of the preoperative and postoperative interviews of other patients who displayed a moderate level of preoperative fear, it seems likely that differentiated reassurances which are cued to perceptible features of the postoperative stress situation can contribute to the individual's ability to cope with stress stimuli. The two case studies which follow are presented primarily to illustrate the apparent continuity of symbolic defenses, which was noticed among cases in the moderate anticipatory fear group. We shall examine the reassurances verbalized before the operation in relation to the way in which the patient reacted to subsequent crisis situations during the postoperative period. The subjective responses of the patients, including dreams and daydreams, will be reported in some detail. This material will furnish a background against which one can perceive more sharply the deviant character of the symbolic defenses that predominated in the low fear cases. The contrasting features will be discussed more fully in the next chapter, when we examine material bearing on the maladjustive consequences of the blanket immunity type of reassurance among patients with low anticipatory fear. By noting the characteristics of successful inner preparation in some of the moderate fear cases, we shall be able to discriminate more sharply the contrasting disadvantageous characteristics of denial defenses, which appear to play such a significant role in setting the stage for subsequent aggrievement reactions.

The relationship between modes of reassurance and adequacy of postoperative adjustment cannot be unambiguously tested by the available interview data. However, the following observations of patients in the moderate group help to explain the ways in which danger-cued reassurances can facilitate postoperative adjustment.

INTERVIEW CASE M–2

Mrs. R., a 62-year-old housewife, was intensively interviewed before and after surgery (esophageal diverticulectomy). Prior to the operation, her fears were concentrated on specific dangers associated with the surgery, and she appeared to have developed a highly differentiated set of reassuring attitudes and expectations. After the surgery, she was able to tolerate a painful convalescence with no apparent emotional disturbance and, according to the nurses' daily notes, consistently maintained a cheerful, optimistic, and affable manner.

In the preoperative interview she verbalized numerous apprehensions about her health and about the impending operation. She told the interviewer that she had been acutely ill for many weeks and that a recent bronchiogram had revealed that the wall of her esophagus was breaking. The operation was needed, according to her account, "to get rid of the terrible obstruction or whatever it is" and to avoid "living a life of agony." She asserted that she had already experienced a great deal of physical discomfort from the condition; even more distressing was "the mental agony from knowing it won't get better but might get worse if I don't have the operation." The operation itself, however, was a source of worry—her "old T.B. condition" might become activated or other "complications" might occur and "I even sometimes think I may not come through it alive." But these negative statements were promptly followed by reassuring notions which apparently helped her to allay the fearful doubts:

> My T.B. condition has been holding good for many years and then, again, I feel I'm in real good hands. . . . If I have complications I might need a transfusion but that is within easy reach.

A similar balanced presentation of specific threats and corresponding reassurances could be discerned in her comments about postoperative suffering, although the reassuring statements did not always occur immediately after the threat statements. If we examine all the other pertinent comments that this patient made about anticipated postoperative occurrences, we find that they can readily be sorted into the two categories, and that each threat content is matched with a corresponding reassurance content:

Threat Content	Corresponding Reassuring Content
1. In the operation I had 24 years ago they gave me gas and ether; I know that isn't good for my lungs and might cause trouble afterwards.	1. The fact that I had that operation [24 years ago] and came through it all right makes me feel better about this one. . . . Science is further ahead now so I expect they have better ways of giving the anesthetic.
2. I recall feeling terribly sick when I awoke after that operation [24 years ago] . . . When I awaken this time I expect pain and nausea.	2. I don't expect to be allowed to suffer too long.
3. For about two or three days or more I suppose I will have pains and feel very sick.	3. Everything is so much better nowadays, maybe the pain will last only for two days.
4. I expect I'll have to stay in the hospital for about two weeks or maybe even more.	4. When I leave the hospital I expect to be healthy again . . . The operation will put me in an excellent frame of mind and will give me back a reasonably normal life again.
5. [From what the doctor said] I've guessed and surmised that it [the success of the operation] depends on what my condition is. He said it wouldn't ever get better by itself.	5. I have a friend who had the same condition. She had the operation and it came out good. That's very encouraging to me.

In addition to the relatively specific reassurances quoted above, there was also a more general form of reassurance which was repeatedly mentioned in many different contexts throughout the preoperative interview, viz., *reliance on the skill of the staff physicians.* The following typical comments convey something of the intensity of this reassuring attitude:

I'm very partial to this institution, and I feel I'm a very fortunate woman with doctors because I have the cream of the very best. . . . I think of what a good surgeon I have and then all my black thoughts go down.

The patient's statements about the nurses were not, however, as enthusiastically positive. She asserted that she had confidence in most but not all of them: "It depends on their character, some are sympathetic and some are not."

Throughout the postoperative period this patient was highly cooperative in conforming with all demands made by the nursing staff. In the follow-up interview, her comments about the physicians remained as glowingly favorable as before the operation (e.g., "I've been very fortunate in having doctors that are the tops. . . . The young doctors here are a marvel at using new methods of saving patients from pain"). Her attitude toward nurses was also essentially unchanged, with perhaps a few less qualified remarks than before: "Considering everything, I got very good attention and care from them. . . . They're very sympathetic and alert. . . . Some are better—more efficient—than others, but they are all good."

This patient reported that when awakening from the anesthetic she had considerable pain and nausea, but, nevertheless, felt pleased and relieved that the operation was over. The only unpleasant episode during the entire convalescent period, she asserted, was the initial tube feeding, which took place on the first postoperative day. She had not known anything about this treatment and found it to be rather distressing at first. However, after the doctor explained the necessity for it, she was no longer bothered by it, because she thought to herself, "It must be one of the new advances in technique that are wonderful for the patient."

In this case, it seems plausible to assume that the moderate level of anticipatory fear operated as a motivation for mental exploration of many important features of the impending surgical experience. From the wealth of specific anticipations discussed by the patient in the preoperative interview, it is apparent that she had done a considerable amount of mental rehearsing of the potential dangers and deprivations that were awaiting her. Such rehearsal seemed to have led to a high degree of awareness of *reassuring* features as well as threatening ones. Thus, the patient developed a set of reassuring beliefs and expectations which *took account of specific features of the danger situation.* For some specific threats, she had developed specific reassurances which referred to mitigating factors (e.g., "There will be pain but it won't last long"), while other threats were countered by her general attitude of reliance on the danger-control authorities. An outstanding characteristic of these reassurances is that they explicitly or implicitly assume that there will be *only partial immunity* to the impact of stress, in contrast to a crude, over-all invulnerability conception which assumes *blanket immunity*. This difference is emphasized because, according to the theoretical assumptions stated earlier in this chapter, when actual stress stimuli are subsequently encountered, the latter type of reassurance is much less likely to be effective than the former. For example, if Mrs. R. had reduced her anticipatory fears by developing the belief that the physicians would protect her from experiencing *any pain at all*, she might have felt somewhat less fearful before her operation but, at the time when the postoperative pain actually occurred, this reassuring belief would no longer have been effective in reducing fear, and the recollection of this falsified expectation might even have created strong feelings of disappointment.

There are some indications in the interview material which suggest that during the postoperative period of stress, the patient was able to make use of some of the specific reassurances she had developed before the operation. For example, from her comments about the distressing tube feeding experience which occurred on the first postoperative day, it seems that her acceptance of the physician's demands was facilitated by adding to his remarks her own concept of "new techniques," which she had developed beforehand, perhaps as a quasi-magical form of reassuring belief.

A central point concerning the *partial* immunity type of reassurance is that it is less likely to be refuted and extinguished by the realities of the subsequent stress experience than the *blanket* immunity type of reassurance. The more differentiated the reassuring belief with respect to taking account of the environmental features of the actual stress experience, the higher the probability that it will survive the crucial reality test and, therefore, remain effective in reducing fear. This does not mean, of course, that a reassuring belief must necessarily be verifiable or empirically validated in the danger situation in order to be effective. A partial immunity concept may be quite unwarranted, or far-fetched, or even wholly irrational from the standpoint of meeting the rigorous empirical tests that a careful scientist might demand. A reassuring belief presumably will continue to be effective as long as it is *not obviously incompatible with any salient perceptions in the stress situation.* For example, many of Mrs. R.'s reassuring beliefs were the product of wishful thinking and some of them were rather superstitious and unwarranted from a medical point of view (e.g., her belief that because she survived a different type of operation 24 years earlier, her chances of surviving this one were very high). Moreover, the main reassurance on which she relied most heavily—her belief that the staff physicians were highly skilled and of the "very best" quality—may well have been correct, but involved a complex issue about which she had neither the professional knowledge, the opportunity, nor the inclination to judge adequately.

The pertinent assumption here (which will be discussed more fully in Chapter 25) is the following: Although a reassuring belief may be unverifiable and even quite irrational, once it has been initially accepted and reinforced by a temporary reduction in anticipatory fear, it will tend to persist unless it is: (*a*) directly counteracted by authoritative refutations, disagreement on the part of one's friends, or other forms of social pressure; or (*b*) falsified by one's direct perceptual experiences.

It may often happen that only the latter type of refutation will exert any corrective influence. For example, a surgical patient may quietly go on accepting whole-heartedly a variety of blanket immunity notions based on superstitions, magical protective formulae, or grossly erroneous assumptions about his medical prognosis, which, if verbalized to a physician, would be sharply counteracted. Although such total invulnerability reassurances may often escape from the first type of reality test (social validation) they, nevertheless, would be sharply refuted by the second type (experiential validation), since any direct exposure to stressful occurrences would fail to be consonant with the content of the belief. A partial immunity belief, on the other hand, even if based on equally erroneous assumptions, would be less likely to be refuted by the second type of reality test because such beliefs are compatible with the occurrence of danger exposure and suffering.

The next case study provides some additional examples of partial immunity beliefs which, although sometimes the product of personal fantasies, were apparently capable of functioning as effective reassurances during the period of maximal postoperative stress.

INTERVIEW CASE M–4

Mrs. F., a 30-year-old housewife, was hospitalized for the repair of a hernia which had first become apparent a year earlier but had recently become enlarged, producing increasing physical distress. This woman expressed a slight degree of preoperative worry concerning the usual risks of undergoing surgery, but she asserted that her main fear was the possibility that the surgeon might discover a tumor. As she spoke about many different sources of danger and deprivation, the patient made additional comments in which one could again discern a corresponding set of reassurances of the type designated as *partial immunity* concepts. After the operation, the patient was highly cooperative, and was able to tolerate postoperative suffering without developing any visible emotional disturbance. She appeared to have been highly successful in maintaining emotional control by means of the reassurances she had evolved prior to the operation.

In the preoperative interview, this patient asserted that she had not been concerned about the hernia until the past month, during which time she had noted that the "lump" on her abdomen was rapidly growing larger and that her backaches and other pains were occurring more frequently. When the examining physician told her that an operation was necessary, she accepted his recommendation and wished to have it done as soon as possible.

As long as the doctor said it had to come out, I decided right then. I don't believe in having anything stay in you that's bad for you. . . . I thought maybe it might not be a hernia but a tumor, and I'd just as soon get rid of it right away so my mind could be at rest. . . . I just hope they do it as soon as they can; I don't want to wait around . . . I'm worried about letting it stay in me too long, that's why I want it out right away.

Throughout the interview she returned to this source of worry time and again, sometimes apparently using it in combination with reassuring concepts to counteract her apprehensions about the prospects of postoperative suffering. For example, she asserted: "I'll take any kind of suffering and any ailment as long as I know it will heal; it's the ones that don't heal that would really bother me."

Like the patient discussed above (M–2), this woman gave indications of having thought concretely about the implications of the surgery, taking account of the unpleasant events that were in store for her. She spoke explicitly about expecting to be groggy, nauseated, and in pain upon awakening from the anesthetic; about suffering from severe aches and pains during the first few postoperative days; about being required to get out of bed on the first postoperative day; and about remaining at the hospital, in a weakened condition, for a period of about ten days. She also anticipated some of her own emotional reactions to stress, such as feelings of loneliness and especially the fear of being left alone in an unfamiliar room after the operation. Finally, the surgical procedure itself was frankly referred to as a "serious operation" that required "a very good man to do it."

The patient seemed to be actively struggling to counteract the distressing notion that a hernia operation could be fatal—a notion which had been explicitly conveyed by an elderly woman from her neighborhood who spoke with her shortly before she left for the hospital. The neighbor said that her own daughter had recently died from just such an operation:

I didn't feel so good hearing that; but I don't believe it. Her daughter must have had something else. I have enough troubles of my own so I don't bother to think of it. She was a young girl, though—it's a shame.

Along with her statements about various sources of worry, she expressed highly specific reassuring concepts. For example, one of her references to the seriousness of the operation was followed by a comment about the quality of the hospital staff which took account of the fact that, as a ward patient, she did not know who her surgeon would be:

It doesn't matter to me which doctor does the operation because I know that all of them here are very good. I've always gone to hospital doctors because I think they know more than the specialists who have private offices. Even if I could afford it, I wouldn't want a private doctor. I wouldn't want to take a chance on getting a doctor who doesn't know what he is doing. They don't have any doctors here like that.

Another somewhat more complicated source of reassurance was the recollection that her mother-in-law had undergone a much more serious operation six months earlier. Despite the fact that she and her husband were told at the hospital clinic that the elderly woman might not be able to survive the operation, they gave permission, and the outcome proved to be highly successful:

> It makes me feel good to realize that her operation came out so well. It gives me even more faith in the doctors. . . . My mother-in-law was afraid of dying and we had to talk her into coming here, but she's glad now. If anything happened, I'd have it on my conscience. But I know it wouldn't really have been anyone's fault. I have faith that the doctors wouldn't have done it if they didn't feel it was the right thing.

Thus, the recollection of her mother-in-law's operation seemed to function as a defense against guilt feelings as well as a reminder of the favorable consequences of the great faith she had already placed in the hospital physicians.

The patient also appeared to be able to bolster her self-confidence by taking account of her familiarity with the hospital procedures, acquired not only from observing her mother-in-law's surgical experiences but also from her own personal surgical experiences. Speaking about certain postoperative procedures, the patient asserted: "I know about that from what they did for my mother-in-law; they'll probably do the same with me." And, then, later on in the interview:

> Everybody is a little nervous about going through an operation. But I think I can control my emotions because I've had two operations before—one five years ago and the other one seven years ago. It's nothing new to me.

In connection with the fear of being left alone in the hospital, which she had explicitly mentioned several times, the patient expressed the following hope:

> When I come from the operating room I'd like to go to the room I'm in now. I don't like to be alone and I think my husband will be here waiting for me.

After referring to the mutual affection between herself and her husband, she indicated that one of the compensatory gains she hoped to derive from the surgery was an improvement in her marital relationship:

I haven't been able to have any relations with my husband because it hurts me and I hope the operation will fix that up. It's important for my husband too; it's bad for him when I'm this way.

She also asserted, with some display of positive affect, that she derived a great deal of emotional support from her husband:

He left the decision [to have the operation] up to me. He doesn't want to see me suffer. He says I have lots of nerve. I've got to have because we have two children. . . . My husband explained to them about my operation and, when I left, they said, "Mommy hurry up and come home."

From these comments, it seems highly probable that awareness of the affectionate family bonds functioned as one of the major sources of reassurance for this patient.

In the operating room and throughout the entire postoperative period, according to the nurses' and physicians' records, this patient behaved in a relatively calm and affable manner. There were no instances of resistant behavior and the patient's morale was consistently high. The same positive picture emerges from what the patient reported in the postoperative interview. She gave a detailed account of her subjective experiences, describing how she felt as she was being brought up to the operating room, during the administration of the anesthetic, after awakening, and during various painful phases of the convalescent period. Her descriptive account indicates that the various reassuring concepts she had expressed in the preoperative interview continued to be effective at moments of acute crisis, although sometimes functioning in purely magical or irrational ways.

As she was being wheeled down the corridors and taken up in the elevator to the operating room, she felt "slightly jittery." At this time she thought of the fact that her last operation, five years earlier, had been successful and she recalled that just as she had been entering the operating room, the orderly had crossed her fingers for good luck.

When I thought of that I crossed my fingers, and I really kept them crossed all the time I was in the operating room. I just thought I'd do it again, but I'm not really superstitious and I don't believe in it. I just did it because that's what I did in my last operation. Maybe it made me feel more comfortable.

While lying on the table, the patient felt somewhat frightened but, just as during the preoperative period, her worry was focused primarily on the possibility that when the surgeon looked to see what was inside her, it might turn out to be a cancer rather than a hernia. This frightening thought was again followed by a series of fear-arousing and fear-reducing thoughts which formed a sequence remarkedly parallel to that verbalized in the preoperative interview:

The only thing I was worried about was if they'd find a tumor, but I figured if they found it they would just take it out. I really believed it was a tumor and I just left it up to them to get it out. I felt I was just in the hands of the doctors. . . . I was waiting there patiently but I was saying to myself, "Hurry up and take it out." Then I started to think of people telling me not to go through this operation—that woman who had put thoughts in my mind, telling me her daughter died from a hernia operation. I thought it couldn't be that, she must have died from something else. I thought to myself that she's a hell of a friend telling me things like that, making you think crazy ideas instead of telling you good luck, which you need for any operation no matter what it is, because anything might happen. I felt if it was my turn to go then I'd go. But I didn't think it was my turn. I just thought, "I have to get well, I have to go back to my children."

Thus, this patient appears to have made effective use of the reassuring concepts she had developed before the operation. The adequacy of her psychological defenses was put to an even more severe test when something "horrible" occurred while she was on the operating table. She had expected a mask to be placed over her face and a general anesthetic to be given, just as in her earlier two operations. Instead she was given a spinal anesthetic. When she felt the needle in her spine she became tense and apprehensive. The unexpected loss of sensation in her legs disturbed her even more and she asked about it. After being told by one of the physicians that this was the way the anesthetic worked, she relaxed and thought that "this method was pleasanter than gas." But then, suddenly, she felt a jabbing pain in the region of her heart. For an instant she thought that she might be having a heart attack and she became extremely frightened. However, at this point, according to her retrospective account, she again reminded herself that she was in good hands and felt very relieved when the surgeon said that everything was all right and that soon she would be asleep.

Upon awakening, the patient realized that she was back in her room. Although very sick and distressed by the needles sticking in her arms, she nevertheless felt "safe" because "I wanted my husband to be around and he was right there with me." For several days she experienced acute pains and was especially distressed by intense headaches, which she had not expected. Throughout this period, she evidently was able to gain reassurance repeatedly through reliance upon the hospital staff:

I would tell the nurses when I felt bad and they would get something for me. . . . I wasn't ever worried, just uncomfortable. . . . I never lost my faith in the doctors.

She felt especially grateful toward a staff physician who answered her questions about the postoperative headaches and informed her that the operation had not revealed a tumor.

Frequently, during the postoperative interview, she repeated, with apparently genuine conviction, the motivating formula she had evolved before the operation, viz., that she must get well in order to go back to her family. Her children and her husband, she informed the interviewer, missed her very much:

They are dying for me to come home. They miss a mother not being around to do for them. . . . A man can't do for them what a mother can. . . . My husband will be very happy when I get back. He says he'll wash all the clothes for me and everything, because he wants me to rest. . . . He feels all alone and he's wishing I'm there with him.

Although she repeatedly asserted that she missed her family and would like to be with them, she nevertheless expressed some reluctance about returning home:

I'm not too anxious to get back home until the doctor tells me I'm ready, because I know that at home I won't rest like here. When I had my last operation, I went home too soon—I began work, washing floors, cooking, doing the dishes, and all that. That's not good for anybody in my condition.

The psychological importance of the patient's need for affection and indulgent care is suggested by the patient's associations to a dream which occurred three days after the operation:

[*Dream Text*] I dreamed I heard my dog barking. I didn't see the dog but just dreamt that I heard his barking.

Her first (spontaneous) associations to the dream were as follows:

When I woke up from this dream I heard a fire engine. It makes you feel something is going on. A chill crept up my back. It was frightening.

When asked to give the first thing that came to mind as she thought about the dream elements, her associations were as follows:

1. [*The dog*] My dog is lonesome for me. I keep him in the house, feed him, treat him well, not like a baby but like a dog should be taken care of. He's a pet for my children.
2. [*The barking heard in the dream*] My husband said to me, "The dog misses you so much that he didn't eat anything since you left." My husband told me that on the day before I had the dream.

The passive dependency theme, which is so apparent in the foregoing associations, occurs in juxtaposition to a nameless danger which, according to her first association, is something so frightening as to send chills up her back. It is especially noteworthy that in her dream she transforms an external danger signal (the siren) into a pathetic expression of affection (the barking of a lonely dog).

Although the available evidence concerning this patient's personality is too meager to warrant attempting a detailed interpretation of an isolated dream, it seems probable that the dream work involves a reassurance against some form of danger, and that the latent content of the reassurance has to do with the gratifying notion that she is not forgotten or unloved. The patient's need for such reassurance presumably was highly aroused as a consequence of the physical suffering she was undergoing, while, at the same time, being separated from her family. One source of anxiety in this situation may have been conflictful self-indulgent tendencies within herself. We have noted that in the postoperative interview this patient frequently spoke about her wish to return home to her husband and children, but she also stated emphatically that she did not want to face the demands and burdens of home life too soon. Such comments suggest that she may have been ambivalent about being reunited with her family because of a temporary protective attitude of narcissistic self-indulgence. (Perhaps this attitude, in turn, originated partly as a defense against separation anxiety, i.e., an attempt to counteract painful longings to be back home.)

A marked increase in narcissistic tendencies is repeatedly mentioned in psychoanalytic accounts concerning the effects of illness and physical suffering; the change in attitude is sometimes described as a temporary increase in cathexis of the self, with a corresponding withdrawal of cathexis from love objects and from the outer social world in general (Fenichel, 1945; Schilder, 1938). When an internal change of this kind takes place, whether for defensive purposes or for other psychological reasons, it may be somewhat threatening to the average person because of the implication that he is capable of becoming quite selfish and detached from loved ones and, therefore, may no longer deserve their love. When a patient becomes dimly aware of his self-indulgent tendencies, separation anxiety may be further aroused if he attempts to ward off guilt by projecting such tendencies to love objects, or if he becomes preoccupied with the "talion" notion that, as a punishment for his own narcissistic detachment from others, the love objects will, in turn, lose all interest in him.

Taking account of the foregoing psychoanalytic assumptions in relation to the patient's interview data, we may speculate that the anxiety which the patient is attempting to alleviate in her dream stems, at least partially, from her desire to retain a self-protective narcissistic attitude without incurring the risk of becoming unloved. Perhaps she identifies herself with the poor dog who, like herself, is lonely, has no appetite, and needs to be cared for almost like a baby. Whether or not this speculative interpretation is correct, there is no doubt that the dream refers to intense dependency longings of exactly the same kind that this patient had so gratifyingly attributed to her husband and children whenever she spoke about them during the postoperative interview.

It should be mentioned that the emphasis on dependency longings in this patient's dream associations, as well as elsewhere in the postoperative interview, does not appear to be a unique phenomenon. We have already had occasion to cite the marked increase in affiliative needs which has been repeatedly noted among persons who are exposed to external dangers or deprivations (pp. 90–93). On the basis of the psychoanalytic observations from the case of Mrs. Blake, Hypothesis 5 was formulated as a tentative explanation for this increase. According to the hypothesis, whenever a physical threat situation occurs in adult life, there tends to be a reactivation of childhood fears of being abandoned by one's parents, with a corresponding increase in the need for reassurance that one still possesses the affection of current love objects.

In the present case study series, there were numerous manifestations of augmented dependency needs which strongly suggest that the patients were striving to reassure themselves that they were not being abandoned. Some of the most pertinent material, just as in Case M–4, is provided by the patients' postoperative dreams.

Whenever a patient was able to recall a postoperative dream, the interviewer made an effort to elicit free associations and to record them verbatim. Altogether there were eight patients who gave dream material (four of whom had displayed *high* preoperative fear, three a *moderate* level of fear, and one *low* fear. Seven of the eight gave associations which referred directly or indirectly to the desire to be taken care of like a child by parental figures, or which dwelt upon gratifying memories or expectations of being affectionately treated. (Verbatim records of the dream text and the accompanying associations given by each patient are presented below.)[4]

The high degree of emphasis on being loved by members of one's family may function as an important means of bolstering self-esteem and of preventing reactions of postoperative guilt and aggression. It may be no coincidence that, of the eight patients who gave dream material, the only one whose associations did *not* make any reference to the gratification of dependency longings was the one patient who came from the *low* anticipatory fear group. As will be seen in the next chapter, his associations pointed instead to acute feelings of *uncompensated loss*. In the next chapter some comparative case evidence is also examined which helps to identify the basic forms of reassurance a surgical patient must be capable of delivering to himself if he is to avoid reacting with intense aggrievement.

Notes

1. The following excerpts from the questionnaire survey show the statements about preoperative anticipations of mutilation or death written by thirteen of the twenty-seven students in the high fear group:

SURVEY CASE H–21

"[I was concerned about the possibility that] I might be disabled for life, or that further complications might arise from the operation."

SURVEY CASE H–22

"I wondered if it would be a permanent cure. . . . At times I worried about the chances of something going drastically wrong. . . . I thought about the fact that some people do die on the operating table."

SURVEY CASE H–23

"[On the day before the operation] I was worried about the complete newness of the whole situation—that is, being in a hospital, being operated on, being shaved, taking an anesthesia, being able to be well enough to go back to Yale at the end of my vacation. . . . I was afraid that, if my left testicle was atrophied, the surgeon would cut it off and this might keep me out of the Air Corps, as well as make me different from other guys. I knew that if this happened it wouldn't affect my sexual potency or activity, since one testicle, I was told, could take the place of two. Nevertheless, I didn't want to lose the left one. . . ."

SURVEY CASE H–24

"[Before the operation] my fear was of some kind of complication from the operation which might cause some discomfort or some more serious defect."

SURVEY CASE H–25

"[Before the operation] I was worried because I felt that the surgeon might slip and ruin the nose."

SURVEY CASE H–26

"I cried hysterically as I entered the O. R. I told my mother I would rather die than go on with the operation. . . . I felt relieved and so glad it was all over because . . . I saw that I had no deformations, such as missing eyes, etc."

SURVEY CASE H–27

"[On the day before the operation] I was worried whether or not I would live through it, but my worries were somewhat counteracted by the wish to get rid of awful pain. . . . I was worried about the unknown things that could happen. . . . [One of my main concerns was] that I might become deaf or some complication might set in."

SURVEY CASE H–28

"[Before the operation] I was worried that the knife would slip and damage would be done to my mouth."

SURVEY CASE H–29

"[On the day before the operation] I had a vague notion that the operation would not be successful. . . . I was concerned that it might cause death. Or it might not be successful and cause future trouble."

SURVEY CASE H–30

"[Before the operation, I felt concerned about] destruction or loss of vocal chords during operation due to accident on part of surgeon."

SURVEY CASE H–31

"[On the day before the operation] I had general fear of operation because of lack of experience with them. I was worried about the anesthesia; would I come out of it?"

SURVEY CASE H–32

"[Before the operation] I realized that some people before me had experienced infection from this operation, particularly tuberculosis, and I was somewhat worried over the matter. . . . I was also worried about the anesthesia [spinal]. I knew that one out of 5000 spinals caused some kind of permanent paralysis."

SURVEY CASE H–33

"[On the day before the operation] I was worried about the sensations of going into the operating room, and having the mask put over my face, and also being sick afterwards if ether was used. . . . I had heard of a case where a man had gas and the pressure blew out the incision. . . . I experienced fear and anxiety while entering the operating room, and slight panic when the mask was put on."

In the survey questionnaires, the following three excerpts include the only statements from the moderate fear group referring to preoperative concern about the possibility of being mutilated or killed on the operating table:

SURVEY CASE M–48

"[On the day before the operation] I was concerned that if the doctor punctured the septum I would always have difficulty breathing."

SURVEY CASE M–50

"Probably the most unpleasant aspect was the anxiety I endured between the time I was told there would be an operation and the time I was given the spinal anesthetic. I was anxious about possible physical injury."

SURVEY CASE M–56

"[Before the operation] Since I knew that the operation would be performed under a spinal, and since I knew the mechanism of a spinal anesthetic, I was concerned about the possibility of its improper administration with unexpected results; this could even lead to death if improperly handled and I was aware of this."

Among the patients in the low fear group, all of whom denied feeling any concern or worry *on the day before the operation*, only the following two references occurred:

SURVEY CASE L–31

"Just before the operation I recall having a fear that the doctor might slip and cut a seminal duct instead of the appendix."

SURVEY CASE L–33

"[Before the operation] I wasn't worried about the operation at all. . . . but [when it was ready to start] I wondered if the doctor would make some mistake that would cause some damage to my spine more serious than the cyst."

2. In addition to Case X–1, there were seven other patients whose interview data were incomplete (see p. 238). All such cases were excluded from the sample used to examine the sequelae of preoperative fear reported in Chapters 20 and 21. Nevertheless, some of the observations of these cases are of value for elucidating certain limited aspects of stress behavior. Whenever such case material is used, the patients are designated by the letter X, to differentiate them from the cases used in the three groups designated as H, M, and L.

3. Case X–1 illustrates the fact that anticipatory fear can be stimulated merely by asking a series of interview questions about impending stressful experiences. It is quite conceivable that some of the patients in the moderate fear group might have experienced less anticipatory fear if they had not been interviewed for the research study. In other words, the interview procedure itself might have altered the spontaneous tendency of some subjects. If so, however, this fact would not in itself reduce the validity of the findings. The patients in the low anticipatory fear group were exposed to the same procedure, with the same questions being asked in a roughly constant sequence. Their anticipatory fear was not stimulated by the interview, presumably because other factors in the situation and/or in their personality make-up enabled them to maintain a strong defense against anticipatory fear. By comparing these cases with patients who experienced some noticeable degree of anticipatory fear, whether attributable partially to the interview or not, one can study the relationship between postoperative adjustment and antecedent psychological variables other than the interview stimuli (since the latter were held fairly constant for both groups).

4. The frequent occurrence of the "passive" dependency theme in the series of postoperative dreams becomes apparent only when one examines carefully the associations given to the dreams. As a standard part of the postoperative interview, all patients were asked whether they could recall a dream that had occurred since the operation (see pp. 229–230). Each of the eight patients who were able to report dreams were asked to give free associations and these, together with the text of the dream, were recorded verbatim.

Inferences are drawn from the dream associations obtained from the surgical patients for the purpose of gaining some further clues to the psychological impact of environmental stress stimuli. This is a quite different purpose from that of almost all other research studies which have hitherto made use of dream material. When one examines the voluminous psychological and psychoanalytical studies in which dreams are reported, it becomes apparent that the main uses are for purposes of either understanding the *personality predispositions* of the dreamers or of gaining insight into the *nature of the dream process itself*. But instead of using each surgical patient's dream to understand his unique personality trends or to arrive at an exhaustive account of the latent content, the attempt here is limited to that of observing *what is common in the thematic content* of the obtained associations from the entire sample of patients. This attempt was made with the hope of being able to identify one or more *common latent (or preconscious) reactions to the common situation of environmental stress to which all patients were exposed.*

The author feels that the technique of eliciting dream material, as used in the present study, may prove to be an extremely valuable adjunct to current research methods for investigating the effects of situational variables. The technique appears to be not only a feasible addition to the usual type of directed interview but also quite harmless in that the patients did not show any visible signs of being disturbed by the procedure while the interview was being conducted, or afterwards.

The validity of this unconventional use of dream material must, of course, be regarded as open to question until the results can be evaluated in relation to other types of observations. There are many sources of errors that can influence the findings from dream analyses of the type employed in the present case study research. The data probably are not comparable to those obtained from the psychoanalytic patient whose dream associations were elicited under conditions of a long-established therapeutic relationship and whose symbolic references can be interpreted in the light of an extraordinarily rich backlog of data bearing on the patient's personality and social background.

In order to document the statements made in the text (p. 325), the dream protocols are reproduced in full for each patient who reported a postoperative dream. It will be noted that, although there are considerable individual differences among the patients with respect to the variety and content of the manifest themes in the free associations, there is, nevertheless, a common theme that occurs explicitly in almost very case. The common theme, designated as the "passive dependency" theme, includes references to: (*a*) being helped or taken care of by parents or by parent-surrogates, (*b*) being comforted by the presence of parental figures, and (*c*) giving or receiving affection from members of the immediate family. (Italics are used to call attention to those manifest associations which, in the author's judgment, allude most directly to one or another aspect of the dependency theme.)

INTERVIEW CASE M–5

The dream of a 73-year-old woman which occurred on about the third night after her operation (subtotal gastrectomy).

Dream Text

"The other night I had a dream of my husband calling me. That woke me up. I thought I was home when I had the dream, but when I woke up I looked around and saw I wasn't home."

Associations

1. "[Spontaneous] I haven't slept good, until last night. I'm not sure when I had that dream. . . . I've had no other dreams since that one."
2. "[Associations to *husband calling*] My husband was calling out 'Ma,' just like when I'm home. He has been on my mind while I'm in the hospital. My husband always calls me at night to *take care of him.* I don't know how many times he would call me at night since he became an invalid. I guess I was tired out when I had the dream."

INTERVIEW CASE M–6

The dream of a 50-year-old male which occurred on the fifth night after his operation (colostomy).

Dream Text

"I dreamed of my daughter visiting me and saying, 'Come on Daddy and kiss me, I'm going home.' "

Associations

1. "[Spontaneous] My daughter visited me on the day before the dream."
2. "[Associations to *daughter visiting*] It was a happy reunion, that's all, *a pleasant reunion for a father and daughter.*"
3. "[Associations to *daughter saying 'I'm going home'*] That has no significance at all. In fact this dream didn't have any connection at all with my life. It's just that the last thing I happened to be thinking of was my daughter—I was thinking that *she kissed me before she left.* It was a pleasant dream and I think it was due to the fact that I kept that idea—of her kissing me—in my subconscious mind. My mind kept dwelling on her as she left, and the meaning of it came to my mind in the dream."
4. "[Associations to *the image of his daughter as she appeared in the dream*] I can't think of anything other than the *love of a daughter for Daddy* and whatever else she did *she wanted to be sure to kiss him before she left.*"
5. "[Associations to leaving] I'll be leaving here in another week or two. Then I'll have my convalescence at home. *I think I'm going to my brother's place out in the country and I'll spend two weeks there resting.* After that I'll go to work. My mind isn't really at peace now. I'm just sort of skipping over the bumps of life. But one has to live, and I've got to make a living. Going through this operation experience takes more out of you mentally and physically than a year of work. It uses up more of your energy than maybe 10 years of working. So I have to rest up. Some people here, some of them less well than I, complain that *they want to go home.* But I feel that even if your home is that of a Rockefeller *you can't get the kind of care and facilities you get here—people on hand 24 hours a day. So I'm not going to leave* until they tell me that I am really ready for it."

INTERVIEW CASE H–1

The dream of a 31-year-old woman which occurred on the third night after her operation (hernia repair).

Dream Text

"It's a funny thing, I dreamt my sister-in-law came down from Boston and my husband's cousin and his wife were there too. It seems I was talking to them. They were here to visit me. It seems I was stepping around very lively, ready to go out. I could see myself all dressed up and I felt very happy about it."

Associations

1. "[Spontaneous] People calling on me was on my mind because I told my husband that, when I come home, I don't want him to tell anybody till I am home a day or two because I wanted to relax first. *I just want to be contented being home.* Something might occur if I don't take it easy. If a whole houseful came in, I might get excited. It's *like when you're first married*, everyone comes in, you have to be a host to them, you have to make them feel right at home. I might jump up, go here and there if a lot of people came."
2. "[Associations to *being all dressed up*] I have a picture of myself *going home* and being happy I went through the operation all right. In the dream I was happy, admiring myself, like it was another person, but it really was me. Another thing, I was summing up in the dream was this: it shows you can stand something. I

had thought I would die, and so on, I think the dream was about that; I felt it just goes to show that what you think you can't stand you can."

3. "[Associations to *husband's cousin and wife*] I feel so happy that I would like to get adjusted, so if they come or if my husband can fix up our car so we could go there for a visit, I would like to go and just relax and let nothing worry me. Now I feel free of pain and so I can really enjoy myself—I'd be glad to see them if they come or if we go there."

4. "[Associations to *stepping around lively*] If I use good sense I'll be doing just that. The only thing that pops into my head is, 'Thank God, I'm free and can go out.' I want to wish all the patients left behind the same luck, so they can get out and dress to go out same way as I am."

5. "[Associations to *going out*] I tried to leave the hospital before my operation when they asked me to sign the paper. I felt that I was having something done for my own benefit and it would make me free from what was bothering me, I wouldn't have to worry any more. The thing that worried me was the *upkeep of my youngsters. How would they be taken care of? It might be the end of my life and maybe I'd never see my youngsters again.* I've heard of people being operated on and reports come back that the operation was an ordeal to the doctors, or something turned up and the doctors did all they could but couldn't save him. I knew there was always a possibility of something turning up, something the doctors couldn't help. I thought of that when it was my time to be operated on, and that made me feel that I might die."

INTERVIEW CASE H–2

The dream of a 37-year-old woman which occurred on the sixth night after the operation (lung lobectomy).

Dream Text

"Last night I had a dream that my three kids were talking to me around the house. I woke up laughing, but I don't know what the kids said. I could just hear the sound of their voices."

Associations

1. "[Spontaneous] At first when you asked me if I could remember a dream since my operation, I thought that the last dream I had was about cats. You see, I had a cat and she was going to have a baby. When I went to sleep, I dreamt *she had her baby* and then the next day she actually did. I felt she wanted to have me around. I had to *help her out*. She is just like a human being, *like a mother and she needed me.* I had that dream the week I was home when I was waiting to come in for the operation. Then I remembered last night's dream. I was thinking of my kids before going to sleep last night because *my little daughter wrote me a note*. In the dream I could just hear the sound of their voices as if I was in a fog, but I couldn't see them and didn't know what they were saying."

2. "[Associations to *the kids' voices*] I had read the letter from my daughter and she said, 'Phillip and Bunny (the other two kids) were *asking for you and give you a big kiss.*' "

INTERVIEW CASE H–3

The dream of a 46-year-old woman which occurred on the night after the operation (lung lobectomy).

Dream Text

"I had a dream about Indians on the warpath last night. I was there with a doll.

The Indians were dancing a war dance, pulling down pieces of canvas that almost fell on my head. They were trying to put it over the wagon I was in. It seemed as if I was choking."

Associations

1. "[Spontaneous] I awoke and found the room very warm."

2. "[Associations to *Indians on the warpath*] I think of wars like they used to have, shooting arrows. It's something I have never given much thought to since I read stories as a kid."

3. [Associations to *pieces of canvas being pulled down*] I didn't want to be strangled. I had the idea that as soon as that came over my head, I wouldn't breathe any more."

4. "[Associations to *being strangled by something overhead*] Just death, I guess. I can't think of anything else."

5. "[Associations to *the dream image of standing there with a doll*] I must of been small. Oh yes, my *Mama* is in the dream too. When I dream of her I am so glad, *I've felt lost without her during the past 10 years.* Usually when I do dream of her, she's sad but in this dream she was looking at me and smiling. That makes me think of the fun we had when I was young. She was always smiling. *When I was about 7 years old up until 16 years old, I was with her the whole time.* I had St. Vitus dance and other diseases and people weren't allowed to see me. *It made me feel better to see my mother smiling* in my dream. My mother looked smiling at me after the nightmare about the Indians. My heart was pounding when I awoke, but *the thought of my mother helped calm me down. Just like when I was small and I was frightened; like when I was away from Mother once and broke my arm. I wanted Mama so much and was so happy to get home to Mama.* I used to like to stay with Mother at night rather than to go out with the girls. *I always liked being with Mama*, especially during the last seven years of her life. *Mother would wait up for me* if I went to a dance or something, and I couldn't enjoy myself if I knew she was there waiting at the window. My sister is bossy and I don't like her. She has made me cry more than anyone else. But *I have a good brother* here."

INTERVIEW CASE H–4

The dream of a 43-year-old salesman which occurred on the fourth night after the operation (cholecystectomy).

Dream Text

"I dreamt of my godfather who is in Greece, last night or, rather, the night before. We were in Athens together—he has a son there, he's in the silk manufacturing business and I haven't communicated with them in 25 years. We walked around in Athens and always the number 'two' was in my mind, I don't know what to make of that."

Associations

1. "[Spontaneous] It was a pleasant dream but the nurse woke me up by giving me a needle. I've seen this number 'two' many times, I've dreamed of it all the time. Maybe having two different causes of sickness in my body is what's in my mind. Two weeks ago I dreamt of two camels in a desert in Egypt; I never dreamt like that before. I saw the camels and said to a fellow I thought there were 50 or 60 camels in a caravan, and he said, 'well this is private ownership.'"

2. "[Associations to the number 'two'] Two children. I'm the father of my two

children. Now I get the idea. Yes, that's the idea, maybe that hit it on the head. Well, I think of *the emotional feeling of being a father, I guess.* They were here the day before I was operated on. One time I dreamt of the number 'seven'; that was a long time ago. I don't dream often, or remember them."

3. "[Associations to *Athens*] I always wanted to see those people because I hadn't seen them in years. I don't know in what shape or form they look, how they're getting along."

4. "[Associations to *godfather*] When I was five or six years old, just before I came to this country, *he and his family used to take care of me just as good as their own children.* There were three boys in their family and three in ours, and we always played together. All this family background from beginning to end came to my mind before my operation; I reviewed the whole history of my life the day before the operation. The dream was after the operation. I had thought of my godfather at that time. In my religion, the godfather is an important relationship. *If anything happened to my father, according to the rules of the church, the godfather would take charge of me,* send me to school, whatever he wanted, even if my mother objected. He was a choirmaster in the church. *I even saw my dead father in a dream* long before I came to the hospital—he looked very sick, and I asked him how he came here, and he said, 'I came in a plane.' He said, 'I had to come on urgent business and couldn't notify you.' I remembered incidents since I was three years old on the day before my operation. *I remembered an orchard from when I was three years old and they shook plums down, because we couldn't get up there to get them. So my mother threw a shoe up and knocked them down for me, and I laughed even though I was only three.* I remembered that and a fire we had when I was six years old. My father had a box of shells for hunting that caught on fire. He got some bullets in his flesh and he had to be operated on, and I thought of that. Maybe because I was going to have an operation."

The dream material from two other patients is presented in the text: for Case M-4, see pp. 323–324; for Case L-7, see pp. 342–344.

It will be recalled that a passive dependency theme was noted in the analysis of the postoperative dreams of Mrs. Blake (see pp. 152–157). Her associations to two dreams indicated very clearly a strong need to assuage powerful dependency longings that were apparently activated by the suffering and damage she had experienced after the operation. This was one of many instances, however, where the author felt dubious about generalizing from this particular patient's postoperative reactions because her manifestations of dependency longings might have been quite atypical of how people generally react to actual stress. After all, this patient was known to be especially troubled by chronic dependency conflicts. Frequently, in the past, she had put up an active struggle to ward off affectionate longings, displaying a defensive attitude of callous indifference or of outright hostility toward her parents, husband, children, analyst, and other significant persons. It seemed likely, therefore, that the upsurge of dependency longings in this case might have reflected a special predisposition linked with the patient's neurotic disorder, and that, in this respect, other persons would not be likely to react in any uniform way.

It came as something of a surprise, therefore, that a similar trend was found in the dream associations of seven of the eight patients for whom this additional depth-interview material was available. From this series of case study findings, it seems warranted to draw the tentative conclusion that an upsurge of dependency longing is likely to become a dominant psychological trend during the period when surgical patients are undergoing the stresses of postoperative convalescence. Thus Hypothesis 5 was formulated in such a way as to include the threats of the *postoperative* period as well as those of the *preoperative* period.

A search of the literature revealed that in a few clinical reports similar contents were noted in the dreams of individual surgical patients. For example, H. Deutsch (1942, p. 111) describes a patient whose postoperative dreams ". . . represented longing for the mother and birth situations . . ."; Sutherland and Orbach (1953, p. 957) noted some preoperative horror dreams which were ". . . accompanied in some instances by other dreams in which parents are beseeched for protection . . ."

In the discussion of Case M–4, it was suggested that the heightened need for reassurance about not being abandoned stems partially from the patient's own narcissistic, self-protective attitude which may give rise to some ambivalence with respect to wanting to return home to the family circle. The latter type of ambivalence is occasionally manifested in the associations given by several patients whose dream protocols are presented above. For example, Case H–1, in her first spontaneous association to her dream, explicitly stated that she was concerned that when she returned home she might be unable to relax because of too many responsibilities, and in her next association she openly expressed narcissistic self-admiration. Case M–5 provides a less explicit example: She referred to her concern about being responsible for taking care of her invalid husband when she is at home, and juxtaposed this preoccupation with the notion that she is "tired out." Perhaps the most clear-cut example of a self-protective attitude coupled with ambivalence about returning home is found in the final associations given by Case M–6. After a series of associations concerning the loving gesture of his daughter, he asserts that after what he has been through he deserves a vacation and that he does not want to go home because of the superior care he is getting at the hospital. Thus, the dream association material from four of the eight patients adds to the plausibility of the supplementary hypothesis that during the postoperative period, convalescent patients are likely to experience a conflict-laden increase in narcissistic and self-indulgent tendencies, which contributes to their need for being reassured that they have not lost the solicitude and affection of their loved ones. (It is conceivable, as stated earlier, that the narcissistic detachment itself originates partly as a defense against separation anxiety: a surgical patient might attempt to counteract his strong wish to return home by adopting the belief that he is better cared for at the hospital.)

In evaluating the inferences drawn from the dream material, it is necessary to bear in mind the fact that for each case the data come from only one interview session. We lack the necessary control data, without which we cannot answer the following question: What types of dreams and associations would these same patients have under "normal" conditions, when they are not subjected to the stresses of postoperative convalescence? The investigator also lacks information as to the types of dreams and associations which would be found among the large subgroup of patients in the case study sample who were unable to recall or unwilling to report a postoperative dream. In the absence of supplementary control data, one cannot be at all confident about the inferences made from the common themes noted in the dream material at hand. For example, one of the seemingly unusual features of the series of dreams under investigation is the fact that half the cases refer to *auditory stimuli* in the manifest content of the dream. Case M–4 hears her dog barking, Case M–5 hears her husband calling, Case M–6 hears his daughter talking, and Case H–2 hears the sound of her children's voices. In two of these instances, the patient reports that nothing was seen in the dream, that it was entirely limited to an auditory image. The apparent emphasis on auditory stimuli might lend itself to interpretation in terms of psychoanalytic hypotheses concerning the relationship between the auditory sphere and superego functions. But is such an attempt at interpretation worthwhile if we do not know whether the alleged characteristic is in any way related to the fact that the patients are currently exposed to a stress situation? One cannot be at all sure that the auditory content would not be just as frequent if the dreams of these same patients were elicited at a time when they were not undergoing a special form of stress.

The above considerations apply directly to all the inferences drawn from the dream material. They highlight the necessity for regarding the inferences as suggestive but nonconclusive data. Despite all the shortcomings, however, the dream data supplement the available observations bearing on the psychodynamic processes specified in Hypothesis 5. In future investigations, if the necessary control observations are made, it should be possible to obtain systematic evidence from dream associations. The systematic use of dream association techniques may eventually prove to be uniquely efficient in eliciting important psychological information that other, more superficial, interview methods cannot provide. Dream analysis may eventually prove to be a "royal road" to the relatively transient, unverbalized reactions to environmental changes as well as to the more constant unconscious features of the human personality.

24.

Causes of resentment

In the preceding chapter, we arrived at a preliminary account of the psychological gains in postoperative adjustment which occur when a person anticipates being exposed to stress stimuli and "works through" his fears before the crisis situation is actually at hand. The observational material presented gives us some conception of what may be missing from the psychological preparation of those surgical patients who remain unconcerned about the impending operation. In this chapter, we continue our inquiry into the psychodynamic factors which account for the adverse behavioral sequelae observed in those patients who were relatively free from anticipatory fear—their overt resistance to postoperative procedures, derogatory comments about the hospital staff, occasional outbursts of intense anger, and other manifestations of intense resentment.

Additional evidence is presented bearing on two important features of stress episodes, both of which are pertinent for understanding the causes of postoperative resentment: (*a*) The specific stimuli or events which seem to be most capable of evoking strong aggressive reactions and (*b*) the accompanying subjective state of the patient on the initial occasion when reactions of postoperative resentment were first manifested, and on the subsequent occasions when such reactions were so intense as to create interpersonal disturbances. We first examine the nature of the postoperative complaints made by the men in the survey sample who reported low preoperative fear. Then we return to a detailed examination of material from the series of intensive case studies, and examine the emotional and cognitive processes of several patients in the low fear group whose especially rich interview data make it possible to gain some psychological insight into the sources of disturbance in their postoperative adjustment. The case material is discussed in relation to the psychoanalytic hypotheses concerning aggrievement reactions presented in Chapter 15, and an attempt is made to give a concise formulation of the psychodynamic mechanisms involved in the development of postoperative resentment.

Content of Complaints

By examining the content of the written comments obtained from the low preoperative fear group in the survey research, we obtain some leads concerning the motivational factors that enter into this group's negative attitudes toward the hospital staff. The pertinent survey questions were those used for constructing Table 9 (p. 294), which shows the marked tendency of the low fear group to express blame and to complain against the staff. The open-end questions, described earlier (pp. 292–293), elicited many written statements which were just as outspokenly hostile as the oral statements made by those ward patients who ventilated their anger against the staff in response to postoperative interview questions.

From the subjective standpoint of those who made complaints, what were the main reasons for becoming angry or resentful? In a few instances, the written complaints were focused directly on the alleged infliction of unnecessary pain, accusing members of the hospital staff of having malevolent intentions. The following is a typical example:

SURVEY CASE L–21

The nurses were often late with the bed pan, or else they would leave it in sight. . . . The food was abominable. . . . I had a redhaired nurse who took sadistic delight in ripping the adhesive shroud from around my middle.

Several other men in the low fear group made complaints of criminal negligence, as illustrated by the following accusation:

SURVEY CASE L–22

[After the operation] I was annoyed at the wrong diagnosis and that they would not relieve the pain. . . . I simply cursed the doctors. . . . I think the surgeon who operated on me made the wrong diagnosis because he was drunk and that angered me. I think I was justified in my annoyance.

Others in the low fear group also made accusations which implied that the medical authorities were so grossly negligent as to cause them unnecessary pain and actual body damage.

SURVEY CASE L–23

[After the operation] I was angry that I couldn't move my left arm because I couldn't see any reason for my left arm being affected when my right side was cut. Also, I was extremely angry with the night nurse who was very rough in yanking my arm out of the oxygen tent for a penicillin shot. It caused me terrific pain on the right side, causing me to scream.

SURVEY CASE L–24

For the most part the operation was more nerve-racking than anything else because the Doc operating seemed to play a tune on the muscles of my leg, causing pain the whole length of the thigh. His foolish excuses plus his inability to perform the operation with any degree of skill caused me increasing anxiety. . . . When he answered my questions, it was a lot of double talk. . . .

From what a few men reported, it appears that their distrustful attitude was sometimes accompanied by a conscious fantasy that the authority figure would end up by maiming them rather than by protecting them from body damage, as illustrated by the following excerpt:

SURVEY CASE L–33

I was annoyed at the fact that the spinal wasn't administered correctly the first time. . . . The injection caused extreme pain for a minute or more . . . I wondered if the doctor would make some mistake that would cause some damage to my spine more serious than the cyst.

Occasionally the danger-control authorities were blamed not only for negligence or ineptness in causing unnecessary postoperative pain but also for evoking intense emotional reactions which allegedly would not have otherwise occurred.

SURVEY CASE L–26

A day after the operation I had not urinated since before the operation. They gave me a hypo which was as unpleasant as the perspiration it produced. . . . I wasn't worried about not urinating, but everyone else seemed to be, and that made me become frightened too.

All of the foregoing excerpts contribute to an over-all impression that among the men who denied having any fear of the operation beforehand, there was a marked tendency to deny, later on, that the pains and discomforts caused by the operation were natural or unavoidable consequences of the surgical procedure. Many of these men regarded stress stimulation as an *avoidable accident caused by the malevolence or gross incompetence of the danger-control authorities.*

A Maladjustive Sequence: Denial—Apperceptive Distortion—Resentment

The reactions delineated in the preceding section closely resemble those found in the case studies of surgical ward patients who manifested low preoperative fear. Some important clues as to what lies behind the tendency to perceive members of the hospital staff as hostile or as dangerously incompetent manipulators can be found in the intensive interviews. We begin by re-examining one typical case study for illustrative purposes, adding a few new details which will help to elucidate the psychological sequence that leads to maladjustive reactions during the postoperative period.

The interview material is from Case L–6, a patient who displayed as marked a change in social behavior as any patient in the entire group. Before the operation, this middle-aged man had expressed extremely optimistic expectations that the convalescent period would be a painless, comfortable "vacation" (see pp. 268–270). His postoperative resistance to treatment as well as his intense verbal assaults against the nurses centered primarily upon specific incidents of pain or discomfort —muscular aches, gas pains, urination difficulties, and many other unpleasant sequelae of the surgical operation. These disturbing events came as a surprise to him, not because he was unaware of such sequelae but because he had so optimistically expected that the discomforts would be so slight *in his particular case* as to be negligible. When he actually did undergo acute postoperative pains and discomforts, he perceived them as a series of deprivations inflicted upon him by the hospital personnel. For example, the severe gas pains which kept him awake at night were on one occasion blamed on the fact that "a nurse came in and gave me cascara because she said the doctor ordered it for me and that formed gas and gave me a bad night." On other occasions the discomfort was allegedly due to the improper diet they fed him: ". . . they gave me jelly which was so sweet that it filled me with gas." Similarly, the intense suffering he experienced as the anesthetic wore off was not because of the pain itself:

The pain was severe but I was able to stand it all right. What made me mad was that there weren't nurses there when I needed them. They didn't check me hardly at all. That's why I was suffering so much.

On the night after the operation his "neck muscles and nerves hurt," not as a consequence of the incision itself but because the nurses refused his repeated demands to allow his wife to remain after visiting hours, thus producing "excitement and causing me to strain my neck, which prevented it from healing properly." Several days later, the distress he experienced in being unable to pass urine was attributed not to his physiological condition but solely to the ineptness of the "routine nurses they sent around with the bottle." For all these instances of acute discomfort, the patient vociferously maintained that the hospital staff was at fault.

It should be noted that this man directly blamed the nurses and attendants (and by implication the physicians as well) not only for the actual stress he experienced but also for his own emotional reactions to the stress. Many of his rantings against them included the charge that they were responsible for making him feel "upset," "worried," and "disgusted." In this patient we see, therefore, an example of the tendency to react to physical suffering by *projecting blame* onto persons in the immediate environment.

If we permit ourselves to attempt to generalize from the data at hand, the following tentative propositions summarize the psychological sequence depicted by the foregoing case material:

1. During the preoperative period, a very low level of anticipatory fear is accompanied by optimistic expectations which constitute a *denial or minimization of the anticipated danger and suffering that will be produced by the surgery*.
2. When actual suffering subsequently does occur, it comes as an unpleasant surprise and is not accepted as the "natural" consequence of the surgical intervention but is apperceived as a *deprivation inflicted by the environment, caused by the malevolence, negligence, or lack of solicitude of the danger-control authorities*.
3. The tendency to misperceive the danger-control authorities as being the source of unexpected deprivations is then followed by the development of *hostile, retaliatory attitudes* toward them.

These propositions seem to provide an initial framework for explaining why patients with low preoperative fear become resentful and uncooperative. The first of the above propositions is fairly well supported by the case study observations of the entire low fear group. When questioned specifically about their expectations during the preoperative interview, none of these patients indicated that they expected to undergo any noteworthy suffering as a result of the operation. (In Chapter 21, examples of the patients' comments about their expectations were included in the case study summaries.) A few asserted that they expected to have some postoperative pain but, in general, the unpleasant sequelae of the operation were regarded as negligible. Moreover, many of the patients, such as Case L–6, expressed some extremely positive anticipations, which have been referred to earlier as "expectations of compensatory gains" (pp. 58–62). Thus, during the period of maximal postoperative stress, these patients may not only feel resentful about their unexpected suffering but also about their failure to gain the special rewards or indulgences they had hoped to obtain.[1]

Disruptive Episodes

In the preceding chapter it was seen that the differentiated, *partial immunity* reassurances noted in the moderate fear group came into play and helped to alleviate fear during major crisis episodes, when the patient was struggling against feelings of helplessness in the presence of harrowing stress stimuli. In contrast, the patients in the low fear group appeared to be exceptionally vulnerable to postoperative crisis episodes; when their blanket immunity expectations were disconfirmed, they were not able to reassure themselves that "everything will come out all right" nor to accept the reassurances afforded by the presence of protective authority figures.

Interview Case L–7 provides a vivid illustration of the untoward consequences of being unprepared for exposure to stress stimuli (see Chapter 21, pp. 252–254). Before the operation he was unworried and expressed grossly optimistic expectations of the "blanket immunity" type. Then, immediately after the operation, on the first occasion when he experienced unanticipated suffering and physical restraint, his only defense against feelings of helplessness was to engage in a violent physical struggle against the nurses, who were perceived as the agents responsible for the danger. Thus he misinterpreted the situation as a hostile attack by the people who were trying to help him. This episode apparently had a sensitizing effect, producing not only a sustained attitude of resentment but also a neurotic type of phobic avoidance reaction.

Some further indications of the patient's latent attitude with regard to this situation is provided by a dream and its accompanying associations, elicited at the end of the postoperative interview. The dream had occurred on the preceding night (ten days after the operation).

[*Dream Text*] Everywhere I went someone was grabbing me, robbing me, beating me up. It was several kids, I don't know who they were. They were grabbing me.

1. [*Initial spontaneous associations*] They gave me pain pills last night. I was soaking wet with sweat, the pain was so bad. I took them about seven o'clock and then slept until ten. Then they gave me more pain pills and I slept till midnight. I had dreams in between. The dream I just told you woke me up.

When asked to tell the first thing that came to mind as he thought about each dream element, his associations were as follows:

2. [*Someone grabbing you*] I guess they wanted to hurt me. It had something to do with my leg.
3. [*Kids*] Just a tough gang, hanging around the corner someplace. I don't know who they were.
4. [*Being beaten up*] I don't know why they were beating me.
5. [*The whole dream*] Nothing comes to mind. I think they were robbing me, that was the main reason.
6. [Can you remember *what they were robbing you of* in your dream?] Of what little money I had—a dime I had in my pocket.
7. [*A dime in your pocket*] I can't think of anything.
8. [*How did you feel during the dream?*] The dream was very unpleasant. It woke me up and I felt my leg hurting.

From this protocol, it appears that the dream fantasy of being grabbed and beaten is directly linked with sensations of pain in his leg (which in all probability was the immediate stimulus giving rise to the dream). In his associations, he elaborates on the hostile intentions of the persons who were inflicting pain on him. Not only did they want to hurt him but they wanted to rob him of the small possession he had left.

For present purposes, one need only take account of the surface aspects of the patient's associations to conclude that this man displays a tendency to place the blame for the painful sensations in his leg on unnamed persons ("they") to whom he attributes the intent of inflicting serious deprivations upon him. It should be noted that the *nurses* are also regularly referred to as "they" and are spoken about in a related context in his very first comments about the dream. From his associations and from the content of other portions of the interview in which he made critical statements about the nurses, it appears very likely that these intrusive, demanding, omnipresent women constitute the "gang" which does the grabbing and which wants to hurt and rob him.

The psychoanalytic case evidence presented in an earlier chapter led to the formulation of Hypothesis 11, which asserts that the disappointments engendered by unexpected deprivations in adult life tend to reawaken aggrievement reactions that originally had occurred during childhood, at times when the individual had felt that he was being excessively punished by one or both parents (see pp. 204–205). This hypothesis, which emphasizes the adverse effects of a large discrepancy between the amount of suffering anticipated beforehand and the amount of suffering actually experienced, provides a possible basis for explaining the hostile behavior and resentment displayed by the male patient under discussion. From the interview evidence, it seems fairly probable that the patient's irrational refusal to permit the nurses to treat his leg (despite the fact that he continually complained about the pain) was an expression of childlike disappointment and retaliation—an underlying attitude of resentment fostered by the initial sensitizing episode in which he was enraged by the nurses who were administering the unexpected postoperative transfusion and were physically restraining him. It was as though he felt that the nurses actually were responsible for damaging his leg and, therefore, could not be trusted to touch it again.

The latent attitude conveyed by the dream material contrasts sharply with that of the seven patients whose dreams were described and discussed earlier (see pp. 323–325 and 328–335). The latter cases, all of whom had displayed moderate or high anticipatory fear, gave associations which conveyed a high degree of acceptance of their childlike status as passive, dependent convalescents. These patients seemed to have gone through a preoperative phase of doubting and worrying, as a result of which they achieved some degree of inner preparation. After having gone through this process, they obtained a great deal of psychological comfort from being supported and nurtured by the "good" parental figures who were taking care of them. For them, even though their passive, dependent needs were only incompletely satisfied, the dangers of being dependent upon the authority figures apparently were surmounted. With high faith and confidence in the staff, they usually were able to submit their bodies to whatever manipulation the authorities chose to impose.

The statements made by the patient discussed above (Case L–7) convey a latent attitude of the opposite sort—he obstinately refuses to accept maternal support or aid, even though it is proffered under the aegis of the paternal authority of a male doctor; he must constantly guard against being attacked and injured by "bad" maternal figures. Whether or not one accepts the plausibility of an interpretation in terms of "regression to an anal retentive phase," there seems to be little question that much of this patient's postoperative maladjustment, especially his noncompliance and obstinate rejection of medical aid, stemmed from his perception of the nurses' behavior as the cause of his suffering. In response to a situation of unexpected physical suffering, which had evoked intense feelings of helplessness, the patient was unable to reassure himself that help was at hand and that he was receiving the benefit of skilled and sympathetic aid. The patient did not accept the fact that the restraints (e.g., leg binding) and deprivations (e.g., withholding of water when he was acutely thirsty) were being imposed for his own well-being. Instead, he viewed the nurses as the inflictors of deprivation, and he refused to allow himself to become dependent upon them or to accept their attempts to soothe his injury.

The patient's lack of inner preparation for the stresses of surgery may have been partly responsible for his becoming sensitized by the disruptive episode which contributed so heavily to his sustained attitude of hostility. The latter attitude was accompanied by an irrational struggle against the authorities which proved to be self-defeating in that his refusal to permit the prescribed medical treatment resulted in a continuation of severe physical pain which probably could have been alleviated. There is also additional case material indicating that, as a result of his lack of psychological preparation, this patient encountered great difficulty in assimilating the disturbing events which immediately preceded the administration of the anesthetic. When he was brought into the operating room he was surprised to see that the situation was so different from what he had expected. For several weeks thereafter, he repeatedly ruminated about this scene, the main detail in his repetitive recollections being the strange appearance of the doctors and nurses, who were wearing green uniforms rather than the white ones he had expected (see p. 253). Probably this relatively innocuous detail represents a displaced source of fear, as in "screen" memories. The repetitious recall of such a detail seems to be similar to the repetitive memories and dreams frequently observed in cases of acute traumatic neurosis, and perhaps serves the same psychological function—a "belated attempt at mastery" of the danger situation (S. Freud, 1920). In this connection it should also be noted that the patient's dream contains manifest themes of the type reported in psychiatric studies as being characteristic of dreams in traumatic neuroses: In the patient's dream picture of himself, he is *in danger*, he is *beaten*, and he *fails to escape* (see Kardiner and H. Spiegel, 1947, pp. 204 ff.).

Probably it would be diagnostically correct to view this patient's emotional disturbances—his irritability and hostility coupled with rumination tendencies and disturbing dreams—as symptoms of an incipient or transient form of traumatic neurosis. This interpretation of the case evidence appears to be quite plausible because, just as in clear-cut cases of acute traumatic neurosis, the patient's behavioral disturbances began immediately after exposure to a danger episode in which he felt frightened and helpless. To recapitulate: The transfusion episode, and perhaps also the preceding episode of being anesthetized, had a sensitizing effect such that he repeated over and over again essentially the same aggressive and defensive reactions whenever similar demands for passive compliance occurred during his subsequent convalescence.

If the above inferences are correct, it could be said that the patient's denial defense was "pathogenic" in that his lack of psychological preparation fostered the development of postoperative disturbances. One or two dramatic incidents of unanticipated suffering and restraint seemed to be sufficient to produce a generalized emotional disturbance in the form of persistent hostility and phobic avoidance reactions directed toward the people who were trying to help him.

Pathogenic Features of Denial Defenses

Further indications of the adverse consequences of denial defenses are provided by the following case material from a well-educated female patient who gave an exceptionally detailed account of the thought sequences and fantasies that were aroused by her surgical experiences. This case study provides another illuminating glimpse of the inner processes that are set into motion when, at a moment of great crisis, a person's reassuring beliefs in blanket immunity are suddenly at marked variance with the reality situation. The case material bearing on the sensitizing episodes is particularly valuable because it shows how the lack of realistic information and the failure to engage in anticipatory mental rehearsal of the danger situation can augment the tendency to blame the danger-control authorities on occasions when unexpected danger or deprivation occurs.

INTERVIEW CASE L–3

Mrs. B., a 25-year-old social worker, was hospitalized at a time when she was completing her Master thesis for a degree in psychiatric social work. She reported experiencing no worry or fear about the operation (appendectomy) beforehand. There was only one thing about which she admitted feeling slightly concerned, namely, the amount of time she would lose in being unable to work on her thesis. As far as the operation itself was concerned, her general attitude was, "there is really nothing to it." On the morning of the operation she was aware of a slight feeling of tension, but she experienced fear for the first time when she was inside the operating room and suddenly "realized that the operation was real." In this crisis situation she began having some difficulty in reassuring herself that there would be nothing to it. Lying flat on her back, perceiving the surgeons and nurses getting ready, her first thought was, "Is this really me who is going to have the operation?" But this momentary feeling of depersonalization soon gave way to the full appreciation of the fact that a surgical operation on her body was about to begin. At this point, according to the patient's postoperative account:

> . . . I began to feel very bitter and irritable. . . . Little things ordinarily never bother me but there, lying in that room, hostility was ready to crop out at any time. I felt the things they were doing were stupid, and ridiculous, but I tried not to show I was disgusted. Ordinarily I never have that sort of reaction. . . .

The mounting feeling of distrust and hostility appears to have been a direct reaction to the inescapable awareness that a "real" operation can entail some real danger to her body. The patient described her feelings of personal vulnerability in the following explicit terms:

> One of the most unpleasant experiences I ever had was lying there on the table just before the operation began. I still don't like to think about it. I felt all exposed, without clothes on, not knowing what's going on. I just felt vulnerable. I had never visualized myself in that situation. The lights, too, made me feel more vulnerable—lying there all lighted up. . . . I don't know exactly what I felt vulnerable to. I had no specific ideas; I just felt a vague idea of being vulnerable. The feeling applied to the nurses as well as the doctors, particularly the surgeon. I felt he could be sadistic if he wanted to. . . . I guess I was afraid he might do a hysterectomy. I had heard of unnecessary operations on women, and there are a lot of stories about surgeons being sadistic. . . . I didn't think there was a real chance of these things happening. It was a vague fear that they could do anything they wanted on the operating table.

Here we see rather clearly one of the subjective states which mediate emotional disturbances when danger is actually encountered. The irritability and hostility she experienced appear to be a direct consequence of the fact that, for the first time since the operation had been scheduled, she could not maintain her belief in complete personal invulnerability. Having developed no other means of reassuring herself about the danger, she suddenly felt helpless when confronted with the inescapable signs that the surgeon, assisted by the nurses, would drug her and cut open her abdomen. Her feelings of helplessness were immediately followed not only by fearful vigilance but also by the attribution of hostile intentions to those responsible for carrying out the operation. In this situation, the tendency to project sadistic intentions was so strong that she could not even dispel the irrational fantasy, which she knew to be absurd, that the surgeon might destroy her sex organs.

The patient experienced similar subjective reactions during the postoperative period, when she was again confronted with the unexpected physical impact of the appendectomy.

> I guess I had thought that when I came out of the operating room everything would be all over and I'd be recovered from my sickness. I never realized I'd be sick afterwards; I never really had any conception of what the postoperative situation would be like. I had thought about what would happen only up to the operation itself and never thought at all about what would happen after it, except to think of myself as being completely well afterwards. I know that's ridiculous but that's the way I felt. . . . I had been told "there's nothing to it," and I believed that. I was shocked when I discovered there was something to it: When I woke up I was sick—it was the sickest I ever was in my whole life. When the incision began hurting; when I peeked at myself and saw mercurochrome all over my body; later on, when I had trouble walking; when they made a big fuss about the bedpan . . . when all these things happened I began thinking, "What is there about this operation, *what have they done inside me* if it's supposed to cause all this trouble?"

In this case, the patient's sudden realization of personal vulnerability emerges as a crucial reaction which appears to mediate the development of hostile attitudes toward the hospital staff. Prior to the psychological crisis she experienced in the operating room, her image of the operation had been restricted to the compensatory gains she anticipated:

> I would be all better, back to normal and enjoy life again; I regarded the operation as standing between the way I was dragging myself around and a normal life, so my only thought was that I wanted to have the operation.

Although she knew intellectually that undergoing an operation could entail some physical danger and actual suffering, the patient never consciously thought of these unpleasant aspects of the operation as applying to her. The patient appears to have avoided seeking any information about the disturbing features of the operation, and was content to reassure herself with a sense of blanket immunity which was, in effect, a total denial of personal vulnerability. As the patient herself described it:

> I couldn't really imagine myself as having the operation during the weeks before it. I really did believe I'd have it, but, at times when I couldn't avoid thinking about it, the idea would occur that *it didn't apply to me*.

It is this form of inadequate preparation for the operation that provides a basis for explaining her exaggerated reactions to the actual signs of danger. In the operating room, when it could no longer be denied that it was her body that the surgeon was about to cut open, the patient could not maintain the sense of personal vulnerability she had previously built up. After an initial attempt at denial via a fleeting sense of depersonalization (expressed by the thought "Is this really me?"), the patient was faced with the full-blown realization that she was actually in a danger situation. The sudden shattering of her blanket immunity concept apparently gave rise to a profound sense of helplessness, which she described as a feeling of being "all exposed" and "vulnerable." It was at this point that she began to exaggerate the magnitude of the danger by attributing sadistic intentions to the person responsible for performing the operation.

During the postoperative period, as we have seen, she again experienced the same sequence of subjective events: An emotional "shock" when confronted with unpleasant sequelae of the operation accompanied by the sharp realization that "there really is something [dangerous] to the operation and it is now happening to me"; then, exaggerated concern about the threat to body integrity coupled with attribution of blame to the hospital staff ("What have they done inside me?").

As a product of the disturbing episodes, this patient, like the preceding case, developed a sustained attitude of distrust, wariness, and resentment toward the danger-control authorities. Thus, in each case, the occurrence of one or two unanticipated distressing episodes on the day of the operation seemed to have a markedly sensitizing effect which interfered with the patient's adjustment throughout the entire convalescent period.

Attitude Changes Produced by Traumatizing Events

Implicit in the interpretive comments made throughout this chapter is a major theoretical assumption concerning the dynamics of stress behavior which must be added to those already formulated. The assumption is that a person's capacity to assimilate a stressful event without developing residual emotional disturbances depends upon the degree to which he has mentally rehearsed the danger situation in advance and has worked out reassuring concepts which can function effectively to counteract feelings of helplessness. According to this assumption, any given set of frightening events (such as those encountered by the average surgical patient when in the operating room and after awakening from the anesthetic) will be likely to give rise to emotional disturbances if the person has not gone through the process of preparing himself beforehand with effective reassurances with which to control his fear at times when perceptible danger is at hand. The episodes of stress impact may be momentarily frightening, but if the person is psychologically prepared, he is less inclined to develop a residual hypersensitivity to the cues present in the danger situation. Moreover, he is less likely to interpret the behavior of danger-control authorities as punitive, negligent, or sadistic if he has correctly anticipated beforehand the occurrence of pain, discomfort, and the authorities' demands for passive submission to body manipulation.

The very same external stimulus situations, however, will tend to have a sensitizing effect if the person is unprepared. The most extreme forms of sensitizing danger episodes can be regarded as potentially "traumatic" in so far as they are capable of evoking characteristic symptoms of acute traumatic neurosis—irritability, affect spells, sleep disturbances, and constriction of ego functions (Fenichel, 1945, pp. 117–121).

In their theoretical comments about war neurosis, Kardiner and H. Spiegel have singled out as the crucial effect of traumatic events a change in the person's basic attitudes toward himself and toward those persons or groups from whom he had expected aid:

> It is most important to bear in mind that the actual situation in battle is dangerous, without any symbolic elaborations which the individual soldier may make as a result of his own personality makeup. Therefore the condition of fear—fear of injury, capture, loss of intactness—is a normal phenomenon . . . It is the normal affect, and it can exercise a tonic and bracing influence. This normal fear can act in this beneficent way only as long as the relatedness of the individual to his group is vigorous and carries with it the guarantee of mutual aid and cooperation, only as long as this fear is directed toward the external danger. But as soon as the fear is directed inward, in the form of questioning the individual's resources to cope with the external danger, or toward the group, in the form of questioning its ability to be a protective extension of the individual, then a new and more serious danger situation is created for the soldier. This is the matrix in which germinate the seeds of the traumatic reaction.
>
> . . . The accompanying signs of an actual diminution of resources are the symptoms of the break with the group. No other interpretation can be made of the lowering of discipline, the increasing selfishness, the rudeness, explosiveness, and profanity which accompany the irritability and the gradual loss of confident orientation toward the external danger. (Kardiner and H. Spiegel, 1947, pp. 73–74.)

According to the theoretical inferences stated by these authors, the attitude changes which mediate the sensitization effects of traumatic war experiences consist of a profound loss of self-confidence combined with generalized demoralization resulting from loss of confidence in protective persons with whom one is affiliated. For the soldier in combat, the persons upon whom he counts for protection are the group leaders and the other members of his combat unit, all of whom are capable of mutually supporting each other in facing the same danger situation. For the civilian who is exposed to a more personal danger situation, there may be no such group, but usually there are other persons who play an equivalent role as protective, supporting figures. In an earlier chapter, an account has already been given of the surgical patient's increase in affiliative needs, directed toward members of the immediate family and toward the surgeon, which parallels the heightened sense of cohesiveness which the individual soldier develops toward his combat group. (See discussion of Hypothesis 5, pp. 90–93.)

It seems plausible to assume that the attitude changes described by Kardiner and H. Spiegel in cases of war neurosis also underlie the symptoms of traumatic neurosis evoked by peacetime disasters, individual accidents, surgical experiences, and other exposures to frightening stimuli. The case study evidence presented in this chapter suggests that essentially the same types of attitude changes occur even when the sensitization effects produced by disturbing events are not as incapacitating as in the cases of acute traumatic neuroses referred to by Kardiner and Spiegel. Many of the sensitization effects which are exemplified in the surgical case study series can be regarded as instances of what are sometimes called "transient" or "mild" forms of traumatic neurosis (Maslow and Mittleman, 1946). In these instances, there is no single event which is so overwhelmingly traumatizing as to induce an incapacitating neurotic breakdown. Rather, the discrete sensitizing episodes which occur while the patient is in the operating room and during the postoperative period may have only very limited pathogenic consequences. Most often, the dominant consequence seems to be a corroding effect on the person's adjustive capabilities which augments the impact of accumulated stresses. With this consideration in mind, the term "sensitizing episode" has been introduced as a generic concept to refer to the entire class of potentially disruptive experiences, ranging from those which have only a mild corroding effect to those which constitute the most harrowing instances of psychological trauma.

In summary, the observations and interpretations discussed in this chapter suggest that a relative absence of anticipatory fear is pathogenic in that the individual fails to build up effective psychological defenses in advance and, therefore, finds it difficult to ward off feelings of helplessness when the danger actually materializes. Such a failure can give rise to sustained sensitization effects because of basic attitude changes consisting of a loss of self-confidence combined with distrust and resentment toward others from whom he could expect to have protective support.

Notes

1. Anticipations of compensatory gains may sometimes be the product of a reactivation of unconscious fantasies which had originally developed as a substitute for forbidden gratifications. In the psychoanalytic case study of Mrs. Blake, it was found that many of her preoperative fantasies were centered upon unconscious wishes for infantile satisfactions, and that she was consciously looking forward to being treated indulgently, "like a baby." (See pp. 66–67.) In several psychoanalytic sessions when Mrs. Blake expressed concern about her leg being cut by the surgeon, she displayed signs of the reactivation of a latent wish to undergo a change of sex; in other sessions, when threats of being rendered weak and helpless were in the foreground, her latent fantasies were centered upon receiving the gratification of an infant being held at its mother's breast. The general formula suggested by such instances seems to be: "Since I am now going to be given a drastic punishment, I should be allowed to do the desirable things that the threat of the punishment has always prevented me from doing." This conjectural formula seems to fit some of the interview data obtained from the series of surgical ward patients. Especially among those in the low fear group, derivatives of various unconscious wishes seem to occur in their statements about anticipated surgical experiences; e.g., the statements quoted from Case L–3 (pp. 346–347) suggest latent fantasies of exhibitionism and rape. If such unconscious gratifications are anticipated before the operation, postoperative reactions of resentment toward the danger-control authorities may be partly attributable to the patient's disappointment that the hoped-for gratifications are not obtained.

25.

Psychological preparation

The theoretical concepts and hypotheses which have evolved from the material presented in the preceding chapters have a number of important implications for the role of warnings, information about impending events, and other types of communications which can influence the adequacy of a person's psychological preparation for stressful life experiences. The case study evidence, as we have seen, suggests that the arousal of some degree of anticipatory fear may be one of the necessary conditions for developing inner defenses of the type that can function effectively when the external dangers materialize. In many of the individual case studies we have examined, the patient had received very little information about the suffering that he would undergo and, in some cases, this lack of information seems to have been a major factor in determining the relative absence of anticipatory fear. One surmises that most people ignore problematical dangers of the future unless they receive specific warnings or predictions from respected authorities. The unpleasant task of mental rehearsal, which appears to be essential for developing effective danger-contingent reassurances, is apt to be shirked, even when a person knows that he is going to be exposed to some form of suffering or deprivation.

If a person is given appropriate preparatory communications before being exposed to potentially traumatizing stimuli, his chances of behaving in a disorganized way and of suffering from prolonged sensitization effects may be greatly decreased. Thus, from the standpoint of preventive psychiatry, it is of considerable importance to determine how preparatory communications can be made to serve an effective prophylactic function. The practical problems of developing emotional inoculation techniques will require for their solution many empirically tested generalizations and also a better set of theoretical concepts than has been developed so far for predicting the consequences of using different types of preparatory communications.

In this chapter an attempt is made to give at least some tentative answers to a number of basic theoretical questions concerning the effects of preparatory communications. The questions are formulated in terms of reactions to the stresses of surgery, concerning which we have some pertinent observations to examine; but the answers may prove to be applicable to a wide range of danger and disaster situations. In what ways, if any, are the postoperative emotional reactions of surgical patients influenced by the information they receive before the operation? What types of information, predictions, persuasive appeals, and recommendations are most effective in facilitating adequate psychological preparation? Under what conditions are preparatory communications likely to have unfavorable effects or fail to dampen the emotional impact of potentially traumatizing events?

First we shall examine evidence from the survey research which points to some of the adverse behavioral consequences of insufficient authoritative information concerning the unpleasant features of surgery. Correlational findings will be presented in which informed and uninformed surgical cases are compared with respect to their preoperative emotional reactions and their postoperative adjustment. Then a number of specific incidents culled from the intensive case studies will be examined to gain a somewhat better understanding of what happens when the preparatory information given by a danger-control authority subsequently turns out to have been incomplete or misleading. Finally, an attempt will be made to give a general theoretical orientation, centered upon a unifying construct ("the work of worrying"), which seems to be useful for integrating all the various observations bearing on psychological preparation reported in this and foregoing chapters. The theoretical discussion will concentrate on what appear to be the major psychological factors which determine whether or not preparatory communications will be successful or unsuccessful in creating some degree of emotional inoculation.

Survey Results: Comparison of Informed Versus Uninformed Patients

The survey questionnaire given to male college students included the following three questions which were designed to determine the amount and adequacy of the preparatory information received by each surgical patient:

QUESTION N: *Before the operation or treatment was started*, did your doctor or one of his assistants tell you about possible unpleasant experiences that you might have during or immediately after the operation or treatment?

____ Was told absolutely nothing about unpleasant experiences.
____ Was told very little.
____ Was told a moderate amount.
____ Was told a great deal.

QUESTION O: Think over in your mind the various unpleasant events that actually did occur during and immediately following your operation or treatment. How many of those unpleasant things had you been told about beforehand by your doctor or by one of his assistants?

____ Was told beforehand about *practically all* of the unpleasant things that actually did occur.
____ Was told beforehand about *most* of the unpleasant things that actually did occur.
____ Was told beforehand about *a few* of the unpleasant things that actually did occur.
____ Was told beforehand about *practically none* of the unpleasant things that actually did occur.

QUESTION P: Before the operation or treatment was started, did your doctor or one of his assistants tell you that it would probably cause some pain?

____ Was *not told anything* at all about pain.
____ Was told that there would probably be *no pain at all.*
____ Was told that there would probably be a *slight amount of pain.*
____ Was told that there would probably be a *moderate amount of pain.*
____ Was told that there would probably be a *considerable amount of pain.*

There were 77 major surgery cases who answered all three questions and these were sorted into the following two groups:[1]

1. *Uninformed* patients: Twenty-six cases consistently reported in their answers to all three questions that they had received *no authorita-*

tive information in advance concerning negative aspects of the operation; i.e., their physicians: (*a*) told them *absolutely nothing* about unpleasant experiences; (*b*) told them beforehand about *practically none* of the unpleasant things that actually did occur (during or immediately following the operation); and (*c*) did not tell them *anything at all* about pain (or else told them that there would probably be *no pain at all*).

2. *Informed* patients: Fifty-one cases reported having received at least a slight amount of authoritative information in advance concerning negative features of the operation. The majority of these cases (65%) reported that they were told about *most* or *practically all* of the unpleasant things that actually did occur.

Background Factors

Before examining the results bearing on the emotional reactions of the informed and uninformed groups, it is important to consider whether there were any differences between the two groups in severity of stress or in other background factors which might give rise to spurious results. There were 9 questions on severity of stress in the questionnaire (see pp. 280–283); analysis of the answers showed that there were no large or significant group differences on any of them. For example, on a type of anesthetic, almost the same percentage of the informed and uninformed groups reported having a general anesthetic (55% versus 54%), and a spinal anesthetic (18% versus 15%); the remainder of each group (27% versus 31%) reported having a local anesthetic. Similarly, there were only very small differences in the percentage who reported having undergone an appendectomy (39% versus 35%), surgical removal of a tumor (22% versus 31%), ENT surgery (21% versus 15%), and miscellaneous other surgical procedures (18% versus 19%). Moreover, the two groups proved to be well matched on a variety of other indicators of severity of stress (see page 391 below) and on temporal and contextual factors such as: (*a*) length of time since the operation took place; (*b*) the time interval between being informed that the operation was necessary and being taken to the operating room; and (*c*) type of hospital in which the operation was performed. The absence of any differences on background factors increases the degree of confidence that can be placed in the correlational findings derived from comparing the emotional reactions of the informed group with the uninformed group.

Relationship Between Information and Preoperative Fear

The first main question is whether the level of anticipatory fear is a function of differences in preparatory information. Does the informed group show a higher level of preoperative fear than the uninformed group? The pertinent results are shown in Chart 6 for the three main questions concerning preoperative fear reactions. (The exact wording

Chart 6. Comparison of the Informed and Uninformed Groups on Level of Preoperative Fear*

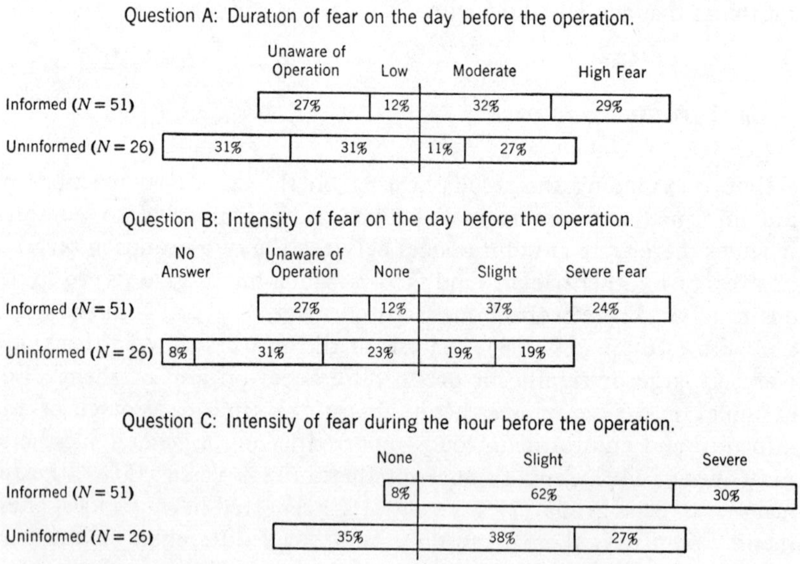

* The data are based on the sample of all major surgery cases.

of the fear questions is given on pp. 277–278.) For each of the three questions, there is a large and significant difference in the expected direction ($p > .05$).[2] These results, therefore, increase the plausibility of the assumption that when people know that they are going to be exposed to approaching danger or deprivation, the tendency to ward off anticipatory fear (e.g., by denying the magnitude of the danger) can be significantly influenced by authoritative information about the unpleasant aspects of the impending stressful events.

It is noteworthy that for all three questions in Chart 6, the incidence of high preoperative fear is about the same for the informed and uninformed groups, with the large differences occurring only in the moderate and low fear categories. This finding is compatible with the hypothesis that the patients with high anticipatory fear are mainly those who are psychoneurotically disposed to overreact to external threats and who remain relatively unaffected by authoritative communications. (See Hypothesis 7, page 201.) For such persons, the mere awareness that they are going to have a surgical operation is presumably sufficient to stir up repressed fears of body damage, abandonment, or annihilation. Thus, their exaggerated anticipatory reactions would tend to occur whether or not they are given some fear-arousing information about the nature of the danger. Among patients with very low anticipatory fear, on the other hand, there is assumed to be a sizeable number of persons capable of being responsive to preoperative information. When given unequivocal information about the threat, the effectiveness of such a person's denial defenses will be reduced and, consequently, he will display a rise in anticipatory fear. Thus, although preoperative information may bear little or no relationship to the occurrence of high anticipatory fear, it seems to make a sizeable difference as to whether a person will experience a moderate degree of anticipatory fear or practically none.[3]

Relationship Between Preoperative Information and Postoperative Emotional Disturbance

In view of the relationship between preoperative information and anticipatory fear described in the preceding section, it seems plausible to expect that *poor preparation* in the form of insufficient or inadequate information from the medical authorities is a major determinant of the unfavorable behavioral sequelae of low preoperative fear. If this expectation is correct, we should find that there are marked differences between the informed and uninformed groups in the occurrence of postoperative emotional disturbances and, moreover, the differences should closely parallel those for the low versus moderate fear groups, as described in Chapters 21 and 22. In order to investigate these predictions, the informed group was compared with the uninformed group on the three objective items dealing with postoperative reactions. (See Chart 7.) These items were the three objective questions which, according to the results in Chapter 22, yielded differences in the expected direction between the low and moderate fear groups.[4] The specific measures were as follows:

QUESTION F: Percentage reporting that they felt disturbed at the present time when thinking about the operation (see p. 289).

QUESTION H: Percentage responding "very angry" or "extremely angry" when asked whether they had felt angry or annoyed on the day of their operation (see p. 292).

QUESTION K: Percentage reporting only an intermediate or low degree of confidence in the surgeon at the present time (see p. 300).

Chart 7. Comparison of Informed with Uninformed Groups on Three Measures of Postoperative Adjustment

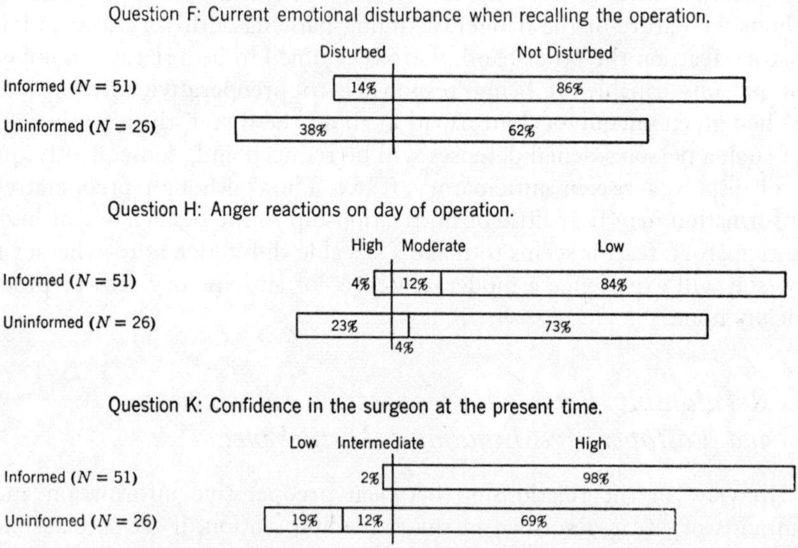

The results in Chart 7 show the comparisons between the informed and the uninformed groups on the three criteria measures. For each measure the difference is significant at beyond the 5% level. (Probability values were computed for two-by-two tables, with each dichotomization based on the cut-point shown by the dividing line in the chart.) The findings bear out the predictions derived from the assumption that the occurrence of acute emotional disturbances during exposure to stressful circumstances depends partly upon whether or not the person has been exposed to preparatory information beforehand. If we are willing to accept the surgical patients' retrospective reports as valid evidence, it appears that those who were told practically nothing about the unpleasant aspects of the operation beforehand were more inclined than the others to display intense anger reactions on the day of the operation, to develop unfavorable attitudes toward the surgeon, and to experience sustained emotional disturbances.

As an addendum to the quantitative data in Chart 7, the fact should be mentioned that the write-in answers by a few men in the uninformed group contain some explicit complaints about inadequate information, along with resentful condemnations of the medical authorities for having misled them. For example, one man in the uninformed group gave the following explanation for his anger reactions:

> I was so mad at the doctor after the operation and after the anesthetic wore off, I couldn't say anything except a few choice bits of profanity in a low voice. . . . I was annoyed at the pain I experienced which *he led me to believe would be small.* After the anesthetic, I was never given a sedative and the pain was extreme and continued for days. . . . Now I know what to expect at the hands of an amateur.

Implications of the Survey Results

To obtain clear-cut evidence for testing the behavioral consequences of psychological preparation, it would be necessary to procure data from controlled experiments in which postoperative comparisons are made between one group of patients who have been given certain types of preparatory communications and an equivalent group of control cases who have not. Unfortunately, there are many special problems involved in conducting research with patients on surgical wards which make it difficult to carry out systematic experiments of this kind in sufficiently controlled fashion as to yield unambiguous findings.[5]

A number of experimental and quasi-experimental studies have been reported by several different investigators, especially concerning psychological preparation of children for surgery (Jackson et al., 1953; Prugh et al., 1953; Winkley, 1953). The results of these studies suggest that when children are given accurate information along with various reassurances, they are less likely to become emotionally disturbed during the postoperative period. However, the effects of the various preparatory communications used in these experiments are confounded with the effects of a variety of other variables which were also included in the same experimental programs. For example, in these studies one cannot tell whether the beneficial effects found in the experimental group were entirely due to noncommunication factors, such as the fact that the mother was allowed to remain in the child's room throughout the hospitalization period. Consequently, up to the present time, no clear-cut experimental evidence is available concerning the influence of preparatory communications on the reactions of children or adults to surgical experiences.

Correlational findings, such as those presented in Chart 7, do not permit one to draw any dependable conclusions about a causal sequence. The evidence can nevertheless be characterized as giving tentative support to hypotheses derived from the theoretical analysis presented in earlier chapters, which attributes a causal role to preparatory information. The main assumptions pertain to the ways in which authoritative statements about an impending danger situation can counteract pathogenic defenses against anticipatory fear. The dominant tendency of most persons is assumed to be that of denying problematical dangers; they attempt to bolster their sense of personal invulnerability by developing blanket immunity expectations and, thus, almost completely ward off anticipatory fear (see Hypotheses 3 and 4, pp. 198–200). Once anticipatory fear is stimulated by an authoritative communication, however, the attitudes and the defences against fear adopted by these same persons may be markedly changed. They can no longer avoid thinking about what might happen to them and, as they mentally rehearse the potential dangers, they gradually build up a new set of partial immunity reassurances which take account of specific features of the danger situation. This new set of reassurances is assumed to have a much better chance of remaining effective in the actual danger situation than the blanket immunity defenses.

Case Study Observations: Consequences of Inadequate Preparation

The case study material obtained from intensive interviews and from behavioral records of the hospitalized surgical patients helps to elucidate some of the implications of the theory of psychological preparation. In the following discussion we shall take account of some hitherto unreported case study data, and we shall also re-examine some case material from patients whose behavior has already been described. This will be done for the purpose of indicating how preparatory communications might help people to develop effective psychological resistances for withstanding external stress.

From the case summaries presented in Chapters 21 and 24, it is apparent that, at the time of their preoperative interviews, the patients who displayed low anticipatory fear were generally uninformed about the unpleasant experiences that were in store for them. We have seen, further, that their comments in the postoperative interviews suggest that subsequently, when unexpected stress episodes occurred, they tended to be much more surprised, disappointed, and aggrieved than patients who had displayed a moderate degree of fear. In the present discussion, the reactions of the latter group are of major interest. The earlier chapters have already presented and discussed a large number of examples of the apparent consequences of the inadequate preparation of the low fear group. What is especially noteworthy here is that a similar lack of psychological preparation seems to be at the root of the isolated episodes of postoperative emotional upset which occasionally occurred among those patients who had experienced a moderate level of anticipatory fear. The implications of this assertion will become clear after we look at some illustrative case material from patients in the moderate fear group.

INTERVIEW CASE M–1

Mrs. C., a 29-year-old housewife, was exceptionally well prepared for her operation (lung lobectomy) inasmuch as she had already been through the same operation a year earlier. Before the operation she felt "a little nervous" from time to time because of the chest pains and the distressing postoperative procedures she knew were in store for her. Mrs. C. was also somewhat worried that there "might not be enough lung left for breathing during the operation," but her fears subsided after discussing the question with her physician, who made some reassuring comments. She felt that since her surgeon recommended the operation, she wanted to have it as soon as possible, despite the unpleasantness and the risks involved.

When reinterviewed on the sixth postoperative day, this patient was extremely optimistic about her recovery and expressed unequivocally favorable attitudes toward the hospital staff. Mrs. C. reported that she had experienced acute pain for four days following the operation, but she felt able to "take" it better than the earlier surgical experience:

> I think I had less pain than after my first operation, but maybe it was because I was expecting pain this time and for the first one I didn't know what to expect. For that first one I asked for hypos all the time, but this time I didn't ask for a hypo once, even though I had a lot of pain.

Although the patient was able to tolerate quite well most of the major unpleasant experiences, there were several unexpected events which had a markedly disruptive effect, evoking considerable agitation and even some momentary resistance to the demands of the medical authorities. The first unexpected episode took place as she was awakening from the anesthetic. The situation was quite different from what she had experienced after her last operation, and she felt that something must have gone wrong:

> As soon as I came out of the anesthetic, I realized that there was something different from last time. That upset me because I hadn't expected it

to be like that. . . . I was sick to my stomach and realized I must have had gas or ether, and also I was having a drain in me and I didn't know they were going to give that to me after the pentathol. It upset me because they hadn't told me anything about it. I thought: "Gee, I'm sicker than last time. I wonder why. After the last operation I didn't feel this way." Then I thought to myself, "I wonder why they didn't tell me I'd have a drain in me." Then I thought, "Maybe they just figured I'd get upset if I knew I was going to have a drain in me." I had enough confidence in them to feel they knew what they were doing. Once I realized that it was a drain there, I felt it must be necessary. But I was also sort of scared at that time by the fact that they left me in the recovery room. I was kept in the recovery room overnight—I thought maybe my case was especially bad because I was not taken back to my own room. I though to myself, "I must be awful sick if they're keeping me there." At first I didn't know where I was—but then I felt it was nice and quiet and the nurses were all treating me well, and so I felt it was O.K. Then I quieted down and just accepted it.

Something wholly unexpected and even more disturbing occurred on the following day. A physician came to Mrs. C.'s room, carrying a drainage tube and asked her to open her mouth. In contrast to her usual passive acceptance of medical procedures, she felt extremely antagonistic on this one occasion. She had never been asked to swallow a drainage tube before, did not know what the procedure was like, and was so surprised that she assumed the strange staff physician must have made a mistake and had come to the wrong room. After being informed that there was no mistake, she begged the physician to let her alone. Under his insistent pressure, she tried to swallow the tube but for about ten minutes was unable to get herself to relax sufficiently.

I knew if I could relax it would help, and I tried not to resist. But I didn't have any confidence in the doctor and I wanted somebody else to come instead of him keeping on trying while I was feeling sicker and sicker. The poor fellow, he knows that I asked for another doctor, and when the doctor came I got the tube down right away. That first doctor practically killed me, he did it so badly. Maybe that's the way you look at it when you are sick. I was in pain but I had expected that. This thing was so awful because I hadn't expected it and I thought something must have gone wrong. I know the things they do here are for my own good. That's why I try hard to cooperate. But I couldn't that time. I think it took as much out of him as out of me.

One cannot be sure how much of the problem stemmed from ineptness on the part of the physician, but it seems quite probable that the psychological factor of surprise contributed greatly to the patient's agitation. During this brief postoperative episode, she was obviously unable to dispel unfavorable thoughts about the physician and could not allow herself to give in to his demands. At no other time during her long and painful convalescence did Mrs. C. display any such overt resistance or express any such doubts about the competence of anyone on the staff.

A number of other patients in the moderate fear group also showed isolated instances of momentary agitation in response to unexpected stressful events. Like Mrs. C., some patients developed a paniclike apprehensiveness that something might have gone wrong when, in a somewhat dazed state after awakening from the anesthetic, they found themselves undergoing pain or bodily confinement which they had not known about in advance. Such unexpected experiences, even in patients who are relatively well prepared for their surgical experiences, seem to exert a demoralizing influence and place a strain on the patient's adjustive capacities.

INTERVIEW CASE M–9

Another clear-cut example of the way in which unexpected suffering is apt to be misinterpreted occurs in the material from Case M–9. This 42-year-old man was relatively free from emotional disturbance during the entire postoperative recovery period, except for a brief period immediately following his chest operation (thoracoplasty). Upon awakening, he felt sharp, piercing pains in his chest which were much worse than any he had ever experienced before. He became extremely frightened because he thought that the operation had failed and "there was some new illness inside of me there." His agitation continued for several hours, but he calmed down immediately after a staff physician told him that he was experiencing the usual postoperative symptoms caused by unavoidable nerve injury. It seems probable that the magnitude of his emotional disturbance during the first postoperative hours could have been markedy lessened had he been given some preoperative information about the piercing chest pains.

Additional instances of the same type were encountered among other patients in the moderate fear group when the case summaries were presented in Chapter 23, but these instances were mentioned only as exceptions to the patients' general way of reacting. We saw that Case M–2, who almost always behaved like a "model" patient from the hospital's standpoint, became momentarily distressed on the first postoperative day when she was unexpectedly given a tube feeding (see pp. 316–317). Case M–4 developed a paniclike reaction on the operating table when she experienced an unexpected jab of pain in her chest after the spinal anesthetic; she thought she might be having a heart attack. The same patient also was very disturbed on her third postoperative night when a new surgical patient, who was brought into her room, began breathing in a loud and uncanny manner (endotrachial aspiration).

The unusual gasping noises made by the new patient shocked and frightened this woman to such a degree that she was "upset" all night and was unable to fall asleep, although ordinarily she slept quite well.

The last example illustrates the fact that the unexpected events which can have a shocking effect are not always a matter of experiencing pain and suffering but may involve the perception of suffering in others. Weird and unfamiliar medical phenomena sometimes evoke acute fright reactions, which, like those elicited by unexpected physical suffering, might be much less severe if the patient were given sufficient information to enable him to work through the distressing occurrences before they materialize. When a patient is wholly unprepared for what is usually seen and heard on a surgery ward, the perception of mutilation and agony in other people seems to be capable of producing acute emotional shock, sometimes rudely disrupting the individual's sense of personal invulnerability at a time when he is struggling to maintain his composure. One of the most serious consequences of such perceptions is that the person may begin to question the trustworthiness of the medical authorities and, thus, find himself deprived of a major source of reassurance. A temporary reaction of this type is exemplified by the following case material from a female patient in the moderate fear group.

INTERVIEW CASE M–3

Mrs. E., a 26-year-old teacher, was hospitalized for the surgical excision of a cyst on her left breast. After she learned that an operation was necessary, she felt slightly worried but was able to maintain consistently high preoperative morale, up until the time a horrifying perceptual experience occurred. On the day she came to the hospital, Mrs. E. had only a vague feeling of anxiety accompanied by the somewhat melancholy thought, "Everything happens to me!" Nevertheless, she was eager to "get the operation over with," and looked forward to a satisfactory recovery. Her emotional equanimity was rudely shaken, however, as a result of being brought into close contact with a seriously ill patient who had undegone major surgery the night before. There were four beds in the room, and Mrs. E. was in the bed across from the acutely ill patient. There was also another woman in the bed next to Mrs. E. who was very talkative and who volunteered the information that the sick lady was a cancer patient in a very critical condition. This information had a powerful effect on Mrs. E., and heightened the disturbing impressions created by witnessing the cancer patient's suffering and the obvious signs of physical crisis.

> The woman who had just been operated on looked so terribly ill, lying there at the foot of my bed. And she had visitors who were crying, so it was a very pathetic sight to see, especially knowing how serious her condition was. . . .

For about half an hour Mrs. E. lay in her bed awaiting her own operation, but she was unable to get her mind off the terrible implications of the ordeal going on in the other bed. She began to feel increasingly concerned about the possibility that the same fate might be in store for her. After all, the surgeon might find that the cyst really turned out to be a breast tumor or, perhaps, he already knew that it was a tumor. The talkative neighbor had mentioned that the cancer victim was told nothing about her malignancy. For the first time, Mrs. E. began to wonder if her own surgeon might also be withholding something.

> I began wondering if they told me the truth because they didn't tell this patient about her tumor. The more I thought about it, the more nervous and upset I became. . . . When my husband came up to my room I asked him if the doctor told him anything he didn't tell me. I had the possibility of a tumor in mind. . . . My husband smiled, and I thought that might confirm my suspicion. Then my husband explained he didn't know anything more than I did. I wasn't really satisfied, but I more or less accepted it. I kept telling myself, "I'm going to the operating room anyhow, so what difference does it make?" When the attendants came, I felt delighted to be wheeled out of the room because . . . seeing that woman lying there was contributing to my distraught feelings. . . . The hour I was in that room was really the worst part of my operation experience.

The period of emotional disturbance in the above example lasted only a short time and apparently had no untoward long-run effects. After the operation, Mrs. E. displayed no extreme emotional symptoms nor did she resume her ruminations about the possibility that the surgeon might be withholding information concerning some dire aspects of her medical condition. This case material, nevertheless, serves to illustrate the degree to which an intelligent person's appraisal of his or her own danger situation can be negatively influenced by the perception of the suffering of others. Apparently, under stress conditions, it is easy to indulge in analogical thinking of the type displayed by Mrs. E., and to identify with those who are in agony.

The disturbing events which we have examined so far have been limited to perceptions of overt suffering or deprivation in either oneself or in others with whom one comes in direct contact. But there are also a number of other types of disturbing perceptions which are aroused by vague or indirect signs of *potential* loss. Chief among these signs are unanticipated changes in the appearance of one's body. A number of surgical patients experienced mild but persistent emotional tension as a result of noticing discolored portions of their skin or other superficial somatic changes, even though there was no accompanying discomfort or impairment of function. Unfamiliar self-perceptions which alter a person's body image seem to be capable of evoking ruminating puzzlement and a low level of gnawing apprehensiveness, especially if the person has no information as to how or why the change in the appearance of his body occurred. The following case material illustrates the rather subtle ways in which this minor type of disturbing perception can affect a patient's postoperative adjustment.

INTERVIEW CASE M–5

Mrs. R., a 73-year-old woman, like others in the moderate fear group, had freely expressed some preoperative concerns about the dangerous and unpleasant aspects of her abdominal operation (subtotal gastrectomy). After the operation she was extremely friendly toward the hospital staff and was generally regarded as a highly cooperative convalescent. In the postoperative interview, as might be expected, she expressed very positive attitudes toward the doctors and nurses. However, the interviewer, while hearing her make these comments, had the impression that there was something a bit forced about her effusive praise. After the session was over, just as the interviewer was about to say goodbye, Mrs. R. pointed to a large black-and-blue spot on her arm and somewhat embarrassedly made the following comments:

> Just look at that! I don't know how I could have got that. Looks like I was fighting with Joe Louis or something. I have no idea how I got that; I noticed it after my operation and I've been wondering about it. I don't know of any struggling or anything. I can't think of anything that could have caused it while I was under.

In order to evaluate the possible significance of this comment, it is necessary to consider what it was that had aroused the interviewer's suspicion that the patient was giving a somewhat distorted account of her feelings about the staff. The interview had been filled with an extraordinarily high frequency of positive statements to the effect that both she and the hospital staff had behaved beautifully. Time and again this patient had made rather saccharine comments such as, "The doctors and nurses are certainly lovely"; "I have complete confidence in all of them because they're all so awfully nice"; "The doctors here think I am wonderful because I don't give them any trouble." It seems probable that the inexplicable bruise on her arm tended to evoke some mild distrust of the staff and perhaps also a lowering of self-confidence with respect to her ability to control herself. Evidently, she was able to suppress these unpleasant implications of the unexplained bruise and to behave in exemplary fashion, controlling her emotional impulses and conforming with all medical demands. But one surmises that this inner control was not achieved without exerting some special efforts to reassure herself repeatedly that there was nothing but mutually high regard between herself and the doctors. One wonders whether she would have found it so easy to set aside the unwelcome thoughts about her unaccountable bruise if a few more such unexplained events had occurred.

Degree of Tolerance for Disturbing Perceptions

Every surgical patient undoubtedly encounters many puzzling and potentially threatening occurrences similar to those described in the preceding illustrations. Quite aside from the physical pains and discomforts, which may at first be the major source of emotional tension, there are a host of other events—including unfamiliar organic sensations, restrictions of body functions, and enforced hygienic routines—many of which are quite ambiguous, but in one way or another convey that "all is not going well with me." These ambiguous perceptions are likely to place a continual strain on the adjustive capacities of each individual. Thus, to be a well-adjusted surgical convalescent, it is necessary, among other things, to be somehow able to maintain a high tolerance for the series of ambiguous and threatening stimuli that occur each day.

From the behavioral evidence in earlier chapters, it can be said that an essential difference between the moderate and low anticipatory fear groups lies in the sphere of stress tolerance. Perhaps one reason for the difference is that the patients with moderate anticipatory fear, having greater motivation to seek information and to mentally rehearse the coming events, are in a better position to ignore a host of potentially distressing perceptions which they are able to explain away as being in the "normal course of events." Witnessing one or two distressing sights of the type which momentarily had upset Mrs. E. and discovering one or two unexpected minor changes in one's body of the type which had puzzled Mrs. R., might be well within the tolerable range for the average person. A *few* such events during the period when the average person is hospitalized for surgery may have little effect on his self-confidence or on his attitudes toward the danger-control authorities and, thus, may create no long-run impairment in morale. But if there is a *large accumulation* of unexpected and unexplicable events, the morale damage may become considerable. Even when the unpleasant surprises are of a rather minor character, such as Mrs. R.'s painless bruise, a high frequency of them may greatly reduce the person's capacity for reassuring himself. After a series of unpleasant, *minor* surprises, each additional *major* instance of unexpected pain or distress may then evoke much more fright and aggrievement because the patient may have already begun to doubt whether he will manage to remain invulnerable to further onslaughts in his present predicament ("Why is everything happening to me?"). At the same time, the numerous unexpected occurrences may lead the patient to question the power and the willingness of the authorities to protect him. Thus, the higher the incidence of minor surprises, the higher the probability of being sensitized or traumatized when the major danger episodes occur.

The pathogenic consequences of warding off anticipatory fear by means of blanket immunity defenses, therefore, are not limited merely to the direct effects of being unprepared to cope with clear-cut danger stimuli but also include the indirect effects of lower tolerance for ambiguous threat stimuli. This theoretical notion carries some specific implications for psychological preparation for stress. In order to be maximally effective, preparatory communications should presumably have the goal of giving as complete a cognitive framework as possible for appraising the potentially frightening and disturbing perceptions that the person might actually experience, so as to prevent the type of surprise and ambiguity that generates unproductive, energy-consuming reactions of hypervigilance. Provided that the material is not presented in a lurid or threatening manner, and is accompanied by impressive reassuring comments, specific forecasts about future stressful experiences can probably influence most persons to engage in an imaginative mental rehearsal of the type that promotes the development of effective danger-contingent reassurances.[6]

On the basis of clinical experience in preparing children for surgical operations, K. Wolf (1957) has suggested that a crucial effect of making correct predictions to the child is that it facilitates the development of favorable attitudes toward authority figures. When the child arrives at the hospital, he finds that everything happens just the way he had been told it would—he is taken to the admission office, then he is seated with his parents in the waiting room, next he is taken up the elevator to his hospital room by a nurse dressed all in white, etc. As these elementary predictions are confirmed, the child begins to feel that the counselor who made the predictions and other authority figures as well, know what is going to happen and can be trusted to take care of him.

This may be one of the ways that favorable contact between the child and a counselor can contribute to the development of a trusting attitude toward the hospital staff in general. In so far as the child regards the doctors and nurses as wise and trustworthy authorities, he will tend to endow them with the protective attributes of "good" parents. (M. Fries, 1946; E. Jackson, 1942, 1945a, 1945b; Pearson, 1951).

Probably a similar attitude develops among adult surgical patients as a consequence of being given correct predictions by a physician or counselor who is a member of the hospital staff. If so, it would be of value to communicate not only the basic information about the unpleasant events that are to be expected but also some predictions about relatively *neutral* and *unimportant* events (e.g., details about the daily hygiene routines). Just as with children, impressive confirmations of the predictions may contribute to a more trusting attitude toward the physician or counselor (and toward the entire group of hospital authorities of which he is a representative). Furthermore, there are other positive effects than can come from giving information which conveys a realistic picture of what postoperative life will be like. First of all, it is somewhat reassuring for a patient to realize that he is at least partially familiar with some features of the strange hospital environment and to have a sense that events are not proceeding in a random, whimsical, or unforeseen fashion ("nothing unusual is happening"). The latter attitude, having been built up by repeated confirmations of a physician's or counselor's predictions, may help the patient to reassure himself on those occasions when an unexpected stressful event occurs. Secondly, when realistic information is given before an operation, it may help to correct the patient's unwarranted or irrational anticipations of compensatory gratifications and, thus, reduce the chances of his becoming disappointed in the authorities for failing to grant him various unobtainable indulgences he had hoped to receive (see page 351). Thirdly, the severity of subsequent frustration may be reduced if the patient, by virtue of the authoritative information he is given about his medical condition, begins to compare himself with other patients who have similar problems. As the patient gets to know others who are suffering from the same illness or who are facing the same operation, he may shift his entire frame of reference for judging "normality," using the additional information he obtains from his interaction with fellow sufferers to evaluate whether his own suffering is greater or less than "normal" (Barker, et al., 1946; Merton and Kitt, 1950).

Probably the most effective preparatory communications would be those which give a detailed factual account of the *outstanding perceptual experiences that are most likely to occur*, concentrating especially on the vague and ambiguous events that are most likely to be misinterpreted. Communications of this type are currently being given, presumably with some success, to prepare pregnant women for the stresses of childbirth (Freedman et al., 1952; Javert and Hardy, 1950). For surgical patients, however, it is much more difficult to predict in advance the outstanding crises that may arise (e.g., unusual organic complications may drastically interfere with the normal course of recovery). Nevertheless, the patient could be told in advance about all those pains, discomforts, and unpleasant treatments which invariably do occur. And then, if unpredictable events were to take place, the patient might be given additional information early enough so that the processes of inner preparation could reduce the shock of surprise. For example, when a surgical incision turns out to be much more extensive or creates more of a cosmetic defect than the surgical staff had originally anticipated, it may be possible to give the patient appropriate information about it during the early phase of the postoperative period, before he makes the shocking discovery himself (see Rosen, 1950). Even for relatively minor complications, such as Mrs. R.'s discolored bruise, the patient can probably be spared some unnecessary emotional tension if information about the unexpected injury is presented and discussed as soon as the patient is capable of engaging in conversation.

Inappropriate Preparatory Information

The foregoing discussion has emphasized the probable advantages of giving detailed preparatory information to surgical patients so that they can anticipate correctly and become emotionally prepared for distressing stimuli which they will subsequently perceive. But this emphasis should not be construed as indicating that there is any special advantage to telling surgical patients about the medical aspects of the operation—details about the surgical procedures that will be carried out while the patient is unconscious, the potential risks from the anesthesia, the unusual complications that occasionally arise, and the factors that make for a poor prognosis. In general, there is probably little or no gain from giving any technical information which is not essential for conveying a realistic picture of what the patient will actually perceive. A small amount of background information about the medical aspects may sometimes have a beneficial effect, but only if it serves to correct a patient's misconceptions or if it subsequently contributes to the patient's understanding that nothing untoward is happening to him.

The available evidence suggests that when a physical crisis occurs, prior familiarity with the fear-arousing stimuli tends to lower the chances of emotional shock. But there are some indications in the case study material that detailed medical knowledge does not necessarily help a patient's postoperative adjustment. On the contrary, he may find it much more difficult to feel reassured if he knows a great deal about the dire complications and potential risks which the surgeon is taking into account.

Too much information about the medical aspects of one's own case can create an attitude of sustained hypervigilance that serves no constructive purpose and that may increase one's sensitivity to adverse events. These negative consequences are suggested by the case study material from a number of well-informed and well-educated surgical patients. The most outstanding example comes from the postoperative interview of the 45-year-old physician who had been hospitalized for the repair of an intervertebral disc (see pp. 242–243). We shall reexamine the material from this patient for the purpose of attempting to gain some leads concerning the essential differences between effective and ineffective preparatory information.

INTERVIEW CASE H–5

Dr. N. was unquestionably the best-informed patient in the entire case study series. As a physician who had treated others for the very same condition from which he was suffering, he knew all about the risks entailed by resorting to surgery. Keenly aware of the suffering and adverse complications that could arise from trying to repair a ruptured disc, he knew that the operation was often unsuccessful. He told the interviewer, "I had sent some patients to the hospital for this operation; none of them got much better, and some got worse." In addition, his discussions with numerous colleagues led him to conclude that there was relatively little scientific knowledge about methods of correcting a ruptured disc.

At the time Dr. N. entered the hospital, the unfavorable aspects of the operation were especially salient because of what he had just been told by a medical colleague he had consulted. The colleague was a friend who also was suffering from the same disorder, and his advice was to avoid surgery at all costs on the grounds that there was too much danger that an operation might transform him from a partial invalid into a total invalid. Other physicians had also told Dr. N. that he was a "damn fool" for subjecting himself to surgery. And yet, he decided to take the gamble, because he could no longer tolerate the excruciating pains which were becoming worse every day.

With all the dire information he had acquired constantly in mind, this patient's anticipatory fears were extremely intense and he hoped for some authoritative reassurance from his surgeon. But, both before and after the operation, he found himself being treated as though he were a slightly indisposed colleague who was a full-fledged collaborator in the medical handling of his case.

> During those days after the operation, I thought that I would be a cripple and I wanted the surgeon to treat me differently than he did. He must have assumed that since I was a physician and knew all about it he could treat me rough. In fact, I got very rough treatment from all the doctors. It seemed to me the surgeon was washing his hands of my case—as if to say: "You know the risks, you're taking them." But what I wanted was the surgeon to be forceful and authoritative. I really felt like a six-year-old child, and I didn't want to be treated differently just because I was a doctor. On the day after the operation, the surgeon came in and said: "Come on you lazy bastard, get up on your feet, you know that's the procedure." I didn't want to get up because I felt that there was no real support for my back after the operation. . . . I was afraid getting up would make me crippled. But under his pressure I did get up.

The fact that the hospital staff gave him practically no reassuring statements was felt by this patient to be a severe deprivation. His need for reassurance reached a sharp peak during the first two postoperative days while he was in a somewhat toxic state from pain-relieving drugs. It was during this period that he began to develop the obsessional idea that he might be permanently crippled by the operation. He made some extraordinary demands for reassurance upon a nurse who, from a rational point of view, was not at all suited to be assigned the role of an authority figure.

> The first two days I was quite toxic from the drugs and I went through real anxiety for the first time in my life. I felt convinced that I would be a cripple from the operation. I was so upset that I became like a baby. I wanted a nurse to hold my hand all the time. There was one particular nurse I had seen the night before the operation, and I knew for a fact that she was green and incompetent. But after the operation I felt completely dependent upon her. I wanted her to reassure me a hundred times that everything would be O.K., even though I must have known that she knew nothing about it.

For more than a week, Dr. N. remained in an acutely agitated state. His excessive concern about being crippled persisted until about the tenth postoperative day, by which time there was clear-cut evidence that his condition was much improved by the operation. Thus, it was only after it was quite apparent that he had completely won the gamble that his attitude changed from pessimism to optimism.

In reviewing the case material bearing on Dr. N.'s attitudes and behavior, one can identify three main factors which appear to have contributed heavily to his high level of anticipatory fear and to his subsequent state of unwarranted postoperative apprehensiveness. First, by virtue of his training and experience as a physician, he knew much more than he needed to know for purposes of being psychologically prepared to face the fear-arousing aspects of his operation. The risk of becoming permanently crippled and the related dangers that worried him were actually of relatively low probability; knowing about them certainly could not be expected to have the same beneficial effect as knowing about the postoperative pains or about the other dependable sequelae of the operation that would be perceptually experienced.

Secondly, whether or not this physician knew too much to begin with, he felt a typical need to be given reassuring statements by the medical authority figures, and this emotional need remained almost completely unsatisfied. From what Dr. N. reported, it appears that all the while he was in the hospital his medical colleagues had no hesitation about reminding him of the risks and the medical problems posed by his condition, but none of them were willing to say anything about the mitigating features or to convey the reassuring side of the picture. Retrospectively, Dr. N. was left with the impression that they either wanted to avoid "corny" sentimentality, or else, they were unwilling to "stick their necks out" in case things did not turn out well. Only one person seemed to have been willing to talk to him in a reassuring way—the inexperienced nurse, who probably was quite unfamiliar with hospital tradition.

A third factor, closely related to the second one, was that the surgeon treated this patient as though he were a collaborator, and, evidently, showed by his behavior that he was unwilling to assume the role of a protective danger-control authority. Dr. N., as we have seen, wanted to enter into the usual patient-doctor relationship. He was deprived of the opportunities for reassurance and emotional support that come from being in daily contact with a strong parental figure whose confident, authoritative demeanor, if not his words, conveys the elementary assurance, "No matter what happens, you can count on me to take good care of you." This type of deprivation, which may sometimes give rise to serious psychological consequences, can be expected to ensue whenever the medical authorities fail to realize that, irrespective of age and training, a sick adult has powerful dependency needs. A sophisticated adult facing the hazards of major surgery is more likely to have the emotional status of "a six-year-old child" than of a mature and judicious professional colleague.

The case material which we have just examined highlights the elementary point that effective psychological preparation for surgery has markedly different objectives and, therefore, requires quite different types of communications than those employed in the technical training of medical and nursing personnel. To be well prepared, a patient needs relatively little of the informational and theoretical background of the scientific expert. Rather, the type of information that makes for successful emotional inoculation is likely to be much more superficial descriptive material which conveys a *concrete, personalized picture of the outstanding danger events as the person will actually perceive them.*

There is the further implication that, if a purely intellectual or didactic approach is used, some of the essential objectives of psychological preparation may not be met. In addition to stimulating a realistic mental rehearsal of the anticipated danger experiences, there are at least two other major objectives which may be essential for adequate psychological preparation: (*a*) to correct erroneous beliefs and anticipations which engender either exaggerated fears or exaggerated expectations of indulgent gratifications; and (*b*) to facilitate the development of reassuring concepts that can continue to function effectively when the crisis comes. As will be seen shortly, these and related considerations have some important implications not only for the thematic content that should be emphasized in preparatory communications but also for the social setting in which the communications should be given. One of the most obvious implications is that pamphlets, formal lectures, films, and other prepackaged messages cannot be counted upon to do the entire job. The give-and-take of direct verbal interaction between the person being prepared and the one doing the preparing is probably an essential condition for overcoming emotional resistances and for meeting the specific emotional needs which often determine the way in which information about an anticipated danger situation is perceived and assimilated.

The Work of Worrying

The observations reported in this chapter, together with those in preceding chapters bearing on the pathogenic consequences of denial reactions, converge on a few basic themes, all of which pertain to the adjustive value of engaging in certain types of mental activity during the precrisis period. The general theoretical implications of these observations, and of related research findings reported by numerous other investigators, have been discussed by the author in a separate essay dealing with psychological preparation for danger (Janis, 1956). In the context of examining the potentially constructive and prophylactic aspects of anticipatory fear, the essay proposes, as a central theoretical construct, that there is a "work of worrying," which, like the "work of mourning," enables a person to adjust more adequately to a painful reality situation. The work of mourning, according to Freud (1917), is stimulated by object loss and, therefore, does not begin until *after* a blow has struck. In contrast, the work of worrying is assumed to begin *before* a blow strikes, as soon as the person becomes convinced that he is facing a genuine threat of potential danger.

In order to specify the functional properties of the work of worrying, it is necessary to delineate what occurs in its absence. What happens when, because of lack of opportunity or inadequate motivation, a person remains unworried about an impending danger experience and fails to undergo any inner preparation before it materializes? At the moment when inescapable signs of danger or actual suffering are encountered, efforts at intellectual denial (by minimizing or discounting the likelihood of being personally affected by the danger) will no longer succeed. . . . The person then suddenly finds himself unable to ward off intense fear or fright (which sometimes is experienced as anger or other affects), especially because he has not developed any means for actively protecting himself from the danger. Moreover, the crisis seems to be augmented by the fact that when more danger or suffering is encountered than had been expected beforehand, feelings of helplessness are likely to occur which drastically interfere with the ego's normal reassurance mechanisms. One of the most important sources of reassurance, markedly impaired under these conditions, is the anticipation of being protected from the full impact of the danger by the danger-control authorities or by other benevolent parent-surrogates. . . .

From what has just been said about the dynamics of stress behavior, one can predict that a number of interrelated adverse effects will ensue if, for any reason, a person fails to do the work of worrying prior to being exposed to actual danger or loss:

1. The [normal] spontaneous tendency to ward off anticipatory fear remains unchecked and the person therefore remains relatively unmotivated to engage in the realistic phantasying or the mental rehearsing essential for developing two types of effective defense against fright: (*a*) reality-based cognitions and expectations about opportunities for surviving the impending danger, the subsequent contemplation of which can function as a source of hope and reassurance, and (*b*) reality-based plans for taking protective actions in case various contingencies arise, the subsequent execution of which can contribute to reducing feelings of passive helplessness.

2. The person's overoptimistic expectations and fantasies remain uncorrected and hence the chances are increased that there will be a marked disparity between the amount of victimization expected beforehand and the amount that is actually experienced, increasing the probability of regressive aggrievement reactions (childlike rage and/or depression).

3. When the person subsequently comes to realize that the danger-control authorities failed to predict or give warnings about the suffering that was in

store for him, childhood experiences of resentment against the parents (for unfair or unprotective treatment) are especially likely to be reactivated, thus increasing the likelihood that the danger-control authorities will lose their capacity to give reassurances and will be irrationally blamed for objective dangers and deprivations.

All three reactions to objective danger situations would be expected to occur whenever a person had failed to engage in adequate worry-work beforehand, whether the failure is attributable primarily to the pre-danger environmental conditions or to exceptionally strong personality needs which predisposed the person to deny clear-cut signs of impending danger. (Janis, 1956.)

The propositions in the foregoing excerpt are to be understood as explications of a theoretical model which conceives of the work of worrying as increasing a person's level of tolerance for subsequent stress stimuli. The more thorough the work of worrying, the more adequate the subsequent adjustment to any given type of danger or deprivation. The maladjustive and pathogenic consequences which have been delineated refer to the extreme negative end-point of the continuum, i.e., where there has been a total failure to carry out any work of worrying at all before the onset of a perceptible source of external danger. It is assumed that similar negative effects will ensue, to varying degrees, as a consequence of a person's partial or complete failure to take account of any specific fear-evoking stimulus or event that subsequently occurs during the danger episode.

The above assumptions are intended to apply to all perceptible stressful events, including not only those associated with surgery, military combat, peacetime disasters, and other situations of physical danger but also a wide variety of crisis episodes involving purely social dangers. For example, F. Romalis' (1942) observations of American women who became emotionally upset when their husbands or sons were drafted into the Army during the early days of World War II suggest that failure to engage in realistic worry about an impending separation may have essentially the same psychological consequences as were observed in surgical patients. It frequently happened that a woman was disinclined to acknowledge the threat beforehand, relying upon overoptimistic slogans and fantasies to the effect that the man would be continuously deferred by his draft board, or, if drafted, would be able to spend much of his time at home. Such denial reactions, according to Romalis, were often followed by extreme surprise, resentment, and exaggerated separation fears when the man's military service subsequently became a reality.

What are the main factors that determine whether or not the work of worrying will be carried out to a sufficient degree so as to prevent subsequent maladjustive reactions? According to the statements quoted from the author's essay on emotional inoculation, the adequacy of the work of worrying may depend partly upon environmental conditions (e.g., exposure to information of the impending danger) and partly on personality predispositions (e.g., motivation to pay attention to warnings). Using similar theoretical concepts in an account of the differences between "realistic" and "neurotic" worrying, Marmor (1958) emphasizes the importance of personality factors in determining the way people respond to anticipated separations from loved ones and other threats of personal loss, such as the possibility of failing an examination or of being fired from one's job. Marmor asserts that worry over realistic matters should be regarded as "a defensive function of the ego, the purpose of which is either to ward off an anticipated real trauma or to deal with the painful consequences of one already experienced." When successful, this mental activity leads to action and mastery of the threat situation. But, according to Marmor, some people are "neurotic" worriers who are unable to achieve inner mastery:

> If the ego fails in its integrative task . . . decompensation takes place in the form of ineffective or circular worrying (which is identical with what is usually clinically labelled as obsessional rumination)—or else the effort to deal with the problem at an *intellectual* level is given up entirely, and regression takes place to the *emotional* level, in which anxiety, bound or unbound, is the dominant feature. The clinical picture may then be that of an anxiety state, phobia, or a conversion hysteria. (Marmor, 1958.)

It must be expected that for some neurotically predisposed personalities, any attempt to produce emotional inoculation by giving warnings and preparatory information will prove to be unsuccessful and may actually precipitate an anxiety attack or exacerbate pre-existing neurotic symptoms. (From the evidence discussed in the preceding chapters, it seems probable that unmodifiable neurotics constitute the majority of the high anticipatory fear group but only a minority of the low fear group.) Among less severe neurotics and among normal personalities, the degree to which realistic worrying occurs will probably depend to some extent upon environmental circumstances and especially on the content of authoritative preparatory communications.

In the remainder of this chapter we shall examine some of the main implications of the theoretical model concerning what happens when the work of worrying is incomplete. The purpose of this discussion is to carry the theoretical analysis of psychological preparation one step further by specifying some of the main conditions under which a communicator's efforts to stimulate the work of worrying by giving preparatory warnings and information about the danger will prove to be unsuccessful, or unnecessary.

Personality Deficiencies

One major source of communication failures, as suggested in the statement quoted from Marmor, involves chronic personality deficiencies such that the person's neurotic fears and defenses are powerfully stimulated whenever he is informed about any realistic threat. Two different types of personality deficiencies have been delineated in the case study material presented in Chapters 20, 21, and 24. One type occurred among some of the surgical patients who were relatively free from anticipatory fear, and the other type among those who displayed high fear. A few persons in the low fear group appeared to be chronically incapable of tolerating feelings of apprehensiveness. Their characteristic cognitive reaction to any threat situation seemed to be that of denying as long as possible the notion that they could be personally affected by the potential danger. In such personalities, extreme control over emotional responsiveness is likely to be achieved at the cost of a rigidly compulsive approach to affect-arousing problems and a highly constricted fantasy life.

Whenever preparatory information about danger is given to large numbers of people, the communicator must expect to encounter strong resistance in at least a small percentage of *overcontrolled* neurotics who rigidly defend themselves against anticipatory fear or any related affect. These neurotics will typically fail to begin the work of worrying even when very impressive communications are given. Because they are so strongly motivated to ignore affect-arousing thoughts, they will be inclined to minimize the importance of any warnings. If the warning is so irrefutable as to be taken seriously, they will tend to be quite inhibited with respect to imagining how the danger could affect them.

At the opposite extreme from the constricted, overcontrolled neurotic personalities are the *undercontrolled* neurotics, whose symptoms have already been described in earlier discussions of the high anticipatory fear group. When confronted with a warning, they do not ignore its implications and have no inhibitions with respect to worrying about the horrible things that may happen to them; their difficulty is, rather, that they cannot stop worrying. These hyperanxious persons, to whom Marmor is referring when he speaks of neurotic worriers, characteristically display obsessional ruminations about real or fantasied traumatic events, or react with hysterical anxiety attacks and related phobic symptoms. One of the main implications of the case studies is that when preparatory communications are given to *undercontrolled* neurotics, the threat content is likely to be excessively stimulating: These persons are capable of actively engaging in the apprehensive thought processes of worrying to some extent, but their neurotic type of worrying involves daydreams that are qualitatively different from normal anticipatory fantasies about realistic dangers. The encroachment of unresolved neurotic conflicts prevents them from bringing the work of worrying to satisfactory completion.

Parenthetically, in line with earlier comments about parallels between the work of worrying and the work of mourning, the intriguing question should be raised as to whether the undercontrolled and overcontrolled neurotic responses to external threats are equivalent to two contrasting types of neurotic reactions to the death of a loved one: At one extreme are those persons incapacitated by prolonged grief, whose exaggerated symptoms reflect an inability to complete the work of mourning because of repressed conflicts mobilized by the loss; at the other extreme are neurotics who behave in a rigid, constricted manner, remaining pathologically indifferent to the loss, presumably as a consequence of chronic affective inhibitions which prevent them from initiating the work of mourning (Fenichel, 1945; Lindemann, 1944).

The modifiability of the two types of personality deficiency, neurotic underreaction and overreaction, carries some implications concerning the conditions under which preparatory communications can successfully stimulate the work of worrying and foster inner preparation for danger. Among the underreactors, there are likely to be some pathological personalities who are almost totally impervious to social influence—severe obsessional neurotics, withdrawn schizoidal characters, and patients with related disorders who continually ward off affect by means of an isolation mechanism. But there is probably also a sizeable proportion of neurotic underreactors who are sufficiently intact personalities to be able to correct their misconceptions of reality and to develop more or less appropriate affective responses, when given the opportunity to find out what other people are saying and doing about an external danger situation. Can preparatory communications succeed in preventing such persons from relying exclusively on blanket denial conceptions? That is, can their spontaneous isolation tendencies be counteracted so as to instigate some effective work of worrying? Insufficient evidence is available to answer such questions conclusively, but the impression derived from most of the intensive interviews of surgical patients in the low anticipatory fear group makes an affirmative answer seem quite plausible. (See especially the following case studies:

Case L–2 [pp. 267–268], Case L–3 [pp. 345–348], Case L–6 [pp. 268–270], and Case X–1 [pp. 308–310].)

At the present time, it is probably unwarranted to be either very pessimistic or very optimistic about developing highly effective techniques for influencing the majority of persons with low anticipatory fear. Perhaps during the next decade, we shall see the development of a variety of new and imaginative communication devices which will prove to be highly effective when tested experimentally. To give a purely speculative example of the type of communication device that should be investigated: It might turn out to be feasible and effective for a skilled interviewer to introduce into the form and content of his preparatory communications some of the basic technical features of "resistance" analysis as currently applied in psychoanalytically oriented psychotherapy; for instance, during one or two sessions, the interviewer might ask a series of nonthreatening, factual questions which would gradually lead the patient to discover for himself that he was displaying a noticeable lack of emotion in the face of circumstances which would make most people quite fearful.

For people with overreactive tendencies, there is a similar need to develop effective quasi-therapeutic methods. If it can be solved at all, the problem of giving adequate preparation to overreactive persons will probably require communication techniques that are quite different from those appropriate for people with underreactive tendencies. Again, we cannot be certain that anything constructive can be done—short of intensive psychotherapy—to break up the spontaneous neurotic pattern with which these people react to signs of external danger. Can some form of brief psychological treatment be developed which will achieve the limited goal of temporarily keeping their worrying within bounds (without making any attempt to "cure" the underlying neurosis)? Can a technique be worked out which will help the hyperanxious person to shift his neurotic fantasies to some other sphere, so that he can orient his anticipations toward the reality situation of impending danger in such a way as to develop some effective reassurances?

It is quite conceivable that a physician or counselor could decrease the intrusion of neurotic fantasies in a patient's conception of surgical and postoperative medical procedures by conducting a series of interviews before the operation: In the first, the patient might be given preparatory information as to what to expect; in the second, he might be encouraged to ventilate his fears; and then in the third, he might be given additional realistic information which is "hand-tailored" to correct his own uniquely distorted conceptions and to reduce the plausibility of those particular fantasy elements or derivatives which were present in the manifest content of his verbalized expectations.

Obviously, if any quasi-therapeutic techniques are evolved for dealing with neurotic personalities, psychological preparation may have to become a specialized professional activity to be carried out by clinically trained personnel who are sensitive observers, skilled in dealing with emotionally distraught people. As interviewers who might be encouraging people to report about their current affective states, and who might sometimes be eliciting derivatives of personal fantasies, they would often evoke intense transference reactions. (See discussion of transference phenomena under conditions of stress, pp. 136–138.) Thus, they would need to meet rigorous personal qualifications required for dealing with the positive and negative transference reactions which they would encounter during and after the interviews.

The above considerations apply to some extent to any deliberate effort to stimulate and guide the work of worrying, whether the client is neurotic or normal. Even relatively healthy personalities have their defensive blind spots and their special sensitivities which can make for emotional underreaction or overreaction to one or another aspect of an impending danger situation. Among surgical patients, for example, we have seen that there are wide individual differences among "normal" persons with respect to the sources of emotional disturbance. In one person, the events that are most disturbing and that must be worked through in advance may be those involving physical incapacitation and the state of passive helplessness during the postoperative period. But in another, equally "normal" person, who is facing essentially the same type of surgical operation, the major source of potential trauma may be limited to the occurrence of severe postoperative pains; in still another the most distressing aspects of the surgical experience may not be the incapacitation, passivity, or pain *per se*, but the necessity for undergoing suffering in a strange place, among strange people, without being in continuous contact with members of his immediate family. Individual differences with respect to *what* is feared will make for individual differences in reactions to preparatory communications. A routine descriptive statement to the effect that the doctors and nurses will give appropriate drugs for the relief of pain may be highly reassuring to a patient who is apprehensive about the possibility that he may be neglected while undergoing prolonged agony. But in another patient with a strong preconscious fear of being seduced into drug addiction, the very same statement may have the opposite effect and require an additional preparatory communication to alleviate the apprehensiveness which is inadvertently aroused.

It is exteremely expensive, of course, for any institution to provide "hand-tailored" communications designed to meet the special requirements of each person. Much more economical would be the use of illustrated pamphlets, recorded lectures, filmstrips, and movie shorts that could be given to large groups without requiring the services of professional personnel to conduct private interviews. Perhaps some standard preparatory communications can be devised that will successfully facilitate the work of worrying, especially among those normal persons who lack information about on-coming dangers. But from what has been said about the complex problems of psychological preparation, it seems probable that substantial numbers of the normal population as well as the vast majority of neurotics cannot be expected to acquire effective reassurances unless they have the opportunity to discuss their reactions to preparatory communications with an authoritative advisor or a professional counselor.

Even when the content consists of facts which are unequivocally regarded as reassuring by all patients—for example, statements about the skill and training of the danger-control personnel—the message may be assimilated by one patient in a way that fosters the development of an effective reassuring concept but in another patient it may reinforce a pre-existing conception of the authorities as godlike beings with magical protective powers, which, in extreme instances, can turn out to have pathogenic consequences. The first type of person may benefit from having his doubts about the dependability of the authorities allayed by additional information concerning their positive attributes; whereas, the second type may benefit only from a realistic picture of the authority figures as human beings with human limitations, so that the myth of being endowed by them with blanket immunity will be replaced by a more differentiated conception—one that allows the authorities to be fallible persons who, nevertheless, can be relied upon to do a good job in living up to the demands and obligations of their protective role.

Only a few illustrations have been sketched out to call attention to the different ways in which a given preparatory communication may be interpreted and assimilated, depending upon the personality predispositions and pre-existing attitudes of the recipient. These examples should suffice to convey the most essential point, which is that whoever attempts to carry out the task of helping people to become psychologically prepared for danger must himself be prepared to deal not only with typical patterns of misunderstanding and emotional resistance but also with the highly unique emotional needs of each individual.

Many of the same interpersonal skills and strategic judgments that are essential for successful work in individual and group psychotherapy are undoubtedly required for successful work in emotional inoculation on the part of would-be practitioners of preventive psychiatry. It is probably a serious mistake to assume that all that is needed to expand this type of activity in modern society is to communicate a set of simple guiding principles to all interested professional workers who are in a position to make use of them, irrespective of their psychological talents, training, or experience. But, on the other hand, it would probably also be a mistake to assume that the amount of talent, training and experience necessary for becoming a good practitioner in this field will prove to be of the same order of magnitude as that required for qualified practitioners of psychotherapy, who must be equipped to deal with the neurotic conflicts and disturbed behavior of chronic mental patients. In any case, a great many more systematic research studies will have to be carried out to test and develop theoretical propositions concerning the effects of preparatory communications before we can expect to have a dependable set of specific guiding principles for producing emotional inoculation. (Janis, 1956.)

Appropriate and Inappropriate Stimulation of Worry-Work

The preceding discussion has illustrated a number of different types of content which would presumably be included in a preparatory communication designed to facilitate effective worry-work. One essential type of content consists of purely factual statements which describe the danger experiences that the person is likely to undergo. From the case material concerning isolated instances of fright reactions among fairly well-prepared surgical patients, one surmises that the work of worrying is apt to be incomplete to the degree that any unfamiliar and distressing occurrence in the danger situation is omitted from the descriptive account presented in preparatory communications. It seems likely that the more precisely every potentially frightening perceptual experience is described, the lower the chances that the given experience will have a traumatizing effect.

A second major type of content consists of fear-reducing statements designed to facilitate the development of reality-oriented reassurances which will subsequently prove to be effective at the time when the danger materializes. Two subtypes of fear-reducing statements should be differentiated because they might facilitate adjustive behavior in somewhat different ways: (*a*) optimistic statements which call attention to the positive side of the picture—references to the limited amount of time that the unpleasant experiences will last and to the mitigating aspects of the situation which will help make the stressful events bearable, and (*b*) hopeful recommendations which urge the recipient of the communication to engage in various physical and mental activities in order to reduce the distressing impact of the potential danger. If presented in a convincing manner, the effect of reassuring predictions and recommendations may be not merely to reduce the recipient's anticipatory fears at the time he receives the communication but also to increase the recipient's ability to cope with the subsequent danger situation. The latter effect can ensue if a preparatory communication encourages the person to try out and to practice various anticipatory thought sequences which enable him to ward off feelings of helplessness and to maintain emotional control in the presence of fear-provoking stimuli. Of special importance are those recommendations which help to build up a sense of *active* control by informing the person about overt actions he can execute (e.g., how to move around in bed in such a way as to minimize muscular aches and pains), and about *decisions* that will be left up to him (e.g., how to judge when to request a sedative).

In earlier chapters a great deal of discussion was devoted to the patient's emotional dependence upon the danger-control authorities (see pp. 134–138 and 306–312). For every surgical patient a crucial part of the work of worrying probably consists of "working through" his ambivalence toward the man who will wield the knife in the operating room and toward the women who will take care of his physical needs afterwards. The case studies of patients who displayed a moderate level of preoperative fear have suggested that there may be at least two separate steps involved in developing a firm conviction in the protective role of the surgeon and the nurses: First, the patient must become aware of the undercurrent of fear and distrust that coexists with his overtly positive attitude toward the authorities, and, second, he must engage in reflective thought as to whether his suspicions and negative feelings toward the authorities are warranted or unwarranted. The latter process involves a combination of *current reality testing* (e.g., seeking information about the actual persons who currently occupy the authority role) and *memory processes* (e.g., recalling past experiences with his parents or other authorities in danger situations which are associatively linked with the present one). Thus, the work of worrying may lead the person to obtain information that may correct his inappropriate views of the power and intentions of the people upon whom he will be dependent and, also, at a less rational level, to build up a more favorable image of the authorities by taking account of past experiences in which he was genuinely helped by his parents or by parent-surrogates ("They will take good care of me"). It seems likely that in some cases this process might be greatly facilitated if the person were to have a series of sessions with a skilled counselor who is sensitive to the problems of conveying accurate information in such a way as to help people to develop confidence in trustworthy authorities.[7]

Research findings from experiments on the effectiveness of communications about potential dangers suggest that the "dosage" of fear-arousing material plays a considerable role in determining the incidence of repudiation and hyperdefensiveness among normal personalities (Hovland et al., 1953, pp. 77–89). Elsewhere, the author has discussed some of the implications of the research findings for the selection and spacing of fear-arousing and fear-reducing statements in preparatory communications (Janis, 1956). One central point, which is pertinent to the present discussion, is that if fear is very strongly stimulated, disruptive effects tend to occur. For maximal effectiveness, the communications probably should be devised in such a way as to elicit a gradual, stepwise increase up to, but not beyond, a moderate level of fear. If the threat content markedly overbalances the reassurance content within any given communication, the recipient is likely to be left in a state of high emotional tension, as a result of which he may become strongly motivated to minimize the threat and to avoid thinking about it. It is conceivable that in circumstances where the threat of future danger cannot be ignored, an overdose of fear-arousing content in a preparatory communication could create a boomerang effect of hypervigilance. In other words, the person might become so sensitized to the frightening aspects of the impending danger that his chances of being subsequently traumatized would be increased rather than decreased.

The possibility that preparatory communications might give an *overdose* of fear-arousing material leads to a more general problem concerning the advisability of exposing people to emotionally disturbing information. What are the main factors that should be taken into account in determining whether or not a person will benefit from being given warnings and preparatory information? It cannot be expected that all stressful life situations warrant the energy expenditure involved in stimulating the work of worrying. Here it is not merely a question of the expense in time and effort on the part of the skilled personnel whose services may be essential for conducting the interview sessions in which preparatory communications can be effectively presented. There is also likely to be a certain amount of energy expenditure on the part of the recipient of a fear-evoking preparatory communication. Whenever someone is stimulated to engage actively in the work of worrying, his thought processes involuntarily become concentrated on the task of anticipating and mastering the threat, leaving him relatively little inner freedom to concentrate on normal daily activities. As long as the emotional task remains unfinished, the worrier may suffer a marked loss in general mental efficiency combined with a strong tendency to indulge in momentarily distracting activities so as to suppress disturbing fantasies about failing to cope with the uncertain future.

Some degree of *neurotic anxiety* is probably always present as a subdominant accompaniment to reality-oriented worrying. Daydreams of being mutilated or annihilated are quite unproductive with respect to gaining emotional control and can be regarded as a form of neurotic worrying. Even in emotionally healthy personalities, such horror fantasies generally cannot be completely suppressed at times when anticipatory fears of potential body damage are aroused. Thus, the normal worrier can be expected to experience sporadic moods of uneasiness or subjective malaise. For the same reason, he may also display a temporary increase in regressive forms of defensive behavior. From descriptive accounts of the behavior of large numbers of people at times when they were worried about realistic threats of an imminent natural disaster or of a wartime bombing attack, it is apparent that a variety of transient anxiety symptoms frequently occur, including sleeplessness, nightmares, obsessional thoughts, and compulsivelike ritualistic actions (Glover, 1942; Janis, 1951; Mira, 1943; M. Schmideberg, 1942; M. Wolfenstein, 1957).

The foregoing discussion highlights some of the major risks that are deterrents to the indiscriminate use of preparatory communications for the purpose of stimulating the work of worrying in advance of all potentially stressful experiences. Everyone can be expected to suffer a short-run personal loss because of his transient maladjustive reactions which accompany realistic worrying. In addition, there is always at least a remote chance that the long-run effects may be the opposite of what is intended—sometimes a recipient's latent neurotic tendencies may be exacerbated by fear-arousing communications. These considerations give sharp emphasis to the importance of specifying the conditions under which the work of worrying is not essential.

The study of surgery cases suggests that there are at least two main types of postoperative stress episodes for which psychological preparation is of relatively little value and, hence, can be dispensed with. One type consists of those episodes in which the *entire* stressful experience is so mild, or of such short duration, that severe fright reactions are unlikely to be evoked, even in wholly unprepared persons. Illustrative examples were given in Chapter 21 of two patients in the low fear group who displayed no subsequent emotional disturbances, apparently because the postoperative stresses to which they were subjected proved to be comparatively mild and psychologically bearable. (See discussion of Cases L–4 and L–8, pp. 258–261.)

A second type of stressful event for which advance preparation seems to be relatively unessential is one during which specific reassurances can be given in a highly effective manner by an authority figure at the crucial time when the fright-evoking stimuli are present. For example, convalescent patients often seem to find it quite easy to tolerate certain unanticipated treatments of a distressing nature—blood tests, penicillin injections, catheterization procedures, etc.—provided that the doctor or nurse who is administering the procedure expresses an encouraging attitude and takes the trouble to notice and to assuage the patient's fear of being injured. When told about such procedures beforehand, however, the patient may visualize the event as a horrible ordeal and may develop vivid fantasies—e.g., of losing huge quantities of blood, of being mutilated by an injection needle, or of undergoing genital damage from a catheter. And then, especially if he is somewhat reluctant to verbalize his apprehensions, the exaggerated notions he has evolved may prevent him from being responsive to the usual reassurances that he is given at the time when the treatment is being carried out. Thus, for certain types of treatments, it may turn out to be much more difficult to reassure a patient after he has spent a good deal of time imagining what the threatening procedure might be like than if he remains unconcerned until the moment when the procedure is about to begin.

Detailed descriptions of certain physical threats—such as those involving the forcible intrusion of a bodily orifice—readily lend themselves to symbolic fantasy elaboration and are especially likely to touch off irrational, infantile fears. An illustrative example was encountered in the psychoanalytic case study of Mrs. Blake. Shortly before going to the hospital, she expressed a high degree of concern about the fact that she would be given an enema. Her mental image of the procedure was connected, in her free associations, with reminiscences of childhood dangers which she had experienced or fantasied during her struggles against toilet training. Subsequently, when the enema was administered, she involuntarily resisted it to such an extent that it was a complete failure.

Like Mrs. Blake, some surgical patients in the case study series seemed to become inordinately concerned when told about routine enemas beforehand. Because a patient's emotional tension can affect his muscular activity in such a way as to interfere with the normal physiological effects of an enema, it becomes a matter of practical medical administration to determine whether or not the average patient is better off if told nothing at all about it in advance.[8] This is only one of many examples that could be cited to illustrate the potentially unfavorable effects that might need to be taken into consideration in order to make an adequate judgment as to whether or not an attempt should be made to stimulate the work of worrying in people who are going to be exposed to a given type of stressful experience.

Whenever it is feasible to do so, it would certainly be worth while to base such policy decisions upon the results of systematic investigations that are devised specifically to find out: (*a*) whether the gains in personal adjustment that come from giving preparatory communications to the average person do, in fact, generally outweigh the potentially adverse effects, and (*b*) whether there are certain identifiable types of persons whose reactions deviate from the average to such a degree that a different policy should be adopted for them. The answers obtained from carefully designed empirical investigations should prove to be not only of immediate practical value from the standpoint of preventive psychiatry but also of more general scientific value. Ultimately, such investigations should lead to the establishment of empirically validated laws and generalizations about the conditions under which preparatory communications will be effective in increasing stress tolerance.

Notes

1. Twelve major surgery cases failed to answer one or more of the three key questions about the preoperative information they had been given, and all of them were eliminated from the present study. Also excluded from the present study were all cases of *minor* surgery. These cases were excluded because, when sorted into two groups, according to the same procedures used for the major surgery cases, it was found that there were large and significant differences between the informed and uninformed cases on a number of important background factors, including type of minor operation and type of anesthetic. It was not felt to be worth while to execute the cumbersome analysis necessary for attempting to control statistically for the differences in background factors. Inspection of the raw data (uncorrected for background differences) showed that the differences between informed and uninformed cases of *minor* surgery were roughly parallel to those obtained from the more dependable analysis of *major* surgery cases (presented in Charts 6 and 7).

2. Question A was the key item used in Chapter 22 to sort the patients into the high, moderate, and low preoperative fear categories. Included in the analysis of this question were those patients who had been unaware of the operation on the day before it occurred. (But it should be borne in mind that all accident victims and emergency cases who did not know beforehand that there would be an operation were systematically eliminated from the sample.) All patients who were included reported that they knew about the operation at least a few hours before it took place. Some of them reported having been given information about the unpleasant aspects of the impending surgery during the preoperative hours when they

were waiting to be taken to the operating room, whereas others reported having been given no such information. Therefore, the pertinent comparisons for our present inquiry could be made. The presence of these "Unaware" cases does not account for the large difference between the informed and uninformed groups on Question A because there is only a small difference between the two groups in the percentage *unaware of the impending operation* on the day before it took place (27% versus 31%).

In order to show how the breakdowns in Chart 6 are related to those in the charts and tables of Chapter 22, a special table was prepared for Question A (Table 14). This table is organized in terms of the original high, moderate, and low

Table 14. Distribution of Cases Entering in the Relationship Between Preoperative Fear and Preoperative Information

Rating Based on Three Key Questions Dealing with Information Received from Medical Authorities	Level of Preoperative Fear: Low (N = 15)		Moderate (N = 21)		High (N = 27)		Unaware (N = 26)		Total	
	No. of Cases	Percent	No. of Cases	Percent	No. of Cases	Percent	No. of Cases	Percent	No. of Cases	Percent
Informed	6	**40**	16	**76**	15	**56**	14	**54**	51	**57**
Uninformed	8	**53**	3	**14**	7	**26**	8	**31**	26	**29**
Indeterminate (no answer to one or more key questions)	1	**7**	2	**10**	5	**18**	4	**15**	12	**14**
Total	15	**100**	21	**100**	27	**100**	26	**100**	89	**100**

groups, showing the percentage in each group who were informed, uninformed or indeterminate. It can be readily seen that the strong relationship between the amount of information and the level of preoperative fear is not attributable to the inclusion of patients who were unaware of the operation on the day before it took place. Of the 15 cases in the original low fear group, 53% were uninformed; whereas, of the 21 cases in the original moderate fear group, only 14% were uninformed. This 39% difference is statistically significant ($p > .05$) and is wholly independent of any data from the "Unaware" group.

Chart 6 shows that on Question B, 61% of the informed group as against only 38% of the uninformed group reported some degree of anticipatory fear (slight or severe). But 12% of the 23% difference comes from the "Unaware" and "No Answer" categories. Hence the results on this question cannot be regarded as clear-cut evidence. There is no such ambiguity, fortunately, in the findings based on Question C. The informed and uninformed groups differ by 27% in the incidence of cases reporting no fear during the hour preceding the operation. Here there were no instances of failure to answer the question and, during the time period in question, all patients in both groups, according to their own statements elsewhere in the questionnaire, were fully aware of the fact that they were scheduled to undergo the operation.

3. The fact that the presence or absence of preparatory information about unpleasant aspects of the operation is positively related to the presence or absence of preoperative fear would not necessarily imply that such information makes for

more fear in the operating room or during the postoperative stress period. An analysis was made of the answers given by the informed and uninformed groups to questions dealing with the severity of fear reactions: (*a*) during administration of the anesthetic; (*b*) during the first few hours after the awakening from the anesthetic; and (*c*) during the day after the operation. No consistent or significant differences were found. The uninformed group reported a somewhat higher incidence of severe postoperative fear reactions than the informed group, but the differences were not large enough to approach statistical significance.

4. Significant differences between the moderate and low fear groups were also reported in Chapter 22 for two other measures, which were obtained not from *objective* questions but from a *content-analysis* of write-in answers concerning blame reactions and complaints against the hospital staff. The present analysis of the informed and uninformed groups was arbitrarily limited to the objective questions merely because of the ease of obtaining the necessary data. The two content-analysis measures were not used because of the great amount of additional time it would have taken to carry out the systematic content-analysis coding of the questionnaires for those patients who were not included in the earlier analysis (i.e., the 22 cases who reported being unaware of the operation on the day before it occurred). Inspection of the content-analysis results from all cases whose questionnaires had been coded showed that there were differences between the informed and uninformed groups in the expected direction. Therefore it was assumed that if the entire content analysis were carried out, the outcome would not alter the overall picture conveyed by the results presented in Chart 7.

5. When the author was conducting research studies on the surgical wards, he planned to carry out a controlled experiment on the effects of preparatory communication. There were several factors, however, which made such an experiment unfeasible to execute. The main source of difficulty stemmed from the fact that the author wished to give correct information to each patient about: (*a*) what he would perceive in the operating room, and (*b*) the pains and other unpleasant occurrences he would experience during the postoperative recovery period. In order to give such information, it is necessary to design the preparatory communications on an individual basis, and this requires the close collaboration of each patient's physician or surgeon. But it was soon discovered that some physicians tended to encourage extremely optimistic views and some used various euphemisms to withhold unpleasant information. Thus, if an outsider (the experimenter) attempted to give the preparatory communications, it would be of great importance to avoid contradicting what the patient's physician or surgeon had told him and to make sure that the information would not in any way undermine the patient's confidence in his doctor. This consideration, again, pointed to the need for setting up the experiment in such a way that each patient's physician or surgeon would contribute his time and energy, at least with respect to determining what detailed information should be given. In a private hospital like the one where the author's research was conducted, many collaborating medical personnel would be required for this purpose because, at any given time, the patients on the surgical wards are under the care of a large number of private and staff physicians. It would not be satisfactory to have only one or two staff physicians who were willing to cooperate give the preparatory communications to all their patients, and then to compare the informed patients with those treated by other physicians who gave no such preparation. This procedure would confound the personal characteristics of the physi-

cian with the main experimental variable (the preparatory communication). Because of the heavy demands for time and effort on the part of a large number of medical personnel, the experimental study turned out to be unfeasible in the private hospital setting. Perhaps such an experiment would be more feasible in a military or government hospital where all the physicians on the staff might be more easily organized to form a coordinated research team for this purpose.

In the absence of experimental evidence, it is necessary to rely upon correlational data. But a major weakness of correlational data of the type presented in Charts 6 and 7, as previously noted, is that they cannot be unambiguously interpreted as demonstrating the effectiveness of preoperative information. There are several possible types of artifacts that could give rise to the observed correlations. In the discussion which follows, an attempt is made to take account of important factors that could conceivably alter the way in which the results should be interpreted.

One obvious possibility is that the men who experienced the most pain, suffering, and incapacitation were those who were most unpleasantly surprised and emotionally upset by the operation. When recalling the operation, these men might retrospectively report that they had been inadequately informed beforehand about the unpleasant postoperative experiences. This interpretation seems quite improbable, however, in the light of the evidence bearing on severity of stress. No consistent or significant differences were found between the informed and uninformed groups in self-ratings on any of the following eight factors: (1) degree of incapacitation from preoperative illness or injury; (2) duration of physical pain on the day before the operation; (3) intensity of the most severe pain on the day before the operation; (4) the type of anesthetic; (5) the type of operation performed; (6) the number of days the patient was kept in bed after the operation; (7) the number of weeks before the patient was able to resume work and engage in usual daily activities; (8) the number of days before postoperative pains subsided.

The absence of any differences between the informed and uninformed groups on the eight factors appears to preclude the following two possible sources of spurious differences: First, the obvious possibility that differences in actual stress exposure might account for the differences in emotional reactions; second, the more subtle psychological influence of a "halo effect." The latter term refers to the possibility that, irrespective of the actual magnitude of stress, the men who were left with the most unpleasant impressions of their surgical experience might tend to make complaints about *all* the negative features of the operation and thus be inclined to allege that their physicians misinformed or failed to give them sufficient information. If either of these two interpretations of the data in Chart 7 were correct, one would expect to find significant differences in at least some of the answers given to the eight items listed above.

Another possible source of misleading conclusions concerning the correlational results in Chart 7 is the possibility that the outcome may merely reflect differences in the patients' *preferences* to be informed or uninformed rather than the actual amount of preoperative information that was made available to them. Those who rated themselves as uninformed might have been given just as much information by the physician, but might have failed to assimilate it or might have forgotten it as a result of defensive personality needs. If so, the differences between the informed and uninformed groups would reflect only *predispositional* differences and the results could not be construed as supporting the hypothesis that postoperative emotional reactions can be influenced by giving the patients preparatory information beforehand. There is, of course, no decisive way to preclude this possibility, but there are some additional findings which seem to imply that the preference for avoiding preparatory information about surgery is no more prevalent in the uninformed group than in the informed group. The following question was asked for the purpose of assessing the patients' preferences with respect to being informed about the unpleasant aspects of surgical experiences.

QUESTION Q: "Suppose that you were going to have a major operation performed (for example, removal of your gall bladder), and several days before it was to take place the doctor or surgeon offered to tell you all the specific details about the *unpleasant experiences you could normally expect to have* in connection with the operation. How much would you actually want him to tell you? (Select the one answer that comes closest to showing how much information of this sort you would want to be given several days before the operation was to take place.)

Table 15. Comparison of the Informed Group with the Uninformed Group on Preference for Being Told Beforehand About the Unpleasant Aspects of a Surgical Operation

Preferred Amount of Preoperative Information	Informed Group ($N = 51$)	Uninformed Group ($N = 26$)
Would want to be told nothing about the unpleasant experiences.	6%	15%
Would want to be given a general idea about the unpleasant experiences to expect, but would *not* want to be told any of the specific details.	22%	15%
Would want to be told the specific details about some of the mildly unpleasant experiences, but would not want to be told the details about the more extreme ones.	4%	4%
Would want to be told the specific details about some of the most unpleasant experiences, but not about all of them.	12%	12%
Would want to be told the specific details about all of the unpleasant experiences.	56%	54%
Total	100%	100%

The Check-list of five alternative answers is reproduced in Table 15. The data in this table show how the answers by the uninformed group compare with those by the informed group. Since there are negligible differences in expressed preferences with respect to being informed about future operations, it seems unlikely that the two groups differ with respect to any manifest or verbalizable desire to avoid being exposed to such information. It is noteworthy that approximately two-thirds of each group indicate a preference to be told "everything" or to be given specific details about "some of the most important unpleasant experiences" beforehand. The possibility remains, of course, that there may be some latent personality differences between the informed and uninformed groups which do not show up at all in self-ratings on desire to be informed.

6. The case material also indicates that surgical patients often have an intense "hunger" for information, which, if not satisfied by the medical authorities, will lead them to seek elsewhere. The observations suggest that one of the goals of

preparatory communications should be that of preventing certain types of misconceptions and disappointments which are apt to arise during the hospitalization period as a result of receiving misleading information from visitors and fellow patients. Numerous comments made by men in the survey research, as well as by the patients in the hospital interview studies, suggest that informal statements from roommates, friends, and other nonauthoritative sources frequently exert a marked influence on surgical patients' apperceptions and judgments. Hospitalized patients seem to derive some marked benefits from informal conversations with each other, but sometimes the information picked up in this way is misleading. A typical example from a survey research questionnaire is the following:

"I was disappointed that I was forced to spend almost 48 hours completely in bed suffering from rather severe pain; this feeling was the result of discussions of similar operations with people who progressed more rapidly."

7. In addition to conveying appropriate information about the surgeon and the nursing staff, there are other functions that might also be fulfilled by a well-trained counselor who may be in a position to help the patient to "work through" his ambivalence toward the danger-control authorities: (*a*) encouraging the patient to verbalize his negative feelings (at least to himself); (*b*) stimulating the patient to have reminiscences of favorable past experiences with his parents; and (*c*) behaving during the interviews in such a way that, in his role as a representative of the hospital authorities, the counselor alleviates some of the patient's doubts about the trustworthiness of the authority figures.

There are a number of other personality factors which may have to be taken into account if it turns out that overcoming latent distrust of the authorities constitutes a crucial part of the work of worrying. One would expect that among persons who have erected powerful reaction formations against hostility toward their parents, many would be too rigidly defensive to be capable of becoming readily aware of negative feelings toward parent-surrogates. Other types of personalities may also have great difficulty in arriving at a basic attitude of confidence in the authority figures because they are unable to muster reminiscences of positive relationships with their own parents. For example, relatively poor adjustment to wartime dangers has been noted among men who had few favorable experiences with their parents to fall back upon (Grinker and Spiegel, 1945a).

8. Some radiologists who give barium enemas to hundreds of people every year are keenly aware of the psychological problems created by telling the patients about the procedure. One radiologist privately communicated to the author that he had worked out a practical solution which consisted of never mentioning the word "enema," until after it had been administered. He used to inform patients, before the session when the lower bowel was to be x-rayed, about the fact that they would be given a barium enema. He noticed that despite his efforts at giving reassurance, a sizeable percentage behaved very apprehensively, became very tense while the enema was being administered, complained vehemently about being unable to retain the fluid while the pictures were being taken, and sometimes even prevented the x-ray series from being completed by jumping off the table to run to the lavatory. After many years of trying to avert such reactions, the radiologist hit upon a different way of handling the situation, which he claims to be quite successful. His technique is as follows: He says nothing at all about the enema and when the time comes to administer it, he tells the patient that he is trying out a simple exploratory procedure which involves inserting a tube in the

rectum. He mentions that this tube can be removed if it becomes uncomfortable, and he asks the patient to tell him if there are any sensations of discomfort. Under these conditions, the radiologist finds that his patients are much less tense. Very few of them complain about having difficulty in retaining the fluid for the requisite time period, and, if they do complain, they are generally quite responsive to his request to allow the tube to remain in place for "just a little while longer." Most of the patients, as the radiologist describes them, are genuinely surprised when they learn that they received an enema. Even the more sophisticated ones who know that an enema is a standard part of the procedure, usually do not recognize what is happening when the enema is being given, and end up being just as surprised as the others when they learn that it is all over.

The stress situation with which the radiologist is dealing appears to be a prime illustration of the conditions under which it is unwarranted to give preparatory communications to stimulate the work of worrying. First of all, the perceptual experiences produced by the physical stimuli evidently are not inherently painful or frightening if the patient is prevented from seeing the apparatus and is not given the emotionally charged verbal label. Secondly, the doctor is right on hand to give encouragement and reassurance. Moreover, part of the radiologists' technique consists of allowing the patient to have a sense of being in control, since he is told that the tube will be removed if he announces that it is distressing. Finally, no matter how objectively and reassuringly the enema is described by the doctor beforehand, the patient's mental picture of it is likely to be distorted because of associative linkages with repressed conflicts, fantasies, and memories of anal experiences. It seems likely, therefore, that for a short, mild stress episode of this type, most persons might react more favorably if given no preparatory communications at all; but there might, nevertheless, be a sizeable minority of persons who would be less upset by it if they were told exactly what was going to happen.

26.

Summary of part II: Conclusions from behavioral research

Among the main propositions derived from the psychoanalytic study (reported in Part I and summarized in Chapter 17) are a number of hypotheses concerning interrelationships between the *level of anticipatory fear and subsequent adjustment to stress.* These interrelationships are the focal point of the behavioral research reported in Part II, the main results of which are summarized in this chapter.

For the purpose of understanding how preoperative emotional reactions are linked with postoperative adjustment, a combination of research techniques was used:

1. A small series of hospitalized patients was studied intensively before and after surgery, using data obtained from: (*a*) intensive preoperative and postoperative interviews conducted by the author, and (*b*) daily behavioral records made by the hospital staff.
2. A questionnaire survey, dealing with the emotional impact of surgical experiences, was conducted among several hundred male adolescents who had undergone an operation within the past few years.

The method of controlled comparisons was used in analyzing the observational data from the case study series as well as from the questionnaire survey in order to assess the following general hypothesis:

Hypothesis 15. *Persons who display a moderate degree of anticipatory fear before being exposed to physical stress stimuli (pain, bodily discomforts, and severe deprivations) will be less likely to develop emotional disturbances during or after the stress exposure than those persons who display either a very high degree or a very low degree of anticipatory fear.*

According to this hypothesis, postoperative adjustment can be predicted from the level of anticipatory fear, but the relationship is a curvilinear one. Reactions of anticipatory fear are assumed to form a continuum ranging from almost complete absence of any fear symptoms ("low" level of fear) through a wide band of intermediate degrees of fear ("moderate" level of fear) to an extreme state of agitated apprehensiveness ("high" level of fear). In Hypothesis 15, the term "emotional disturbances" refers to any form of maladjustive reaction to stress such as: (*a*) demoralization; (*b*) reactive depression; (*c*) acute anxiety symptoms; and (*d*) hostility or resentment. The latter two categories appeared to constitute the most frequent types of manifest "problem" behavior among convalescing surgical patients and were investigated in relation to the two extremes of the anticipatory fear continuum. The available observational data on postoperative anxiety and hostility were used to test the following two descriptive hypotheses, which supplement Hypothesis 15 by specifying more precisely what is likely to happen when a person displays either very low or very high anticipatory fear:

Hypothesis 16. *Persons who display an extremely high level of anticipatory fear or anxiety during the "threat" period will be more likely than others to display intense fear of body damage during the subsequent crisis period, when exposed to actual stress stimuli.*

Hypothesis 17. *Persons who display an extremely low degree of anticipatory fear or anxiety during the "threat" period will be more likely than others to display reactions of anger and resentment toward danger-control authorities during the subsequent crisis period, when exposed to actual stress stimuli.*

The findings from the case studies and the survey research support the three hypotheses. It was found to be necessary, however, to specify a proviso for Hypothesis 17, namely that persons with low anticipatory fear will tend to display a higher incidence of subsequent reactions of anger and resentment only if they are exposed to relatively *severe* stress stimuli, such as intense pain or an accumulation of harassing deprivations. It was observed that when postoperative stress stimuli turn out to be comparatively mild (as is usually the case with those "minor" surgical operations which do not require opening the abdomen or the chest wall), patients displaying a low level of preoperative fear do not differ appreciably in their subsequent postoperative behavior from those displaying a moderate level of preoperative fear. However, for "major" surgery cases, large and consistent differences were observed, indicating that patients who are relatively free from fear before the operation are more likely than others to become angry and resentful during the recovery period after the operation.

A number of important psychological variables, in addition to those specified in Hypotheses 15, 16, and 17, were found to be closely linked with the adequacy of the patient's adjustment to postoperative stresses. Additional observations were made which contain numerous indications of how the low, moderate, and high fear groups differ with respect to: (*a*) modes of reassurance and defensive efforts which the patients use to control their emotional reactions; (*b*) exposure to authoritative information and to other communications which can affect both the level of anticipatory fear and the emotional impact of subsequent stressful events; (*c*) postoperative fantasies, dreams, and verbal reports about subjective moods which may reflect latent motives aroused during the convalescent period; and (*d*) personality predispositions which may be determinants of individual differences in responsiveness to danger stimuli.

In the following sections, a detailed summary is presented of the main findings and inferences concerning the overt behavior and psychological mechanisms of patients with low, moderate, and high anticipatory fear. The primary purpose of the summary is to provide a composite picture of each of the three groups, bringing together the empirically derived generalizations and interpretive hypotheses that are scattered throughout the preceding eight chapters.

For each group, the generalizations will be classified into the following categories: (1) preoperative behavior; (2) postoperative behavior; (3) reassurance mechanisms; (4) major causal factors; and (5) problems of psychological preparation. No attempt will be made, however, to repeat the statements already made concerning the nature of the evidence bearing on each conclusion. Suffice to say, the statements in all five categories are to be regarded as more or less tentative conclusions, none of which have as yet been rigorously verified. The first two categories deal with preoperative and postoperative behaviors that are directly observable, and the findings are based on relatively systematic comparative data. The findings in these two categories may therefore be regarded as the most reliable ones. Somewhat less dependable are the generalizations in the third category, which state inferences about intervening reassurance mechanisms derived from: (*a*) a content analysis of the men's comments in the survey questionnaires, and (*b*) qualitative features of the intensive interviews which provide suggestive leads as to how different individuals attempt to cope with their fears at times of crisis. Most tentative of all are the statements in the last two categories, dealing with causal factors and problems of psychological preparation. A few of the conclusions are supported by systematic correlational data showing that the absence of preoperative information is related to postoperative disturbances. Most of the propositions, however, are speculative inferences based on an attempt to piece together a coherent explanation from the over-all array of case study and survey findings. Such propositions are offered merely as suggestive hypotheses which are capable of being tested—and which warrant being tested—by means of longitudinal "panel" studies, systematic correlational research, and controlled experiments.

For the reader who wishes to trace back and assess the evidence supporting the main generalizations, page references are given which designate the places where pertinent observations have been described in earlier chapters.

Low Anticipatory Fear

Preoperative Behavior*

A surgical patient is said to have a "low" degree of anticipatory fear if he displays practically no perceptible signs of fear or emotional disturbance during the period when he knows that he is scheduled to have an operation. Thus the patients in the low fear group are those who remain consistently calm and unperturbed while receiving routine preoperative care. They have no special sleeping disturbances at night. When interviewed, they report feeling quite unworried about the impending surgical operation and show no symptoms of emotional tension. In response to intensive questioning, they will at most admit being mildly concerned about their financial affairs or about other extraneous matters, but they will deny any apprehensiveness about the potential dangers or deprivations that may ensue from undergoing surgery. Consistent with

* See pp. 251–253; 262–268; 304–310; 345–347; and 356–357.

their subjective reports is the fact that they make little or no effort to seek information about the operation, although when authoritative information is offered, they do not ignore it. By and large, these patients appear to spend little time thinking or fantasying about the operation. In so far as their physical condition permits, they engage in their usual daily activities with no apparent loss in mental efficiency and without noticeable changes in their everyday social behavior.

Postoperative Behavior*

Upon being subjected to the pains and other stresses of the postoperative period, patients in the low anticipatory fear group tend to react with angry resentment, combined with varying degrees of anxiety and depression. They are more likely than others to display a prolonged mood of irritable grouchiness along with occasional outbursts of belligerent protest. Although it rarely happens that a surgical patient refuses to conform with the postoperative medical procedures administered by nurses or physicians, a uniquely high incidence of such refusals occurs among patients in the low fear group. Moreover, this group of patients is more likely than others to express complaints against the hospital staff, including serious charges that doctors, nurses, and orderlies are deliberately sadistic, grossly negligent, or wholly incompetent. The strongly negative attitudes which develop during the stressful recovery period persist long after convalescence is over. These patients look back upon the operation as having been an unnecessarily disturbing experience and they retain an attitude of relatively low confidence in the surgeon.

Reassurance Mechanisms†

While awaiting the operation, the dominant mode of reassurance of patients with low anticipatory fear consists of optimistic denial of potential dangers and deprivations. Their view of what is in store for them seems to be quite different from that of patients with moderate fear, most of whom develop a rather differentiated conception of their personal invulnerability, involving the expectation of surviving intact *despite* undergoing pain and suffering. In contrast, the patients with low anticipatory fear tend to feel convinced that they will remain wholly unaffected by the surgical experience, and sometimes also expect

* See pp. 253–261; 263–272; and 276–301.

† See pp. 304–308; and 337–350.

to obtain unusual gratifications. They are apt to adopt a joking or facetious attitude and often make use of simple slogans, such as "there's nothing really to it," to bolster their belief that the stressful occurrences will prove to be of a very trivial nature. When actual suffering occurs, it comes as a somewhat shocking surprise and is frequently interpreted as meaning that someone has failed to treat them properly. The usual pains, discomforts, and unpleasant postoperative treatments tend to be regarded as unnecessary accidents caused by the hospital staff. Thus, instead of regarding their suffering as an unavoidable consequence of surgery, they are inclined to place the blame upon danger-control personnel, who are now apperceived as being inept, unprotective, or malevolent. By becoming distrustful and resistant toward danger-control personnel, these patients may succeed in warding off apprehensiveness to some degree, but their level of postoperative emotional disturbance nevertheless tends to be comparatively high, the symptoms of which include low frustration tolerance and externalized rage, as described in the above section on postoperative behavior.

Major Causal Factors*

Among patients in the low fear group there are marked individual differences in the degree to which emotional reactions are determined by predispositional and situational factors. In some surgical patients, low anticipatory fear seems to be largely attributable to personality predispositions which incline the person to deny signs of impending dangers and to ignore the explicit as well as implicit warnings made by medical authorities. This subgroup probably includes a variety of severe neurotics and prepsychotics—severe obsessionals, withdrawn schizoidal characters, and patients with related types of disorders who are chronically disposed to use denial and isolation mechanisms for warding off disturbing affect. But there are other patients in the low fear group who appear to be relatively normal personalities, highly responsive to emotional stimulation from the environment. For such persons, exposure to specific information about unpleasant aspects of impending surgical experiences has a marked influence, shifting them from a calm, unworried attitude to a moderate degree of apprehensiveness. However, if given no such information, these same patients are likely to remain free from preoperative fear. Thus, a tentative answer can be given to the question: Do environmental factors play a significant role in causing the presence or absence of anticipatory fear? In

* See pp. 261–273; 308–310; 336–360; 379–380; and 389–392.

a sizeable minority, if not in the majority of cases, the relative absence of preoperative fear is partly attributable to environmental circumstances which prevent the person from being exposed to impressive information about the impending stresses of surgery.

It is a separate question whether low anticipatory fear plays any causal role in producing postoperative reactions of anger and resentment. The available evidence suggests that a major consequence of low anticipatory fear is a general lack of psychological preparation for coping with subsequent episodes of stress. This generalization may apply to the entire low fear group, whether the patient's lack of fear is attributable primarily to predispositional or to situational factors. The unworried person is inclined to develop spontaneously a sense of *blanket immunity* which is readily shattered by the impact of actual stress stimuli; whereas, if motivated by anticipatory fear, he is more likely to develop *partial immunity* reassurances which take account of the actual dangers to which he expects to be exposed. The latter type of reassurances continues to be effective in preventing feelings of helplessness at moments of acute crisis, thereby reducing the probability of emotional shock and aggrievement reactions when personal suffering subsequently occurs. A low degree of anticipatory fear can, therefore, be regarded as *pathogenic* in that subsequently, if exposed to severe stress stimuli, the unworried person tends to lose emotional control and becomes adversely sensitized because of his lack of effective inner defenses.

Problems of Psychological Preparation*

The evidence bearing on the relationship between preoperative information and postoperative emotional reactions forms the basis for the following inferred generalization concerning the probable effects of preparatory communications: If a person's anticipatory fear is stimulated to a moderate degree by impressive warnings or by other forms of information, the probability that he will subsequently overreact emotionally to actual stress stimuli and develop sustained attitudes of resentment toward danger-control authorities will be markedly lower than if his anticipatory fear is not at all stimulated during the precrisis period.

For the purpose of conceptualizing the normal processes of inner preparation, the "work of worrying" has been introduced as a construct which is analogous to the "work of mourning." The prophylactic goal

* See pp. 353–360; and 376–380.

of preparatory communications can be described in terms of guiding the surgical patient's affective processes as well as his thought sequences in such a way that he will carry through the "work of worrying" to completion before being exposed to the actual stresses of the postoperative period. Carefully planned communications, individually "hand-tailored" in private interviews conducted by the patient's physician or by a professional counselor, will probably be required in order to take account of individual differences in personality tendencies which make for evasion of the "work of worrying."

The problem of devising effective preparatory communications to *initiate* the work of worrying applies most directly to the low anticipatory fear group and especially to that subgroup which consists of chronic, overcontrolled neurotics who rigidly defend themselves against affect and, hence, remain unresponsive to authoritative communications about impending dangers. For such persons, it may be essential to develop quasi-therapeutic techniques to reduce internal resistances to the point where the person will begin thinking over the implications of the threatening situation, become affectively involved, and, hence, be motivated to replace his blanket immunity expectations with reality-oriented reassurances.

Within the low anticipatory fear group there is probably also a sizeable subgroup of more or less normal personalities who will spontaneously develop and cling to pathogenic attitudes of denial unless their anticipatory fears are deliberately stimulated by impressive communications. For such persons, no special psychological devices may be necessary for successful emotional inoculation beyond conveying purely factual statements from a prestigeful source. In order to guide the work of worrying in such a way that the person will end up with an effective set of reality-oriented reassurances, it will probably prove to be advantageous to present well-balanced communications with respect to two general types of content: (*a*) fear-arousing statements which describe the impending dangers and deprivations in sufficient detail so as to evoke a vivid mental rehearsal of what the crisis situations will actually be like, thus reducing the chances that subsequent adverse events will be frighteningly ambiguous or surprising; and (*b*) fear-reducing statements which describe realistically the favorable or mitigating aspects of the threat situation, calling the person's attention to the ways the authority figures will help him and to the things he can do for himself.

Moderate Anticipatory Fear

Preoperative Behavior*

Surgical patients with a *moderate* degree of anticipatory fear have minor symptoms of emotional tension but do not display outbursts of acute, paniclike apprehensiveness. They appear to be "part-time worriers," occasionally preoccupied with fretful forebodings but quite capable of suppressing disquieting thoughts about the dire crises that may be in store for them. At night they sometimes suffer from insomnia but usually respond well to a mild dose of a sedative. During the day, their outward manner is relatively calm and well-controlled, punctuated only infrequently by visible signs of inner agitation. These patients generally engage in their usual daily tasks and recreational activities, if circumstances allow them to do so; but they are likely to become restless from time to time. Their work efficiency is occasionally reduced as a result of sporadic episodes of heightened uneasiness, usually precipitated by external signs which remind them of the grim events ahead.

Postoperative Behavior†

Although they appear to be experiencing just as much postoperative pain and deprivation as those in the other two groups, the patients in the moderate fear group show a relative absence of emotional disturbance throughout the entire recovery period. Rarely, if ever, do these patients display any overt signs of resentful attitudes, anger, depression, or apprehensiveness during their convalescence. Many of them are regarded as "model" patients by the hospital staff because they are so affable, cooperative, and conscientious. They generally conform uncomplainingly to all authoritative demands.

Reassurance Mechanisms‡

During the preoperative period, patients in the moderate fear group generally ask for and pay attention to information about the nature of

* See pp. 278–279; 304–308; and 314–321.
† See pp. 255–258; 274–301; 315–325; and 360–367.
‡ See pp. 304–335.

their impending surgical experiences. They use the information available to them to develop a set of reassuring concepts which take into account some of the objective characteristics of the dangers and deprivations to which they will be exposed. Their reassuring concepts frequently include references to mitigating features of the stress situation, focusing especially on the skill and availability of the surgeon and other members of the hospital staff who are regarded as protective authority figures. In arriving at these reassuring notions, the patients seem first to have a few disquieting fantasies about being physically helpless and being at the mercy of the powerful authority figures who may inflict hazardous procedures or withhold essential aid. Their imaginative rehearsal of these and other potential dangers leads them to counteract the frightening features of the impending stress situation by arriving at plausible fear-reducing anticipations to the effect that: The authorities have genuinely benign intentions; effective aid will be available; the intensity and duration of pain will be within tolerable limits; and some compensatory gains or rewards will ensue from undergoing suffering. Thus, as a result of taking account of available information and "working through" the impending dangers in advance, the patients develop some reality-tested reassurances. Such reassurances continue to function effectively in warding off disturbing feelings of helplessness when the objective stress situation actually materializes.

Major Causal Factors*

Persons who react with a moderate level of anticipatory fear are less likely to have a history of psychoneurotic disorder than those who react with low or high anticipatory fear. They appear to be normal personalities whose emotions are highly responsive to external stimulation. Thus, when facing a threat of body damage, their level of anticipatory fear is markedly influenced by the information available to them. The mere knowledge that an operation is scheduled may produce very little fear in such persons if they are led to believe that it is a safe, routinized procedure; but additional information about the temporarily distressing effects of the surgery will tend to increase anticipatory fear to a moderate level. The arousal of anticipatory fear plays a causal role in the development of psychological stamina because, when the person pictures himself in the danger situation, blanket immunity con-

* See pp. 304–327; 354–367; and 388–392.

cepts are recognized to be inadequate and lose their capacity to reduce emotional tension; the person then seeks to discover more convincing sources of reassurance which take into account objective features of the danger situation. The learning process whereby blanket immunity concepts are gradually replaced by a more effective set of danger-contingent reassurances tends to be facilitated when the person is given concrete information concerning: (*a*) the nature of the potential dangers; (*b*) how the dangers can be surmounted; and (*c*) the mitigating or protective features of the environment.

Problems of Psychological Preparation*

Although surgical patients in the moderate fear group develop more adequate defenses for coping with the crisis phases than those in the low or high fear groups, their psychological preparation may, nevertheless, be incomplete in various ways. During the postoperative period, isolated episodes of fright or emotional agitation occasionally occur among patients in this group, despite the fact that they are reasonably well prepared for the main sources of stress. Disruptive episodes seem to occur mainly when there is a gap in the patient's knowledge about postoperative occurrences (e.g., the patient may be surprised to find that he is required to swallow a stomach tube shortly after awakening from the anesthetic). Thus, systematic efforts to give comprehensive information covering as many distressing events as possible may have the effect of minimizing the subsequent occurrence of fright reactions within the moderate fear group.

In addition to personal somatic experiences of suffering and discomfort, there are numerous other unpleasant events which should be mentally rehearsed beforehand. For example, unless specifically informed in advance, a naive surgical patient is apt to become upset and temporarily demoralized by the "gruesome" sights and sounds of mutilation or agony among other patients on the surgical ward. A subsidiary goal of psychological preparation may be that of building up tolerance for the large series of ambiguous, annoying, and mildly threatening events that occur every day during the recovery period. Thus, it may be useful to let the patient know beforehand about various minor discomforts, restrictions of movement, and unfamiliar body sensations which he will experience during convalescence, even though none

* See pp. 354–367; and 385–388.

of these occurrences are apt to be acutely frightening or severely frustrating. There are some indications that even when stressful events are only mildly unpleasant, if there is a large *accumulation* occurring unexpectedly, the patient tends to lose confidence in the protective capabilities of the danger-control authorities. At the same time, he may find his own psychological capacity for controlling emotional behavior gradually diminishing with each new onslaught of unexpected stimulation. Hence, the lower the incidence of minor surprises, the higher the chances of being able to ward off overwhelming fright or aggrievement when a major danger episode occurs.

However, if vivid descriptions are given of a large variety of potentially frightening and distressing stimuli, the person may develop an exaggerated, anxiety-laden conception of the danger situation which interferes with the normal work of worrying. Accordingly, it may be essential to present the fear-arousing material in small doses, and also to encourage the patient to ventilate his fears so as to devise supplementary communications which will help to correct his mistaken notions about the extent to which he might be victimized.

Since a person's stress tolerance depends to a considerable degree upon his ability to maintain high confidence in protective authority figures, preparatory communications could present some additional contents especially for this purpose. In this connection, it has been suggested that confidence may be fostered whenever a representative of the authorities makes a series of correct predictions, even if they refer to relatively unimportant events. Thus, the communications designed for the psychological preparation of patients may be more effective if they include, along with statements about the major and minor unpleasant occurrences that are to be anticipated, a series of predictions concerning relatively neutral aspects of the daily convalescent routines. In a new environment, such predictions may have an especially reassuring effect by reducing the ambiguity of unfamiliar stimuli and, at the same time, fostering the view that the seemingly strange things which happen are well understood by the authorities.

In general, the "work of worrying" in surgical patients is facilitated by information which conveys a concrete picture of what the patient will himself *perceive*. There is probably little gain from didactic explanations of the nature of surgical procedures or from comments about those surgical risks which will not be directly perceived by the patient. Such material may do more harm than good, and probably should be omitted, except when specifically needed to clear up a patient's misconceptions about what is going to happen.

High Anticipatory Fear

Preoperative Behavior*

Surgical patients with high anticipatory fear display overt symptoms of sustained emotional tension with occasional outbursts or affect spells characterized by trembling, flushing, and agitated weeping. Throughout the day, they are markedly restless and have difficulty concentrating on normal activities; at night they complain about insomnia or other sleep disturbances, and usually require relatively heavy sedation. These patients report feeling continually "jittery" or "nervous" about the impending operation. Sometimes the intense motivation to escape from the threatening situation breaks through into overt action, as when a hyperanxious patient seeks to postpone or cancel the scheduled operation, or actually leaves the hospital against medical advice.

Postoperative Behavior†

Patients with a high level of fear before the operation continue to display a relatively high level of fear after the operation. According to their own reports, they frequently feel apprehensive during the convalescent period, lack confidence about fully recovering from the operation, and are often preoccupied with reminiscences of one or another event that distressed or frightened them. Nevertheless, their attitudes toward the hospital staff tend to be extremely positive and they frequently express gratitude and admiration. These patients make strong efforts to be in frequent contact with members of the hospital staff and to obtain their attention. They also make a strong effort to comply with the demands made upon them in connection with routine convalescent procedures. However, from time to time, they involuntarily delay the administration of injections and other such treatments because of their intense fear of being injured. In general, their convalescence is characterized by friendly and cooperative relationships with physicians and nurses, punctuated by occasional disruptive incidents, stemming from the patient's excessive timidity or hypochondriacal attitudes.

* See pp. 239–243; 304–308; and 326–327.

† See pp. 240–243; 255–258; 277–301; and 371–374.

Reassurance Mechanisms*

Surgical patients with high anticipatory fear make repeated efforts to gain reassurance, but are unsuccessful at putting aside frightening anticipations of being mutilated or killed by the operation. They seem to be more likely than others to make deliberate efforts to: (*a*) engage in distracting mental activities; (*b*) think about the personal gains that will ensue from undergoing the ordeals of surgery; and (*c*) adopt an attitude of resignation or fatalism. But none of these self-initiated efforts at reducing fear are successful for more than a very short period, and the patients repeatedly turn to authority figures for emotional support. They ask many questions about what will happen to them but, even when given highly optimistic answers, their emotional relief is short-lived. It appears that whether the reassurances come from others or are self-delivered, these patients cannot sustain a conception of themselves as being safe and physically intact; any optimistic picture of the future is rapidly replaced by an involuntary image of being helpless and overwhelmed by catastrophic danger. When contemplating the implications of undergoing surgery, these patients are much more likely than others to dwell upon improbable dangers—such as the possibility that the surgeon's knife may make a fatal slip—which appear to be the product of inner conflicts. Thus, although strongly motivated to build up reassuring concepts beforehand, these patients enter into the postoperative phase without any highly effective defenses with which to reduce their emotional tension. They have a low capacity for gaining reassurance when they encounter frightening stimuli during the postoperative period, just as during the preoperative period.

Major Causal Factors†

The most important single factor in accounting for extremely high preoperative and postoperative fear appears to be a chronic psychoneurotic predisposition. The case history data available for a small sample of patients in this group suggest that, prior to the present hospitalization, most of these individuals had suffered from severe neurotic symptoms, including acute anxiety reactions in response to a variety of major and minor danger experiences in the past. Thus the excessive apprehensiveness and timidity displayed before the operation and then

* See pp. 304–308; 326–327; and 330–335.

† See pp. 243–250; 280–285; 354–360; and 388–392.

again afterwards may be attributable to an underlying neurotic predisposition.

The basic predisposition to overreact to surgery is probably not present in all chronic psychoneurotics, but, rather, may be limited to those for whom threats of body damage arouse certain types of intense psychosexual conflicts. The unconscious symbolic significance of the threat may be either of a castration punishment or of a temptation to satisfy latent masochistic strivings. The anticipated dangers of surgery are symbolically elaborated in the patients' horror fantasies of being mutilated or annihilated, which they know are irrational, but which they cannot dispel. Thus, the fact that repressed inner dangers are touched off by the external threat may be responsible for preventing the person from gaining any effective reassurances from factual knowledge about protective features of the environmental situation, and may also account for the person's subsequent inability to correct his exaggerated fears, despite favorable opportunities for emotional relearning provided by successful surgical experiences.

In a minority of patients in the high fear group, the overreactive tendency may be very narrowly confined to only one specific type of threat which happens to resemble a past traumatizing situation; in such instances, the predispositional factor may involve a special vulnerability which does not necessarily imply a chronic neurotic disorder.

Because of the predominance of one or another type of predispositional factor, variations in situational factors play only a limited or subsidiary role as determinants of a high level of fear. Nevertheless, certain features of the threat situation appear to influence the over-all incidence of high fear reactions. Surgical operations are more likely to evoke a sustained high level of fear if the patient knows that: (*a*) the risk of suffering pain, permanent injury, or death is relatively high rather than low; and (*b*) the incision will be near the genital region rather than in the upper part of the abdomen or the chest. Cognitive factors involving detailed knowledge about the potential complications and risks of surgery may also augment the chances of intractible fear reactions. However, the majority of patients in the high fear group tend to be relatively uninfluenced by the authoritative information they are given. Although preoperative information was found to be related to the relative incidence of moderate as against low fear, such information did not have any relationship to the incidence of high fear. Thus, it appears that once a person is aware of the fact that he is required to have a certain type of operation, further information about the nature of the surgical situation probably plays only a small causal role, if any, in determining whether or not he will react with an excessively high level of fear.

Problems of Psychological Preparation*

For excessively fearful persons, the central problem is not that of stimulating the work of worrying but, rather, of reducing emotional excitement to a moderate level so that the work of worrying can be carried out more effectively and brought to successful completion. When a very high level of anticipatory fear persists it implies an inability to develop adequate inner defenses with which to cope with the situation; the person remains in a state of hypervigilance, involving a loss of mental efficiency, lowering of reality-testing capacities, and reduced tolerance for subsequent stress.

In some cases, excessive fear may be evoked primarily because of misleading information or cognitive errors concerning the severity and magnitude of the impending danger. Whenever misinformation plays a major role, the disruptive effects of acute anticipatory fear may be somewhat lessened by means of corrective communications which convey a realistic and concrete picture of the danger situation, with special emphasis on those positive features and protective resources that warrant a more optimistic attitude concerning the chances of surviving intact. However, such information is probably of little value for the majority of high fear cases who react to anticipated surgery and to other external threat situations with paniclike affect spells, severe hypochondria, phobic avoidance reactions, obsessional ruminations about anticipated catastrophe, or related types of acute anxiety symptoms. In so far as these psychoneurotic reactions are attributable to repressed psychosexual conflicts, surgical patients who display such symptoms during the preoperative period cannot be expected to benefit very much from any program of psychological preparation on the part of professional counselors, unless some form of therapy can be included to decrease the pathogenic influence of repressed sources of fear. Perhaps a brief form of psychological treatment can be developed which will help the overreactive patient to gain emotional control by confining his neurotic fantasies to other spheres; so that, even though the underlying neurosis is not "cured," it encroaches to a lesser extent upon his apperception of surgical experiences and no longer blocks so completely the development of reality-based reassurances.

In many normal persons, certain types of information about impending dangers may be capable of evoking excessive fear reactions, i.e.,

* See pp. 243–250; 370–374; and 385–393.

when frightening events are depicted which stimulate fantasies associated with repressed conflicts or which reactivate memories of past traumatic experiences. It may be necessary, therefore, to design preparatory communications for surgical patients in such a way as to avoid giving overdoses of fear-arousing material, especially by eliminating those horror elements which lend themselves most readily to autistic, anxiety-arousing elaborations. This is one reason why preparatory communications should be carefully pretested with a pilot group and rigorously assessed by means of systematic research studies.

The above summary, which emphasizes the major differences between low, moderate, and high anticipatory fear groups, should not be construed as an attempt to formulate a typology. Anticipatory fear, like any other emotional response, should be conceptualized as a continuum ranging from zero intensity to very high intensity. The characteristics specified for each group should, therefore, be regarded as behavioral tendencies or trends that predominate within a given region of the continuum. On every aspect of postoperative adjustment, it was observed that the three groups showed considerable overlap; hence any predictions based on the level of anticipatory fear must be expected to have a wide margin of error. The most that can be claimed for any of the observed relationships between preoperative and postoperative behavior is that they may enable one to predict significantly better than chance.

It must be emphasized once again that all the conclusions pertaining to the behavioral sequelae of different levels of anticipatory fear are based on observations of how people react to one particular type of stress situation. Consequently, it remains an open question whether the same conclusions will prove to be applicable to other types of dangers and deprivations. When a person is facing the stresses of major surgery, many of his emotional reactions, fantasies, and psychological defenses may be influenced by the realization that the danger situation is one which requires passive submission to a direct medical assault at the hands of an authority figure who will cut an opening with his knife and remove something from inside the body. Quite different subjective reactions may be evoked in other physical danger situations, such as those encountered in military combat where a person is expected to participate actively in concerted aggressive action with others who are exposed to a common danger emanating from a malignant enemy; or in a peacetime disaster where the threat emanates from an impersonal natural force, and the most adaptive response may be to flee from the site of danger. But despite all the important psychological differences that may differentiate surgery from other kinds of physical danger situations, it seems probable that there are some general features of stress behavior which regularly occur in all of them. Marked individual differences in the level of anticipatory fear, comparable to those observed in the present study of surgical patients, have been noted in many situations involving a threat of body damage, whether the source of danger is an occupational hazard, an epidemic, a wartime bombing attack, or any other type of disaster. In some of these situations, it should prove to be quite feasible to reinvestigate the above hypotheses derived from the study of surgical patients in order to determine whether the level of anticipatory fear regularly bears the same relationships to subsequent stress behavior.

If the present tentative findings are replicated in other situations of physical danger, the next step will be to conduct further tests of their generality by studying the sequelae of anticipatory fear among persons exposed to threats of defamation, ostracism, loss of status, and other dangers that are purely social in character. Until such studies are carried out, no definite answers can be given as to which of the above hypotheses, if any, hold true for all types of fear-arousing events, and which ones require specifications of limiting conditions. It seems probable, however, that even if many of the specific conclusions prove to be erroneous or of limited applicability, some of the main variables and constructs defined in the present study will turn out to have heuristic value for investigating a wide variety of stress-induced reactions and for developing a general theory of stress behavior. It was with the latter goal in mind that the author devoted a considerable amount of space to discussing the "work of worrying" and the learning processes that are involved when wishful anticipations of blanket immunity are replaced by reality-oriented anticipations of partial immunity. In these discussions a number of general theoretical assumptions and concepts have been introduced which may prove to have broad implications for understanding the psychodynamics of human adjustment under many different conditions of threat and danger.

Bibliography

Abraham, K., 1920a, The narcissistic evaluation of excretory processes in dreams and neurosis. (Trans. by D. Bryan and J. Strachey, 1942.) *Selected Papers.* London: Hogarth Press.

Abraham, K., 1920b, Manifestations of the female castration complex. (Trans. by D. Bryan and J. Strachey, 1942.) *Selected Papers.* London: Hogarth Press.

Abraham, K., 1924, A short study of the development of the libido, viewed in the light of mental disorders. (Trans. by D. Bryan and J. Strachey, 1942.) *Selected Papers.* London: Hogarth Press.

Adler, A., 1943, Neuropsychiatric complications in victims of Boston's Cocoanut Grove disaster. *J. Amer. med. Assoc.*, **123**, 1098–1101.

Affleck, J., 1948, Psychiatric disorders among the chronic sick in hospital. *J. mental Sci.*, **94**, 33–45.

Alexander, F., 1942, *Our Age of Unreason.* New York: Lippincott.

Alexander, F., 1955, On the psychodynamics of regressive phenomena in panic states. *Psychoanalysis and the Social Sciences*, IV. New York: International Universities Press, 104–110.

Allport, G., J. Bruner, and E. Jandorf, 1948, Personality under social catastrophe. *Personality in Nature, Society, and Culture*, C. Kluckhohn and H. Murray (Eds.). New York: Knopf.

Allport, G., and L. Postman, 1947, *The Psychology of Rumor.* New York: Henry Holt.

Anderson, C., 1944, On certain conscious and unconscious homosexual responses to warfare. *Brit. J. med. Psychol.*, **20**, 161–174.

Arnold, M., 1942, A study of tension in relation to breakdown. *J. gen. Psychol.*, **26**, 315–346.

Arntzen, F., 1948, Psychological observations of prisoners of war. *Amer. J. Psychiat.*, **104**, 446–447.

Arp, A., and L. Arp, 1940, Surgery in mentally ill. *J. Internat. Coll. Surgeons*, **3**, 519–523.

Arsenian, J., 1943, Young children in an insecure situation. *J. abnorm. soc. Psychol.*, **38**, 225–249.

Auld, F., and E. Murray, 1955, Content analysis studies of psychotherapy. *Psychol. Bull.*, **52**, 377–395.

Bainbridge, W., 1930, Consideration of psychic factors in surgical diagnosis and procedure. *Psychiat. Quart.*, **4**, 414–424.

Ballard, S., and H. Miller, 1944, Neuropsychiatry at a Royal Air Force center: Analysis of 2000 cases. *Brit. med. J.*, **2**, 40–43.

Bard, M., 1952, Sequence of emotional reactions in radical mastectomy. *Public Health Repts.*, **67**, No. 11.

Barker, R., B. Wright, and M. Gonick, 1946, Adjustment to physical handicap in illness: A survey of the social psychology of physique and disability. *Bulletin* **55.** New York: Soc. Sci. Res. Council.

Barnett, J., 1946, Psychosomatic aspects of problem cases in medicine and surgery. *J. med. Assoc. Georgia*, **35**, 250–256.

Basowitz, H., H. Persky, S. Korchin, and R. Grinker, 1955, *Anxiety and Stress.* New York: McGraw-Hill.

Bassan, M., 1947, Some factors found valuable in maintaining morale on a small ship. *Bull. Menninger Clin.*, **11**, 33–42.

Beier, E., 1951, The effect of induced anxiety on flexibility of intellectual functioning. *Psychol. monogr.*, **65**, No. 9.

Bellak, L., 1950, Psychiatric aspects of tuberculosis. *Social Casework*, **31**, 183–189.

Bender, L., and J. Frosch, 1942, Children's reaction to the war. *Amer. J. Orthopsychiat.*, **12**, 571–586.

Benedek, T., 1948, *Insight and Personality Adjustment: A Study of the Psychological Effects of War.* New York: Ronald Press.

Benjamin, J., 1950, Methodological considerations in the validation and elaboration of psychoanalytic personality theory. *Amer. J. Orthopsychiat.*, **20**, 139–155.

Bernstein, S., and S. Small, 1951, Psychodynamic factors in surgery. *J. Mt. Sinai Hosp.*, **17**, 938–958.

Bettelheim, B., 1943, Individual and mass behavior in extreme situations. *J. abnorm. soc. Psych.*, **38**, 417–452.

Bibring, E., 1953, The mechanism of depression. *Affective Disorders*, P. Greenacre (Ed.). New York: International Universities Press, 13–46.

Bion, W., 1940, The "War of Nerves": Civilian reaction, morale and prophylaxis. *The Neuroses in War*, E. Miller (Ed.) New York: Macmillan, Ch. 10, 180–200.

Bitterman, M., and C. Kniffin, 1953, Manifest anxiety and perceptual defense. *J. abnorm. soc. Psychol.*, **48**, 248–252.

Blain, D., 1950, Psychologic aspects of cancer problem. *Trans. Am. clin. climatol. Assoc.*, **61**, 229–238.

Blanton, S., and V. Kirk, 1947, A psychiatric study of sixty-one appendectomy cases. *Ann. Surg.*, **126**, 305–314.

Bonaparte, M., 1945, Notes on the analytic discovery of a primal scene. *Psychoanalytic Study of the Child*, Vol. I. New York: International Universities Press, 119–127.

Bond, D., 1952, *The Love and Fear of Flying*. New York: International Universities Press.

Bond, D., 1953, The common psychological defenses to stressful situations and the patterns of breakdown when they fail. *Symposium on Stress*. Washington: National Research Council and Walter Reed Army Medical Center, 142–153.

Bondy, C., 1943, Problems of internment camps. *J. abnorm. soc. Psychol.*, **38**, 453–475.

Bornstein, B., 1949, The analysis of a phobic child: Some problems of theory and technique in child analysis. *Psychoanalytic Study of the Child*, Vols. III–IV. New York: International Universities Press.

Bowers, W., 1943, Hysteria and malingering on surgical service. *Military Surgeon*, **92**, 506–511.

Braatoy, T., 1954, *Fundamentals of Psychoanalytic Technique*. New York: John Wiley and Sons.

Brierly, M., 1951, *Trends in Psychoanalysis*. London: Hogarth Press.

Brody, S., 1956, Psychological factors associated with disseminated lupus erythematosus and effects of cortisone and ACTH. *Psychiat. Quart.*, **30**, 44–60.

Bromberg, W., and P. Schilder, 1933, Death and dying. *Psychoanal. Rev.*, **20**, 133–185.

Brosin, H., 1953, The reciprocal relations between incentives, motivation and strain in acute and chronic stressful situations. *Symposium on Stress*. Washington: National Research Council and Walter Reed Army Medical Center, 209–221.

Brown, F., 1941, Civilian psychiatric air-raid casualties. *Lancet*, **1**, 686–691.

Brownlee, A., 1931, Disasters and disaster relief. *Encyclopaedia of the Social Sciences*, Vol. 5, New York: Macmillan, 161–166.

Bruner, J., 1951, Personality dynamics and the process of perceiving. *Perception: An Approach to Personality*, R. Blake, and G. Ramsey (Eds.). New York: Ronald Press, 121–147.

Bruner, J., and L. Postman, 1949, Perception, cognition and behavior. *J. Pers.*, **18**, 14–31.

Brunswik, E., 1952, The conceptual framework of psychology. *International Encyclopaedia of Unified Science*, Vol. I, No. 10. Chicago: University of Chicago Press.

Burgum, M., 1944, The fear of explosion. *Amer. J. Orthopsychiat.*, **14**, 349–357.

Burt, C., 1940, Neurotic symptoms among evacuated children. *Brit. J. educ. Psychol.*, **10**, 8–16.

Bychowski, G., 1944, Personality changes characterizing the transition from civilian to military life. *J. nerv. ment. Disease*, **100**, 289–296.

Cannon, I., 1935, Social and personal problems of surgical patients. *Bull. Amer. Hosp. Assoc.*, **9**, 34–39.

Cantril, H., 1940, *The Invasion From Mars*. Princeton: Princeton University Press.

Cantril, H., 1943, The causes and control of riot and panic. *Public Opinion Quart.*, **7**, 669–679.

Caplan, G., 1951, Mental-hygiene work with expectant mothers. *Ment. Hyg.*, **35**, 41–50.

Carr, L., 1933, Disaster and the sequence-pattern concept of social change. *Amer. J. Sociol.*, **38**, 207–218.

Caudill, W., 1953, Cultural perspectives on stress. *Symposium on Stress*. Washington: National Research Council and Walter Reed Army Medical Center, 194–208.

Clothier, F., 1941, Some thoughts on the psychology of postoperative convalescence. *Diseases of the Nervous System*, **2**, 266–270.

Cobb, B., R. Clark, M. Carson, and C. Howe, 1954, Patient-responsible delay of treatment in cancer. *Cancer*, **7**, 920–926.

Cobb, S., and E. Lindemann, 1943, Neuropsychiatric observations (following the Cocoanut Grove fire). *Ann. Surg.*, **117**, 814–824.

Cohen, R., and J. Delanos, 1945, Subacute emotional disturbances induced in combat. *War Med.*, **7**, 284–296.

Committee on Disaster Studies, 1955, *Some Selected Observations and Case Materials on Psychological and Emotional Reactions to Disaster.* Document prepared for the Conference on Theories of Human Behavior in Extreme Situations. (Mimeo.)

Cooper, E., and M. Jahoda, 1947, The evasion of propaganda: How prejudiced people respond to anti-prejudice propaganda. *J. Psychol.*, **23**, 15–25.

Coriat, I., 1946, Dental anxiety: Fear of going to the dentist. *Psychoanal. Rev.*, **33**, 365–367.

Cottrell, L., 1946, Understanding the adolescent: The adolescent and his emotional reaction to illness. *Amer. J. Nurs.*, **46**, 181–183.

Coverdale, H., 1945, Hysteria in ophthalmology: Experiences with New Zealand troops in the Middle East. *Brit. J. of Ophthalmol.*, **29**, 120–124.

Cowen, E., and E. Beier, 1950, The influence of threat-expectancy on perception. *J. Pers.*, **19**, 85–94.

Cowen, E., 1952, Stress reduction and problem solving rigidity. *J. consult. Psychol.*, **16**, 425–428.

Cramond, W., and D. Aberd, 1954, Psychological aspects of uterine dysfunction. *Lancet*, **2**, 1241–1245.

Crolin, B., 1935, Psychic effects of abdominal trauma. *Med. Clin. North Amer.*, **19**, 837–845.

Culpin, M., 1940, Mode of onset of the neuroses in war. *The Neuroses in War*, E. Miller (Ed.). New York: Macmillan, Ch. 2, 33–54.

Davis, S., 1956, Stress in combat. *Sci. American*, **194**, 31–35.

Deese, J., R. Lazarus, and J. Keenan, 1953, Anxiety, anxiety reduction, and stress in learning. *J. exp. Psychol.*, **46**, 55–60.

Deutsch, H., 1942, Some psychoanalytic observations in surgery. *Psychosomat. Med.*, **4**, 105–115.

Deutsch, H., 1945, *Psychology of Women*, Vol. II. New York: Grune & Stratton.

Deutsch, M., 1954, Field theory in social psychology. *Handbook of Social Psychology*, G. Lindzey (Ed.). Cambridge: Addison-Wesley.

Diamond, B., and A. Ross, 1945, Emotional adjustment of newly blinded soldiers. *Amer. J. Psychiat.*, **102**, 367–371.

Diethelm, O., and M. Jones, 1947, Influence of anxiety on attention, learning, retention, and thinking. *Arch. Neurol. Psychiat.*, **58**, 325–336.

Diethelm, O., 1949, The evaluation of a psychiatric examination. *Amer. J. Psychiat.*, **105**, 606–611.

Diggory, J., 1956, Some consequences of proximity to a disease threat. *Sociometry*, **19**, 47–53.

Dollard, J., 1938, The life history in community studies. *Amer. sociol. Rev.*, **3**, 724–737.

Dollard, J., and F. Auld, 1955, *Development of Quantitative Methods for Detailed Study of Psychotherapy Hours.* Report on Project M-648, U. S. Public Health Service Grant. (Mimeo.)

Dollard, J., and N. Miller, 1950, *Personality and Psychotherapy.* New York: McGraw-Hill.

Dollard, J., L. Doob, N. Miller, and R. Sears, 1939, *Frustration and Aggression.* New Haven: Yale University Press.

Drayer, C., 1952, Relation of civilian and military psychiatry in crisis situations. *Amer. J. Psychiat.*, **109**, 259–261.

Duke-Elder, P., and E. Wittkower, 1946, Psychologic reactions in soldiers to loss of vision of one eye, and their treatment. *Brit. med. J.*, **1**, 155–158.

Dunbar, F., 1934, Physical mental relationships in illness: Trends in modern medicine and research as related to psychiatry. *Amer. J. Psychiat.*, **91**, 541–562.

Dunbar, F., 1942, Symposium on social psychiatry: Relationship between anxiety states and organic disease. *Clinics*, **1**, 879–908.

Ebaugh, F., 1937, Psychiatric complications in surgery. *Bull. Amer. Coll. Surgeons*, **22**, 153–158.

Ebaugh, F., 1939, Psychiatrist in relation to surgery. *Surg., Gynecol. Obstet.*, **68**, 372–376.

Edelston, A., 1943, Separation anxiety in young children. *Genet. Psychol. Monogr.*, **28**, No. 1, 3–95.

Eliot, T., 1943, —of the shadow of death. *Ann. Amer. Acad. polit. soc. Sci.*, **229**, 87–99.

Ellis, A., 1956, An operational reformulation of some of the basic principles of psychoanalysis. *The Foundations of Science and the Concepts of Psychology and Psychoanalysis*, H. Feigl and M. Scriven (Eds.). Minneapolis: University of Minnesota Press, 131–154.

Engel, M., 1947, Reactions to injury. *Nova Scotia med. Bull.*, **26**, 154–159.

English, H., 1937, Symbolic versus functional equivalents in neurosis of deprivation. *J. abnorm. soc. Psychol.*, **32**, 392–394.

English, O., and G. Pearson, 1945, *Emotional Problems of Living.* New York: W. W. Norton.

Erickson, E., 1950, *Childhood and Society.* New York: W. W. Norton.

Escalona, S., 1952, Problems in psycho-analytic research. *Intern. J. Psychoanal.*, **33**, 1–11.

Fahrenkamp, K., 1931, *Der Herzkranke.* Leipzig: Hippokrates-Verlag.

Fahrni, G., 1951, Factors minimizing reaction to operative procedures. *Can. med. Assoc. J.*, **64**, 500–502.

Fairbairn, W., 1936, The effect of the King's death upon patients under analysis. *Intern. J. Psychoanal.*, **17**, 278–284.

Farber, I., 1954, Anxiety as a drive state. *Nebraska Symposium on Motivation.* Lincoln: Nebraska University Press, 1–46.

Federn, P., 1952, *Ego Psychology and the Psychoses.* New York: Basic Books.

Feiling, A., 1937, Nervous and mental postoperative complications. *Practitioner*, **138**, 259–268.

Fenichel, O., 1939a, Trophy and triumph. (Trans. by D. Rapaport and Hanna Fenichel.) *The Collected Papers of Otto Fenichel*, Second Series, 1954. New York: W. W. Norton, 141–162.

Fenichel, O., 1939b, The counter-phobic attitude. *Intern. J. Psychoanal.*, **20**, 263–274.

Fenichel, O., 1941, *Problems of Psychoanalytic Technique.* (Trans. by D. Brunswik.) Albany, New York: The Psychoanalytic Quarterly.

Fenichel, O., 1944, Psychoanalytic remarks on Fromm's *Escape from Freedom. Psychoanal. Rev.*, **31**, 133–152.

Fenichel, O., 1945, *The Psychoanalytic Theory of Neurosis.* New York: W. W. Norton.

Ferenczi, S., 1912, Transitory symptom-constructions during the analysis. *Sex in Psychoanalysis.* Boston: Badger, 1916.

Ferenczi, S., 1917, Two types of war neuroses. (Trans. by J. I. Suttee.) *Further Contributions to the Theory and Technique of Psycho-Analysis.* London: Hogarth Press.

Ferraro A., 1948, Somato-psychic factors in anxiety neurosis. *J. nerv. ment. Dis.*, **107**, 228–242.

Fessler, L., 1931, Psychogene Potenzstörungen nach urologischen Operationen. *Z. für ärztliche Psychoanalyse*, **17**, 125–140.

Ficarra, B. J., 1950, Psychic trauma associated with colostomy. *Geriatrics*, **5**, 219–221.

Flugel, J., 1939, Examination as initiation rite and anxiety situation. *Intern. J. Psychoanal.*, **20**, 275–286.

Flugel, J., 1945, *Man, Morals and Society.* New York: International Universities Press.

Frank, J., 1946, Emotional reactions of American soldiers to an unfamiliar disease. *Amer. J. Psychiat.*, **102**, 631–640.

Fraser, R., I. Leslie, and D. Phelps, 1943, Psychiatric effects of severe personal experiences during bombing. *Proc. Roy. Soc. Med.*, **36**, 119–123.

Freedman, L., F. Redlich, L. Eron, and E. Jackson, 1952, Training for childbirth: Remembrance of labor. *Psychosomat. Med.*, **14**, 439–452.

Freeman, G., and J. Pathman, 1942, The relation of overt muscular discharge to physiological recovery from experimentally induced displacement. *J. exp. Psychol.*, **30**, 161–174.

Fremont-Smith, F., 1949, Discussion of the paper by Jessner and Kaplan. *Problems of Infancy and Childhood.* New York: Josiah Macy Jr. Foundation, 119.

French, J., 1941, The disruption and cohesion of groups. *J. abnorm. soc. Psychol.*, **36**, 361–377.

French, T., 1952, *The Integration of Behavior*, Vol. I. *Basic Postulates.* Chicago: University of Chicago Press.

Frenkel-Brunswik, E., 1949, Intolerance of ambiguity as an emotional and perceptual personality variable. *J. Pers.*, **18**, 108–143.

Frenkel-Brunswik, E., 1954a, Meaning of psychoanalytic concepts and confirmation of psychoanalytic theories. *Sci. Monthly*, **79**, 203–300.

Frenkel-Brunswik, E., 1954b, Psychoanalysis and the unity of science. *Proc. Amer. Acad. Arts Sci.*, **80**, 271–350.

Freud, A., 1936, *The Ego and the Mechanisms of Defense.* (Trans. by C. Baines, 1942.) London: Hogarth Press.

Freud, A., 1953, The bearing of the psychoanalytic theory of instinctual drives on certain aspects of human behavior. *Drives, Affects and Behavior*, R. Lowenstein (Ed.). New York: International Universities Press, 259–277.

Freud, A., and D. Burlingham, 1944, *Infants Without Families.* New York: International Universities Press.

Freud, S., 1904, Freud's psychoanalytic method. (Trans. by J. Bernays, 1940.) *Collected Papers*, Vol. I. London: Hogarth Press.

Freud, S., 1905a, *Wit and Its Relation to the Unconscious.* (Trans. by A. A. Brill, 1938.) *The Basic Writings of Sigmund Freud.* New York: Modern Library.

Freud, S., 1905b, Fragment of an analysis of a case of hysteria. (Trans. by A. Strachey, and J. Strachey, 1943.) *Collected Papers,* Vol. III. London: Hogarth Press.

Freud, S., 1909a, Analysis of a phobia in a five-year-old boy. (Trans. by A. Strachey and J. Strachey, 1943.) *Collected Papers,* Vol. III. London: Hogarth Press.

Freud, S., 1909b, Notes upon a case of obsessional neurosis. (Trans. by A. Strachey, and J. Strachey, 1943.) *Collected Papers,* Vol. III. London: Hogarth Press.

Freud, S., 1910, Psychogenic visual disturbances. (Trans. by E. C. Magne, 1942.) *Collected Papers,* Vol. II. London: Hogarth Press.

Freud, S., 1913, *Totem and Taboo.* (Trans. by A. Brill, 1938.) *The Basic Writings of Sigmund Freud.* New York: Modern Library.

Freud, S., 1914, On narcissism: An introduction. (Trans. by C. M. Baines, 1946.) *Collected Papers,* Vol. IV. London: Hogarth Press.

Freud, S., 1917, Mourning and melancholia. (Trans. by J. Riviere, 1946.) *Collected Papers,* Vol. IV. London: Hogarth Press.

Freud, S., 1918, From the history of an infantile neurosis. (Trans. by A. Strachey, and J. Strachey, 1943.) *Collected Papers.* Vol. III. London: Hogarth Press.

Freud, S., 1919a, Turnings in the ways of psychoanalytic theory. (Trans. by J. Riviere, 1942.) *Collected Papers,* Vol. II. London: Hogarth Press.

Freud, S., 1919b, Psychoanalysis and war neuroses. (Trans. by J. Strachey, 1950.) *Collected Papers,* Vol. V. London: Hogarth Press.

Freud, S., 1920, *Beyond the Pleasure Principle.* (Trans. by J. Strachey, 1950.) New York: Liverwright.

Freud, S., 1921, *Group Psychology and the Analysis of the Ego.* (Trans. by J. Strachey, 1949.) New York: Liverwright.

Freud, S., 1923, Remarks upon the theory and practice of dream interpretation. (Trans. by J. Strachey, 1950.) *Collected Papers,* Vol. V. London: Hogarth Press.

Freud, S., 1930, *The Interpretation of Dreams* (8th Edition). (Trans. by J. Strachey, 1955.) New York: Basic Books.

Freud, S., 1932, Constructions in analysis. (Trans. by J. Strachey, 1952.) *Collected Papers,* Vol. V. London: Hogarth Press.

Freud, S., 1933, *New Introductory Lectures on Psychoanalysis.* (Trans. by W. J. H. Sprott.) New York: W. W. Norton.

Freud, S., 1936, *The Problem of Anxiety.* (Trans. by H. A. Bunker.) New York: W. W. Norton.

Fries, M., 1946, The child's ego development and the training of adults in his environment. *The Psychoanalytic Study of the Child,* **2,** 85–112.

Fritz, C., and E. Marks, 1954, The NORC studies of human behavior in disaster. *J. soc. Issues,* **10,** 26–41.

Fritz, C., and H. Williams, 1957, The human being in disasters: A research perspective. *Ann. Amer. Acad. polit. and soc. Sci.,* **309,** 42–51.

Fromm-Reichmann, F., 1943, Insight into psychotic mechanisms and emergency psychotherapy. *Med. Ann.,* **12,** 107–112.

Garner, H., 1945, Psychiatric casualties in combat. *War Med.,* **8,** 343–357.

Geleerd, E., 1942, Psychiatric care of children in wartime. *Amer. J. Orthopsychiat.,* **12,** 587–594.

Gero, G., 1936, The construction of depression. *Intern. J. Psychoanal.* **17,** 423–461.

Ginsburg, S., 1942, What unemployment does to people. *Amer. J. Psychiat.,* **99,** 439–446.

Girdwood, R., and M. Ballinger, 1949, Factors that commonly worry patients in hospital. *Edinburgh med. J.*, **56**, 247–352.

Glass, A., 1953, Problem of stress in the combat zone. *Symposium on Stress.* Washington: National Research Council and Walter Reed Army Medical Center, 90–102.

Glover, E., 1941, Notes on the psychological effects of war conditions on the civilian population, Part I: The Munich crisis. *Intern. J. Psychoanal.*, **22**, 132–146.

Glover, E., 1942, Notes on the psychological effects of war conditions on the civilian population, Part III: The Blitz. *Intern. J. Psychoanal.*, **23**, 17–37.

Greenson, R., 1949, The psychology of apathy. *Psychoanal. Quart.*, **18**, 290–303.

Grinker, R., 1944, Army Air Forces. *War Psychiatry.* Chicago: *Proc. of the Second Brief Psychotherapy Council*, 6–19.

Grinker, R., and J. Spiegel, 1945a, *Men Under Stress.* Philadelphia: Blakiston.

Grinker, R., and J. Spiegel, 1945b, *War Neuroses.* Philadelphia: Blakiston.

Grinker, R., A. Bradley, A. Fastovsky, and B. Willerman, 1946, A study of psychological predisposition to the development of operational fatigue, I and II. *Amer. J. Orthopsychiat.*, **16**, 191–214.

Gross, A., 1951, The Secret. *Bull. Menninger Clin.*, **15**, 37–44.

Haas, S., 1952, Psychiatric implications of gynecology and obstetrics. *Psychology of Physical Illness*, L. Bellak (Ed.). London: A. Churchill, 90–118.

Hadfield, J., 1940, Treatment by suggestion and hypno-analysis. *The Neuroses in War*, E. Miller (Ed.). New York: Macmillan, Ch. 7, 128–149.

Haggard, E., 1943, Some conditions determining adjustment during and readjustment following experimentally induced stress. *Contemporary Psychopathology.* S. Tomkins (Ed.). Cambridge: Harvard University Press, 529–544.

Haggard, E., 1949, Psychological causes and results of stress. *Human Factors in Undersea Warfare.* National Research Council, pp. 441–461.

Haggard, E., and G. Freeman, 1941, Reactions of children to experimentally induced frustration. *Psychol. Bull.* (abstract), **38**, 581.

Hamburg, D., 1953, Psychological adaptive processes in life-threatening injuries. *Symposium on Stress.* Washington: National Research Council and Walter Reed Army Medical Center.

Hamburg, D., C. Artz, E. Reiss, W. Amspacher, and R. Chambers, 1953, Clinical importance of emotional problems in the care of patients with burns. *New England J. Med.*, **248**, 355.

Hamburg, D., Hamburg, B., and S. de Groza, 1953, Adaptive problems and mechanisms in severely burned patients. *Psychiatry*, **16**, 1–20.

Hamill, R., 1934, Mental factors in traumatic situations, *Internat. J. Med. Surg.*, **47**, 468.

Hammerschlag, E., 1952, Psychology applied to internal medicine. *Psychology of Illness*, L. Bellak (Ed.). London: A. Churchill, 27–44.

Hanfmann, E., 1950, Psychological approaches to the study of anxiety. *Anxiety*, P. Hoch, and J. Zubin (Eds.). New York: Grune & Stratton, 51–67.

Hardy, J., 1951, Changing concepts in supportive therapy of surgical patients. *Penn. med. J.*, **54**, 869–871.

Hargreaves, G., 1940, The differential diagnosis of the psychoneuroses of war. *The Neuroses in War*, E. Miller (Ed.). New York: Macmillan, Ch. 4, 85–104.

Hartmann, H., 1951, Ego psychology and the problem of adaptation. *Organiza-*

tion and Pathology of Thought: Selected Sources (Edit. and trans. by D. Rapaport). New York: Columbia University Press.

Hartmann, H., E. Kris, and R. Lowenstein, 1946, Comments on the formation of psychic structure. *Psychoanalytic Study of the Child*, Vol. II. New York: International Universities Press, 11–38.

Hartmann, H., E. Kris, and R. Lowenstein, 1949, Notes on the theory of aggression. *Psychoanalytic Study of the Child*, Vols. III–IV. New York: International Universities Press, 9–36.

Hastings, D., D. Wright, and B. Glueck, 1944, *Psychiatric Experiences of the Eighth Air Force, First Year of Combat (July 4, 1942–July 4, 1943)*. New York: Josiah Macy Jr. Foundation.

Hebb, D., 1949, *The Organization of Behavior*. New York: John Wiley and Sons.

Hempel, C., 1952, Fundamentals of concept formation in empirical science. *International Encyclopaedia of Unified Science*, Vol. II, No. 7. Chicago: University of Chicago Press.

Hilgard, E., 1952, Experimental approaches to psychoanalysis. *Psychoanalysis as Science*, E. Pumpian-Mindlin (Ed.). Stanford: Stanford University Press, 3–45.

Hill, G., and A. Silver, 1950, Psychodynamic and esthetic motivations for plastic surgery. *Psychosomat. Med.*, **12**, 345–355.

Himmelweit, H., and T. Pear (Eds.), 1950, *Psychological Factors of Peace and War. Frustration and Aggression: A Review of Recent Experimental Work.* London: Hutchinson.

Hitschmann, E., 1948, The history of the aggression-impulse. *The Yearbook of Psychoanalysis*, Vol. 4. London: Imago Publishing Co.

Hoch, P., 1950, Bio-social aspects of anxiety. *Anxiety*, P. Hoch, and J. Zubin (Eds.). New York: Grune & Stratton.

Hogan, B., 1943, Psychiatric observations of Senior Medical Officer on board aircraft carrier U.S.S. "Wasp" during action in combat areas at time of torpedoing, and survivors' actions. *Amer. J. Psychiat.*, **100**, 90–93.

Hogan, R., 1952, A theory of threat and defense. *J. consult. Psychol.*, **16**, 417–424.

Horney, K., 1937, *The Neurotic Personality of Our Time*. New York: W. W. Norton.

Hovland, C., I. Janis, and H. Kelley, 1953, *Communication and Persuasion.* New Haven: Yale University Press.

Huddleson, J., 1932, *Accidents, Neuroses and Compensation.* Baltimore: Williams and Wilkins.

Hudson, B., 1954, Anxiety in response to the unfamiliar. *J. soc. Issues*, **10**, 55–60.

Huschka, M., and O. Ogden, 1938, The conduct of a pediatric prophylaxis clinic. *J. of Pediat.*, **12**, 794–800.

Isaacs, S., 1939, Criteria for interpretation. *Intern. J. Psychoanal.*, **20**, 148–160.

Isaacs, S. (Ed.), 1941, *The Cambridge Evacuation Survey*. London: Methuen.

Jackson, E., 1942, Treatment of the young child in the hospital. *Amer. J. Orthopsychiat.*, **12**, 56–63.

Jackson, K., R. Winkley, O. Faust, E. Germak, and M. Burtt, 1953, Behavior changes indicating emotional trauma in tonsillectomized children. *Pediatrics*, **12**, 23–28.

Jacobson, E., 1946, The effect of disappointment on ego and super-ego formation in normal and depressive development. *Psychoanal. Rev.*, **33**, 129–147.

Jacobson, E., 1953, Contribution to the metapsychology of cyclothymic depression. *Affective Disorders*, Phyllis Greenacre (Ed.). New York: International Universities Press, 49–83.

Jahoda-Lazarsfeld, M., and H. Zeisel, 1932, *Die Arbeitslosen von Marienthal.* Leipzig: Hirzel.

James, W., 1911, *Memories and Studies.* New York: Longmans, Green.

Janis, I., 1943, Meaning and the study of symbolic behavior. *Psychiatry*, **6**, 425–439.

Janis, I., 1945, Psychodynamic aspects of adjustment to army life. *Psychiatry* **8**, 159–176.

Janis, I., 1951, *Air War and Emotional Stress.* New York: McGraw-Hill.

Janis, I., 1954, Problems of theory in the analysis of stress behavior. *J. soc. Issues*, **10**, 12–25.

Janis, I., 1956, Emotional inoculation: Theory and research on the effectiveness of preparatory communications. (Mimeo Report), Yale Communications Research Program. To be published in *Psychoanalysis and the Social Sciences.* New York: International Universities Press. (In press.)

Janis, I., and S. Feshbach, 1953, Effects of fear-arousing communications. *J. abnorm. soc. Psychol.*, **48**, 78–92.

Janis, I., and S. Feshbach, 1954, Personality differences associated with responsiveness to fear-arousing communications. *J. Pers.*, **23**, 154–166.

Javert, C., and J. Hardy, 1950, Measurement of pain intensity in labor and its physiologic, neurologic, and pharmacologic implications. *Amer. J. Obstet. Gynecol.*, **60**, 552.

Jessner, L., and S. Kaplan, 1949, Observations on the emotional reactions of children to tonsillectomy and adenoidectomy. *Problems of Infancy and Childhood.* New York: Josiah Macy Jr. Foundation, 97-117.

Jirasek, A., 1940, Wenn der Kranke nach der Operation nach Hause kommt. *Wien. Med. Wochenschr.*, **90**, 919–924.

John, E., 1941, A study of effects of evacuation and air raids on children of preschool age. *Brit. J. educ. Psychol.*, **11**, 173–182.

Jones, E., 1955, *The Life and Work of Sigmund Freud, Vol. II: Years of Maturity, 1901–1919.* New York: Basic Books.

Kahn, E., et al., 1938, Symposium on anxiety conditions. *J. Conn. State med. Soc.*, **2**, 15–25.

Kaplan, S., 1956, Psychological aspects of cardiac disease (A study of patients experiencing mitral commissurotomy). *Psychosomat. Med.*, **18**, 221–233.

Kardiner, A., 1941, *The Traumatic Neuroses of War.* New York: P. B. Hoeber.

Kardiner, A., and H. Spiegel, 1947, *War Stress and Neurotic Illness.* New York: P. B. Hoeber.

Keats, A., 1956, Postoperative pain: Research and treatment. *J. of chronic Diseases*, **4**, 72–83.

Kennedy, A., 1950, The psychology of the surgical patient. *Brit. med. J.*, **1**, 396–400.

Kennedy, A., 1953, Psychological factors in abdominal surgery. *Management of Abdominal Operations*, R. Maingot (Ed.). New York: Macmillan.

Kennedy, F., 1930, Neuroses following accident. *Bull. N. Y. Acad. Med.*, **6**, 1–17.

Killian, L., 1952, The significance of multiple-group memberships in disaster. *Amer. J. Sociol.*, **57**, 307–314.

Killian, L., 1954, Some accomplishments and some needs in disaster study. *J. soc. Issues*, **10**, 66–72.

Kirk, V., 1949, Anxiety reactions of patients with appendicitis. *Ph.D. Thesis* (unpublished). Chicago: University of Chicago.

Klatskin, E., 1952, An analysis of the effect of the test situation upon the Rorschach record: Formal scoring characteristics. *J. Proj. Tech.*, **16**, 193–199.

Klein, E., 1942, The influence of teachers' and parents' attitudes and behavior upon children in wartime. *Ment. Hyg.*, **26**, 434.

Klein, M., 1952, On the theory of anxiety and guilt. *Developments in Psychoanalysis.* J. Riviere (Ed.). London: Hogarth Press, 271–291.

Kluckhohn, C., 1949, *Mirror For Man.* New York: McGraw-Hill.

Knapp, R., 1944, A psychology of rumor. *Public Opinion Quart.*, **1**, 22–37.

Knight, R., 1953, The present status of organized psychoanalysis in the United States. *J. Amer. Psychoanal. Assoc.*, **1**, 197–221.

Kral, V., 1952, Psychiatric observations under severe chronic stress. *Amer. J. Psychiat.*, **108**, 185–192.

Kris, E., 1941, Morale in Germany. *Amer. J. Sociol.* **47**, 452–461.

Kris, E., 1944, Danger and morale. *Amer. J. Orthopsychiat.*, **14**, 147–156.

Kris, E., 1947, Problems in clinical research. (Round Table, 1946.) *Amer. J. Orthopsychiat.*, **17**, 210–214.

Kris, E., 1952, *Psychoanalytic Explorations in Art.* New York: International Universities Press.

Kris, E., 1956, The recovery of childhood memories in psychoanalysis. *Psychoanalytic Study of the Child,* Vol. XI. New York: International Universities Press.

Kubie, L., 1947, Problems in clinical research (Round Table, 1946). *Amer. J. Orthopsychiat.*, 17, 196–203.

Kubie, L., 1952, Problems and techniques of psychoanalytic validation and progress. *Psychoanalysis as Science.* E. Pumpian-Mindlin (Ed.). Stanford: Stanford University Press, 46–124.

Kupper, H., 1945, Psychic concomitants in wartime injuries. *Psychosomat. Med.*, **7**, 15–21.

Lafler, H., 1906, My sixty sleepless hours. *McClure's,* **27**, 275–281.

Lander, J., 1946, The psychiatrically immunizing effect of combat wounds. *Amer. J. Orthopsychiat.*, **16**, 536–541.

LaPiere, R., 1938, *Collective Behavior.* New York: McGraw-Hill.

Lasswell, H., 1938, A provisional classification of symbol data. *Psychiatry,* **1**, 197–204.

Lasswell, H., 1948, *Power and Personality.* New York: W. W. Norton.

Lawton, G., 1956, *Straight to the Heart.* New York: International Universities Press.

Lazarus, R., J. Deese, S. Osler, 1952, The effects of psychological stress upon performance. *Psychol. Bull.*, **48**, 293–315.

Lazarus, R., N. Lonzo, 1953, The consistency of psychological defenses against threat. *J. abnorm. soc. Psychol.*, **48**, 495–499.

Leavitt, H., 1953, Relationships between conditioned fear patterns and development of anxiety. *Psychoanal. Rev.*, **40**, 27–35.

Lehmann, H., 1952, Stress dynamics in psychiatric perspective. *Psychiatry,* **15**, 387–393.

Leites, N., 1948, Psychocultural hypotheses. *World Politics,* **1**, 102–119.

Levanway, R., 1955, The effect of stress on expressed attitudes towards self and others. *J. abnorm. soc. Psychol.*, **50**, 225–226.

Levy, D., 1945a, Psychic trauma of operations in children and note on combat neurosis. *Amer. J. Diseases Children,* **69**, 7–25.

Levy, D., 1945b, Child patients may suffer psychic trauma after surgery. *Mod. Hosp.*, **65**, 51–52.

Levy, D., 1945c, The war and family life. *Amer. J. Orthopsychiat.*, **15**, 140–152.

Lewin, B., 1950, *The Psychoanalysis of Elation.* New York: W. W. Norton.

Lewin, K., 1935, *A Dynamic Theory of Personality. Selected Papers.* New York: McGraw-Hill.

Lewis, N., and B. Engle, 1954, *Wartime Psychiatry—a Compendium of the International Literature.* New York: Oxford Press.

Liddell, H., 1950, The role of vigilance in the development of animal neurosis. *Anxiety,* (Eds.). P. Hoch, and J. Zubin. New York: Grune & Stratton.

Lidz, T., 1946, Casualties from Guadalcanal: A study of reactions to extreme stress. *Psychiatry,* **9**, 193.

Lidz, T., 1953, Chronic situations evoking psychological stress and the common signs of the resulting strain. *Symposium on Stress.* Washington: National Research Council and Walter Reed Army Medical Center, 116–131.

Lidz, T., and S. Fleck, 1950, Integration of medical and psychiatric methods and objectives on a medical service. *Psychosomat. Med.*, **12**, 103–107.

Liebman, S. (Ed.), 1955, *Stress Situations.* Philadelphia: Lippincott.

Lindemann, E., 1938, Hysteria as problem in general hospital. *Med. Clin. N. Amer.*, **22**, 591–605.

Lindemann, E., 1941, Observations on psychiatric sequelae to surgical operations in women. *Amer. J. Psychiat.*, **98**, 132–139.

Lindemann, E., 1944, Symptomatology and management of acute grief. *Amer. J. Psychiat.*, **101**, 141–146.

Loewenstein, R., 1954, Some remarks on defences, autonomous ego and psychoanalytic technique. *Internat. J. Psychoanal.*, **35**, 188–193.

MacCurdy, J., 1943, *The Structure of Morale.* New York: Macmillan.

Malmo, R., 1950, Experimental studies of mental patients under stress. *Feelings and Emotions,* M. Reymert (Ed.). New York: McGraw-Hill.

Malmo, R., and C. Shagass, 1949a, Physiologic studies of reaction to stress in anxiety and early schizophrenia. *Psychosomat. Med.*, **11**, 9–24.

Malmo, R., and C. Shagass, 1949b, Physiologic study of symptom mechanisms in psychiatric patients under stress. *Psychosomat. Med.*, **11**, 25–29.

Margolin, S., L. Kubie, M. Kanzen, and L. Stone, 1943, Acute emotional disturbances in torpedoed seamen of the Merchant Marine who are continuing at sea. *War Med.*, **3**, 393–408.

Marmor, J., 1958, The psychodynamics of realistic worry. *J. Amer. Psychoanal. Assoc.* (In press.)

Martin, A., 1942, The prevention of panic. *Ment. Hyg.*, **26**, 546–553.

Maskin, M., 1941, Psychodynamic aspects of the war neuroses: A survey of the literature. *Psychiatry,* **4**, 97–115.

Maskin, M., and L. Altman, 1943, Military psychodynamics: Psychological factors in the transition from civilian to soldier. *Psychiatry,* **6**, 263–269.

Maslow, A., 1954, *Motivation and Personality.* New York: Harper.

Maslow, A., and B. Mittelman, 1951, *Principles of Abnormal Psychology.* New York: Harper.

May, R., 1950, *The Meaning of Anxiety,* New York: Ronald Press.

Mayo, C., Jr., 1932, Preoperative preparation and its relation to postoperative complications. *J. Iowa State med. Soc.*, **22**, 73–76.

McClary, A., E. Meyer, and E. Weitsman, Observations on the role of the mechanism of depression in some patients with disseminated lupus erythematosus. *Psychosomat. Med.*, **17**, 311–321.

McClelland, D., 1951, *Personality*. New York: Sloane.

McGraw, R., 1930, Postoperative emotional disorders: Their prevention and management. *Bull. N. Y. Acad. Med*, **6**, 179–188.

McGregor, D., 1938, The major determinants of the prediction of social events. *J. abnorm. soc Psychol.*, **33**, 179–204

McLester, J., 1937, Emotional element in surgical diseases. *Bull. Amer. Coll. Surg.*, **22**, 96–98.

McNeel, B., and T. Darcey, 1945, The personality of the successful soldier. *Amer. J. Psychiat.*, **102**, 337–342.

Menninger, C., 1954a, Psychological aspects of the organism under stress. Part II: Regulatory devices of the ego under major stress. *J. Amer. Psychoanal. Assoc.*, **2**, 280–310.

Menninger, C., 1954b, Regulatory devices of the ego under major stress. *Internat. J. of Psychoanal.*, **35**, 412–420.

Menninger, K., 1934, Polysurgery and polysurgical addiction. *Psychoanal. Quart.*, **3**, 173–199.

Menninger, W., 1946, Modern concepts of war neurosis. *Bull. Menninger Clin.*, **10**, 196–209.

Menninger, W., 1948, *Psychiatry in a Troubled World*. New York: Macmillan.

Menninger, W., 1952, Psychological reactions in an emergency. *Amer. J. Psychiat.*, **109**, 128–130.

Mercier, M., and J. Despert, 1943, Psychological effects of the war on French children. *Psychosomat. Med.*, **5**, 266–272.

Merton, R., and A. Kitt, 1950. Contributions to the theory of reference group behavior. *Continuities in Social Research: Studies in the Scope and Method of "The American Soldier,"* R. Merton and P. Lazarsfeld (Eds.). Glencoe: The Free Press, 40–105.

Michaels, J., 1943, Psychiatric implications of surgery. *The Family*, **23**, 363–369.

Miller, E., A. Wilson, and E. Wittkower, 1940, Clinical case studies and their relationships, including the psychosomatic disorders. *The Neuroses in War*, E. Miller (Ed.). New York: Macmillan, Ch. 3, 55–84.

Miller, H., 1939, Acute psychoses following surgical procedures. *Brit. med. J.*, **1**, 558–559.

Miller, H., and D. Baruch, 1949, Psychosomatic symptoms resulting from the impact of war: Observations in civilian medical practice. *Amer. J. Diseases Children*, **77**, 703–708.

Miller, N., 1944, Experimental studies of conflict. *Personality and Behavior Disorders*, Vol. I, J. McV. Hunt (Ed.). New York: Ronald Press, Ch. 14.

Miller, N., 1951, Comments on theoretical models illustrated by the development of a theory of conflict. *J. Pers.*, **20**, 82–100.

Minski, L., 1942, Psychologic reactions to injury. *Proc. Roy. Soc. Med.*, **35**, 195–199.

Minski, L., 1945, Psychological reactions in the wounded. *Brit. med. J.*, **1**, 444–445.

Mira, E., 1943, *Psychiatry in War*. New York: W. W. Norton.

Mittelman, B., A. Weider, K. Brodman, D. Wechsler, and H. Wolff, 1945, Personality and psychosomatic disturbances in patients on medical and surgical wards: A survey of 450 admissions. *Psychosomat. Med.*, **7**, 220–223.

Moulton, R., 1944, Oral and dental manifestations of anxiety. *Psychiatry*, **18**, 261–273.

Mowrer, O., 1950, Pain, punishment, guilt, and anxiety. *Anxiety*, P. Hoch and J. Zubin (Eds.). New York: Grune & Stratton, 27–40.

Muncie, W., 1934, Postoperative states of excitement. *A. M. A. Arch. Neurol. Psychiat.*, **32**, 681–703.

Murray, H., et al., 1938, *Explorations in Personality*. New York: Oxford University Press.

Musaph, H., 1950, Death instinct, castration complex and depression. (Abstract.) *Dig. of Neurol. Psychiat.*, **18**, 156.

Myers, H., and S. Von Koch, 1945, Reactive depression: A study of 100 consecutive cases. *War Med.*, **8**, 358–364.

Needles, W., 1945, Statistical study of 100 neuro-psychiatric casualties from the Normandy campaign. *Amer. J. Psychiat.*, **102**, 214–221.

Nirembeski, M., 1946, Psychological investigation of a group of internees at Belsen Camp. *J. Ment. Sci.*, **92**, 60–74.

Nunberg, H., 1949, *Problems of Bisexuality as Reflected in Circumcision*. London: Imago.

Ochsner, A., 1950, The importance of psychiatry in surgery. *Dig. of Neurol. Psychiat.*, **18**, 91–96.

Orbach, E., 1948, Psychosomatic aspects of post-traumatic edema and allied states. *Industr. Med.*, **17**, 372–376.

Pardee, I., 1943, Traumatic psychoneuroses versus organic injury: Critical analysis of cases. *Surg. Clin. N. Amer.*, **23**, 589–598.

Parsons, T., 1951, *The Social System*. Glencoe: The Free Press.

Pascales, G., 1933, Préparation des grands motifs aux opérations chirurgicales. *Rév. Gen. Clin. Thérap*, **47**, 263–264.

Pearson, G., 1941, Effect of operative procedures on the emotional life of the child. *Amer. J. Diseases Children*, **64**, 716–729.

Postman, L., and J. Bruner, 1948, Perception under stress. *Psychol. Rev.*, **55**, 314–323.

Powell, J., J. Raynor, and J. Finesinger, 1953, Responses to disaster in American cultural groups. *Symposium on Stress*. Washington: National Research Council, and Walter Reed Army Medical Center, 174–193.

Prince, S., 1920, *Catastrophe and Social Change*. Columbia Studies in Political Science. New York: Columbia University Press.

Prins, S., 1947, Psychological aspects of an escape from occupied territory. *Brit. J. med. Psychol.*, **21**, 30–37.

Prugh, D., 1950, Variations in attitudes, behavior and feeling states as exhibited in the play of children during modifications in the course of ulcerative colitis. *Life Stress and Bodily Disease*, **29**, 692–705.

Prugh, D., E. Staub, H. Sands, R. Kirschbaum, and E. Lenihan, 1953, A study of the emotional reactions of children and families to hospitalization and illness. *Amer. J. Orthopsychiat.*, **23**, 70–106.

Rado, S., 1942, Pathodynamics and treatment of traumatic war neurosis (traumatophobia). *Psychosomat. Med.*, **4**, 362–368.

Rado, S., 1950, Emergency behavior. *Anxiety*, P. Hoch and J. Zubin (Eds.). New York: Grune & Stratton, 150–175.

Raines, G., and S. Thompson, 1950, Suicide, some basic considerations. *Dig. of Neurol. Psychiat.*, **18**, 97–107.

Ramsey, J., 1939, Nervous disorder after injury: Review of 400 cases. *Brit. med. J.*, **2**, 385–390.

Randall, G., J. Ewalt, and H. Blair, 1946, Psychiatric reaction to amputation. *Milit. Neuropsychiat.*, **25**, 94–115.

Rangell, L., 1955, On the psychoanalytic theory of anxiety: A statement of unitary theory. *J. Amer. Psychoanal. Assoc.*, **3**, 389–414.

Redlich, F., B. Moore, and I. Kimbell, 1946, Lumbar puncture reactions: Relative importance of physiological and psychological factors. *Psychosomat. Med.*, **8**, 386–398.

Reichard, J., 1938, Preventing psychic shock. *Mod. Hosp.*, 47–48.

Reik, T., 1949, *Listening with the Third Ear.* New York: Farrar, Straus.

Reiss, E., J. Davis, and W. Amspacher, 1953, Comprehensive clinical management of severe injuries. *Symposium on Stress.* Washington: National Research Center and Walter Reed Army Medical Center, 241–244.

Reznicoff, L., 1938, Emotional factors in rehabilitation of physically disabled. *J. Psychiat.*, **94**, 819–824.

Richter, J., 1931, Postoperative fear. *N. Y. State J. Med.*, **31**, 74–76.

Rickenbacker, E., 1943, *Seven Came Through.* New York: Doubleday, Doran.

Rickman, J., 1937, A discursive review (*Air Raid,* by Langdon-Davies). *Brit. J. med. Psychol.*, **17**, 361–373.

Rickman, J., 1938, Panic and air-raid precautions. *Lancet*, **1**, 1291–1295.

Roberts, D., and E. Torkelson, 1945, Preparing the mind for battle. *Infantry J.*, **56**, 34–36.

Robinson H., J. Finesinger, and J. Bierman, 1956, Psychiatric considerations in the adjustment of patients with poliomyelitis. *New England J. Med.*, **254**, 975–980.

Romalis, F., 1942, The impact of the war on family life. Part I: Reactions to change and crisis. *The Family*, **23**, 219–224.

Rosen, V., 1950, Role of denial in acute postoperative affective reactions following removal of body parts. *Psychosomat. Med.*, **12**, 356–361.

Rosenzweig, S., 1944, An outline of frustration theory. *Personality and the Behavior Disorders.* J. McV. Hunt (Ed.). New York: Ronald Press.

Ross, H., 1944, Group psychotherapy related to group trauma. *Amer. J. Orthopsychiat.*, **14**, 609–615.

Ruesch, J., and K. Bowman, 1948, Personality and chronic illness. *J. Amer. Med. Assoc.*, **136**, 851–855.

Ruesch, J., and A. Prestwood, 1949, Anxiety—Its initiation, communication and interpersonal management. *A.M.A. Arch. of Neurol. Psychiat.*, **62**, 527–550.

Russell, R., 1953, Behavior under stress. *Intern. J. Psychoanal.*, **34**, 1–12.

Saul, L., 1947, *Emotional Maturity.* Philadelphia: Lippincott.

Scheerer, M., 1954, Cognitive theory, *Handbook of Social Psychology,* Vol. I., G. Lindzey (Ed.). Cambridge: Addison-Wesley, 91–142.

Schilder, P., 1938, *Psychotherapy.* New York: W. W. Norton.

Schilder, P., 1942, *Goals and Desires of Man.* New York: Columbia University Press.

Schilder, P., and D. Wechsler, 1934, The attitudes of children towards death. *J. genet. Psychol,* **45**, 406–451.

Schmideberg, M., 1942, Some observations on individual reactions to air raids. *Internat. J. Psychoanal.*, **23**, 146–176.

Schwab, R., and J. Pritchard, 1949, Situational stresses and extrapyramidal disease in different personalities. *Life Stress and Bodily Disease.* Assoc. Research Nervous Mental Disease, 48–60.

Schwartz, S., and B. Winograd, 1954, Preparation of soldiers for atomic maneuvers. *J. soc. Issues,* **10**, 42–52.

Scott, J., 1949, Relative importance of social and hereditary factors in producing disturbances in life adjustment during periods of stress in laboratory animals. *Life Stress and Bodily Disease.* Assoc. Research Nervous Mental Disease, 60–71.

Segal, H., 1954, Initial psychiatric findings of recently repatriated prisoners of war. *Amer. J. Psychiat.*, **111**, 358–363.

Seidenfeld, M., 1949, *Psychological Aspects of Medical Care.* Springfield, Ill.: C. C. Thomas.

Sells, S., 1953, Personnel selection, classification and assignment in relation to stress. *Symposium on Stress.* Washington: National Research Center and Walter Reed Army Medical Center, 275.

Selye, H., 1950, *The Physiology and Pathology of Exposure to Stress.* Montreal: Acta.

Senn, M., 1945, Emotional aspects of convalescence: Fulfillment of child's emotional needs is factor in physical as well as psychological recovery. *Child,* **10**, 24–28.

Shaffer, L., 1947, Fear and courage in aerial combat. *J. consult. Psychol.*, **11**, 137–143.

Shands, H., 1955, An outline of the process of recovery from severe trauma. *A.M.A. Arch. Neurol. Psychiat.*, **73**, 403–409.

Shands, H., J. Finesinger, S. Cobb, and R. Abrams, 1951, Psychological mechanisms in patients with cancer. *Cancer,* **4**, 1159–1170.

Shils, E., and M. Janowitz, 1948, Cohesion and disintegration in the Wehrmacht in World War II. *Public Opinion Quart.*, **12**, 280–315.

Siegel, S., 1956, *Nonparametric Statistics for the Behavioral Sciences.* New York: McGraw-Hill.

Simmel, E., 1944, War neuroses. *Psychoanalysis Today,* S. Lorand, (Ed.). New York: International Universities Press.

Simon, A., and M. Hagan, 1942, Social data on psychiatric casualties in the armed services. *Amer. J. Psychiat.*, **99**, 349–353.

Skinner, B., 1954, Critique of psychoanalytic concepts and theories. *Sci. Monthly,* **79**, 300–305.

Solomon, A., 1933, Clinical classification of post-traumatic mental reactions. *Industr. Med.*, **2**, 72–80.

Sorokin, P., 1942, *Man and Society in Calamity.* New York: E. P. Dutton.

Spence, K., 1948, The postulates and methods of behaviorism. *Psychol. Rev.*, **55**, 67–78.

Spiegel, H., 1944, Psychiatric observations in the Tunisian campaign. *Amer. J. Orthopsychiat.*, **14**, 381–385.

Spiegel, J., 1953, Psychological transactions in situations of acute stress. *Symposium on Stress.* Washington: National Research Council and Walter Reed Army Medical Center, 103–115.

Spiegel, J., 1955, Emotional reactions to catastrophe. *Stress Situations,* S. Liebman (Ed.). Philadelphia: Lippincott.

Steinberg, K., and M. Wittman, 1943, Etiological factors in the adjustment of men in the armed forces. *War Med.*, **4**, 129–139.

Stengel, E., 1944, Air raid phobia. *Brit. J. med. Psychol.*, **20**, 135–143.

Sterba, R., 1946, Report on some emotional reactions to President Roosevelt's death. *Psychoanal. Rev.*, **33**, 393–398.

Sterba, R., 1947, Some psychological factors in Negro race hatred and in anti-Negro riots. *Psychoanalysis and the Social Sciences*, Vol. I, G. Roheim (Ed.). New York: International Universities Press, 411–427.

Stokes, A., 1945, War strains and mental health. *J. nerv. ment. Disease*, **101**, 215–219.

Strassman, H., M. Thaler, and E. Schein, 1956, A prisoner of war syndrome: Apathy as a reaction to severe stress. *Amer. J. Psychiat.*, **112**, 998–1003.

Strauss, A., 1944, The literature on panic. *J. abnorm. soc. Psychol.*, **39**, 317–327.

Strecker, E., and K. Appel, 1945, *Psychiatry in Modern Warfare.* New York: Macmillan.

Strecker, E., F. Braceland, B. Gordon, 1938, Mental attitudes of tuberculous patients. *Ment. Hyg.*, **20**, 529–543.

Stouffer, S., E. Suchman, L. DeVinney, S. Star, and R. Williams, 1949a, *The American Soldier, Vol. I: Adjustment During Army Life.* Princeton: Princeton University Press.

Stouffer, S., A. Lumsdaine, M. Lumsdaine, R. Williams, M. Smith, I. Janis, S. Star, and L. Cottrell, Jr., 1949b, *The American Soldier, Vol. II: Combat and Its Aftermath.* Princeton: Princeton University Press.

Sullivan, H., 1941, Psychiatric aspects of morale. *Amer. J. Soc.*, **47**, 277–301.

Sutherland, A., C. Orbach, R. Dyk, and M. Bard, 1952, The psychological impact of cancer and cancer surgery. I. Adaptation to the dry colostomy; Preliminary report and summary of findings. *Cancer*, **5**, 857–872.

Sutherland, A., and C. Orbach, 1953, Psychological impact of cancer and cancer surgery: II. Depressive reactions associated with surgery for cancer. *Cancer*, **6**, 958–962.

Szasz, T., 1949, Psychiatric aspects of vagotomy. *Psychosomat. Med.*, **11**, 187.

Szekely, L., 1954, Biological remarks on fears originating in early childhood. *Internat. J. Psychoanal.*, **35**, 57–67.

Thouless, R., 1941, Psychological effects of air-raid. *Nature*, **148**, 183–185.

Thurmond, C., 1943, Last thoughts before drowning. *J. abnorm. soc. Psychol.*, **38**, 165–184.

Titchener, J., I. Zwerling, L. Gottschalk, M. Levine, W. Culberston, and S. Cohen, 1956, Problem of delay in seeking surgical care. *J. Amer. med. Assoc.*, **160**, 1187–1193.

Titmuss, R., 1950, *Problems of Social Policy.* London: His Majesty's Stationery Office.

Tolman, E., 1949, Discussion: interrelationships between perception and personality. *J. Pers.*, **18**, 48–50.

Trumbull, R., 1942, *The Raft.* New York: Henry Holt.

Tyhurst, J., 1951, Individual reactions to community disaster: The natural history of psychiatric phenomena. *Amer. J. Psychiat.*, **107**, 764–769.

USSBS Report, 1946, *The Effects of Atomic Bombs on Hiroshima and Nagasaki.* Washington: U. S. Govt. Printing Office.

USSBS Report, 1947a, *The Effect of Strategic Bombing on German Morale*, Vols. 1 and 2. Washington: U. S. Govt. Printing Office.

USSBS Report, 1947b, *The Effects of Strategic Bombing on Japanese Morale.* Washington: U. S. Govt. Printing Office.

Veltfort, H., and G. Lee, 1943, The Cocoanut Grove fire: A study in scapegoating. *J. abnorm. soc. Psychol.*, **38**, 138–154.

Vernon, P., 1941, Psychological effects of air raids. *J. abnorm. soc. Psychol.*, **36**, 457–476.

Volkmann, J., 1936, Erfahrungen mit einer Schwerstbeschädigtenabteilung. *Fortschr. Therap.*, **12**, 743–749.

Wallace, F., 1954, *Human Behavior in Extreme Situations: A Survey of the Literature and Suggestions for Further Research.* Document prepared for Committee on Disaster Studies. (Mimeo.)

Wegrocki, H., 1946, Anxiety and plane flight. *Psychoanal. Rev.*, **33**, 1–36.

Weinstein, E., and R. Kahn, 1955, *Denial of Illness.* Springfield, Ill.: C. C. Thomas.

Welch, L., and T. Rennie, 1952, The influence of psychopathological emotions on psychological test performance. *Relation of Psychological Tests to Psychiatry*, P. Hoch, and J. Zubin (Eds.). New York: Grune & Stratton, 271–289.

Wengraf, F., 1946, Psychoneurotic symptoms following hysterectomy. *Amer. J. Obstet. Gynecol.*, **52**, 645–650.

Werner, H., and S. Wapner, 1955, Changes in psychological distance under conditions of danger. *J. Pers.*, **24**, 153–167.

White, R., 1952, *Lives in Progress.* New York: Dryden Press.

Whiting, J., and I. Child, *Child Training and Personality.* New Haven: Yale University Press.

Williams, D., 1947, Psychological problems in flying personnel. *Brit. med. Bull.*, **5**, 39–42.

Wilson, A., 1941, Reactive emotional disorders. *The Practitioner*, **146**, 254–258.

Wilson, W., 1944, State of men severely wounded in battle. *Lancet*, **246**, 586–589.

Winkley, R., 1953, The Case-Worker's participation in preparation for tonsillectomy in children. *Ment. Hyg.*, **37**, 430–440.

Withey S., 1956, *Reaction to Uncertain Threat.* Ann Arbor: University of Michigan. (Mimeo. report and addenda dated February 1957.)

Wittkower, E., 1949, *A Psychiatrist Looks at Tuberculosis.* London: National Association for Prevention of Tuberculosis.

Wittkower, E., 1952, Psychological aspects of physical illness. *Can. med. Assoc. J.*, **66**, 220–224.

Wittkower, E., and R. Davenport, 1946, War blinded: Emotional, social and occupational situation. *Psychosomat. Med.*, **8**, 121–134.

Wolf, K., 1957, Personal communication.

Wolfenstein, M., 1957, *Disaster.* Glencoe: The Free Press.

Wolff, H., 1953, *Stress and Disease.* Springfield, Ill.: C. C. Thomas.

Wright, D., 1946, Anxiety in aerial combat. *Military Neuropsychiat.*, **25**, 116–124.

Zborowski, M., 1952, Cultural components in responses to pain. *J. soc. Issues*, **8**, 16–30.

Zetzel, E., 1953, The depressive position. *Affective Disorders*, Ph. Greenacre (Ed.). New York: International Universities Press, 84–116.

Ziegler, D., 1948, Amelioration of anxiety symptoms accompanying the healing of a peptic ulcer. *J. nerv. ment. Disease*, **107**, 276–278.

Zilboorg, G., 1936, Differential diagnostic types of suicide. *A.M.A. Arch. Neurol. Psychiat.*, **35**, 270–291.

Author Index

Subject Index